30-Day Revitalization Plan

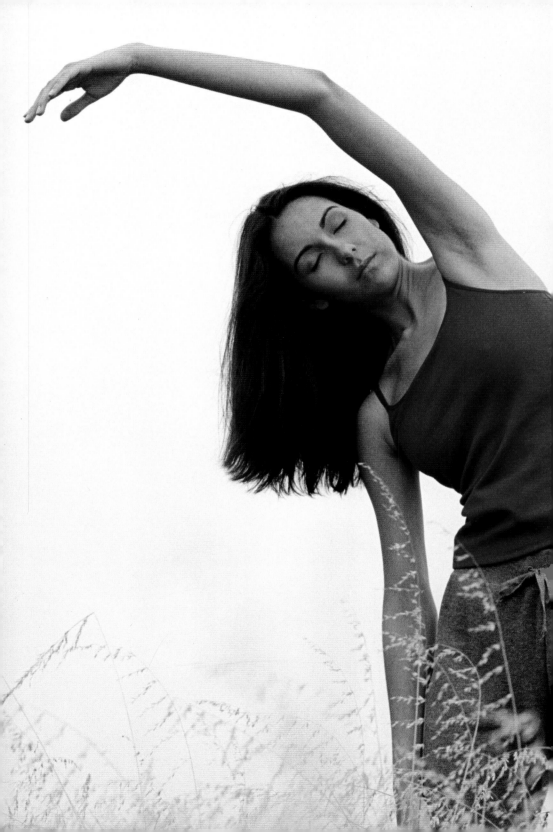

30-Day Revitalization Plan

A Total Rejuvenation for Body & Mind

Edited by Miriam E. Atkins

BARNES
&NOBLE
BOOKS
NEW YORK

Library of Congress Cataloging-in-Publication Data Available

10 9 8 7 6 5 4 3 2 1

Published by Sterling Publishing Co., Inc.
387 Park Avenue South, New York, NY 10016
© 2005 by Sterling Publishing Co., Inc.
Designed by Liz Trovato
Photography © by Getty Images except pages 268 to 308, which contains photographs © by Theresa Raffetto

This book is comprised of material from the following Sterling Publishing Co., Inc. titles:
Aromatherapy for Mind & Body © 1996 by Carol Schiller & David Schiller
Beauty Recipes from Natural Foods © 1974 by Sterling Publishing Co., Inc.
Body-Shaping with Free Weights © 1997 by Stephanie Karony and Anthony L. Ranken
Face-Building, English translation © 1991 by Sterling Publishing Co., Inc.
Giant Book of Super Nutritious Recipes © 2000 by Sterling Publishing Co., Inc.
Healthy Fasting, English translation © 1999 by Sterling Publishing Co., Inc.
Little Giant® Encyclopedia of Meditations & Blessings © 2000 by Nathaniel Altman
Quick Cooks' Kitchen Good-Carb Recipes © 2004 by Sterling Publishing Co., Inc.
Purify Your System for Health & Beauty, English translation © 1998 by Sterling Publishing Co., Inc.
Stretching for Fitness Health & Performance © 1998 by Sterling Publishing Co., Inc.
Yoga for Wimps © 2000 by Miriam Austin

ISBN 0-7607-6212-0

Contents

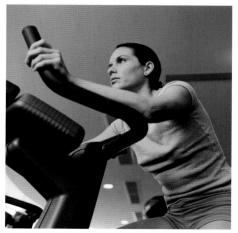

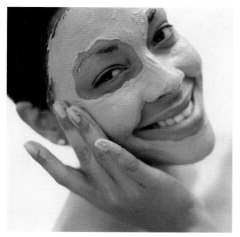

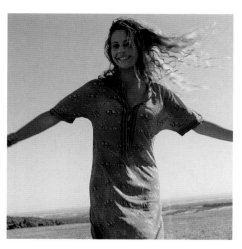

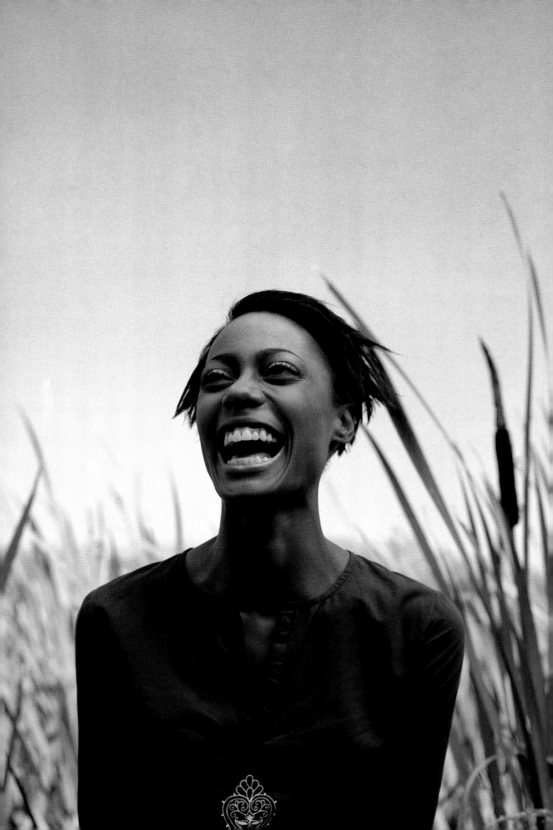

Introduction

The trouble with diets is that they're easy to start but hard to maintain. Most people quickly become frustrated because they focus, understandably, on what they're giving up and not on what they are gaining. This book is not like other diet books; it is not merely about eating less and exercising more. Rather, the *30-Day Revitalization Plan* is about learning to love yourself by

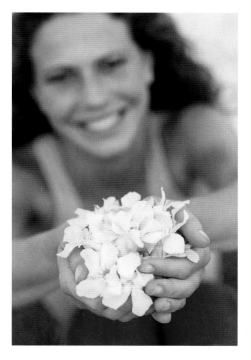

finding peace through meditation, relaxing with aromatherapy, and pampering yourself with luxurious at-home spa treatments, as well as strengthening your core and harvesting your energy through exercise, and purifying your body through healthy eating. The *30-Day Revitalization Plan* will not only change your body, it will change your attitude. Follow the Plan, and you will change your outlook on dieting and exercise and your way of life by learning how to renew yourself emotionally and physically. The topics covered in this book include a full-body purification cure; meditation techniques; aromatherapy recipes; exercise regimens; stretches; weight training exercises; home spa treatments for your face, body, hair, hands and feet; and food and nutrition guidelines.

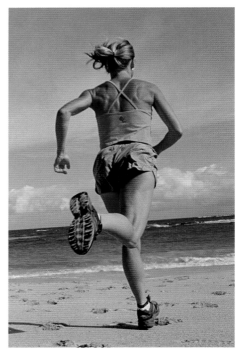

Without a doubt, renewing yourself from head to toe, inside and out, can be an overwhelming experience. To simplify the process and make the information in this book approachable and manageable, the *30-Day Revitalization Plan* is divided into two parts. The first section, the Basics, explains the benefits and importance of each piece that the Plan covers and also offers step by step instructions. The second part, the Plan, takes the information from Part One and applies the pieces on a day-by-day basis, telling you exactly what you need to do each day.

The first step to renewing yourself is to cleanse your body. The purifying process, designed to last seven days, will eliminate the toxins that prevent your body from functioning optimally. During this first week, you will use a curative, a partial fast; exercise; purifying spa treatments; and mentally stimulating activities to clean up your system. As the 7-Day Cure purges unnecessary and potentially harmful toxins from your system, you will feel cleaner, more energetic, and in tune with the rhythms of your body and mind.

In addition to purifying your system, refreshing yourself mentally is an important aspect of the *30-Day Revitalization Plan*. Because increased physical activity will stimulate your mental alertness, the meditation and aromatherapy exercises in this book will help you harness your mental energy, allowing you to develop your emotions as well as helping you to relax. At the same time, the meditation and aromatherapy exercises will help you deal with the increased physical demands and the physical changes that your body will endure over the next thirty days and beyond. Keep in mind that half the battle of looking good is feeling good.

The fitness aspects of this plan cover four essential areas: aerobic exercise, yoga, stretching, and weight training. The effects of these four areas, which complement each other, will produce the combined result of a renewed, improved body. Aerobic exercise will optimize your heart rate, burn off excess calories, and increase your endurance. Stretching your muscles helps increase the effects of aerobic exercise by preparing muscles for a workout, easing the transition from rapid movement to regular motion after a workout, and increasing flexibility, which improves your overall performance. Weight training exercises enhance your metabolism, tone your physique, and build up your strength. Yoga minimizes the intensity of the other fitness components, while emphasizing their more subdued effects. Yoga helps build flexibility, strengthens muscles, and provides a cardiovascular workout. It regulates the internal organs and balances the circulatory, respiratory, and hormonal systems. Moreover, yoga offers the added benefit of emotional comfort; it alleviates stress, aids in the healing of physical injuries and illnesses, and helps us reclaim our general sense of well-being.

In addition to recharging your mind and physique, the *30-Day Revitalization Plan* will also help you rejuvenate your face, hair, hands, feet, and skin with luxurious at-home spa treatments. There are specialized spa

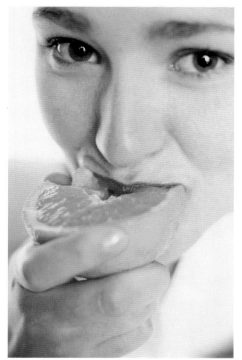

treatments to help with the initial purification cure, as well as other treatments that you will use throughout the plan. The treatments use natural ingredients to help restore a youthful glow to your appearance.

To further reinvigorate yourself, you also need to pay attention to what you eat. With a diet balanced in its vitamins, minerals, proteins, carbohydrates, and other nutrients, you will have the necessary fuel to engage in the mental and physical aspects of the *30-Day Revitalization Plan* without feeling sluggish or weighted down by too much of a particular nutrient and not enough of another. With a balanced diet of moderate proportions and limited in processed foods, you will find yourself refreshed and ready to go. To help you make the most beneficial choices, each day, the Plan offers menu suggestions for breakfast, lunch, and dinner along with the recipes to produce these super-nutritious meals.

The *30-Day Revitalization Plan* values emotional fitness as much as physical fitness. In the long run, one without the other is inconsequential. In order to look good, you must feel good about yourself. With this book you will learn about yourself—your strengths, your goals, your desires, and your ability to persevere. Over the next thirty days, you will work hard, but you will find the rewards of a renewed self wonderfully satisfying and extraordinarily gratifying.

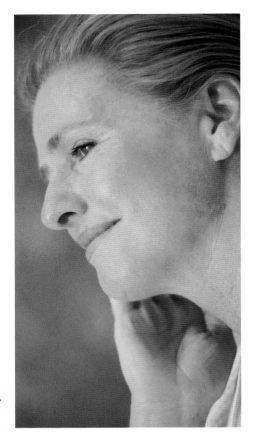

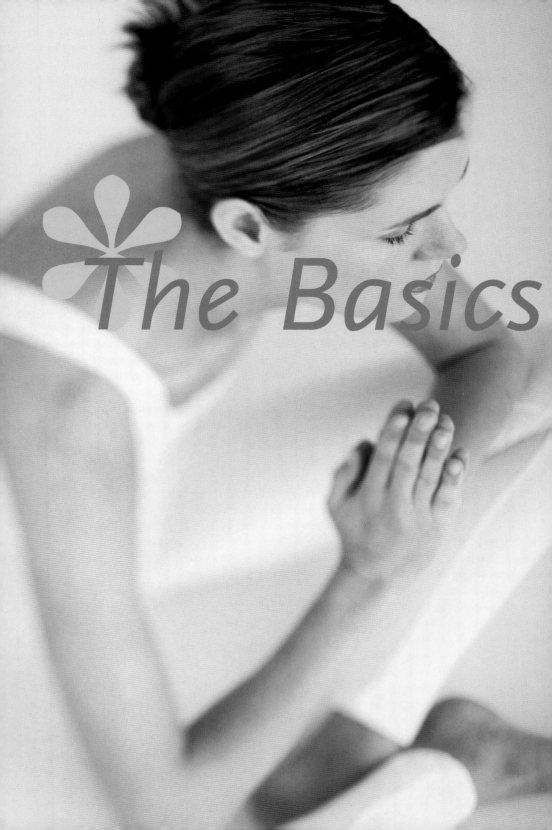

The Basics

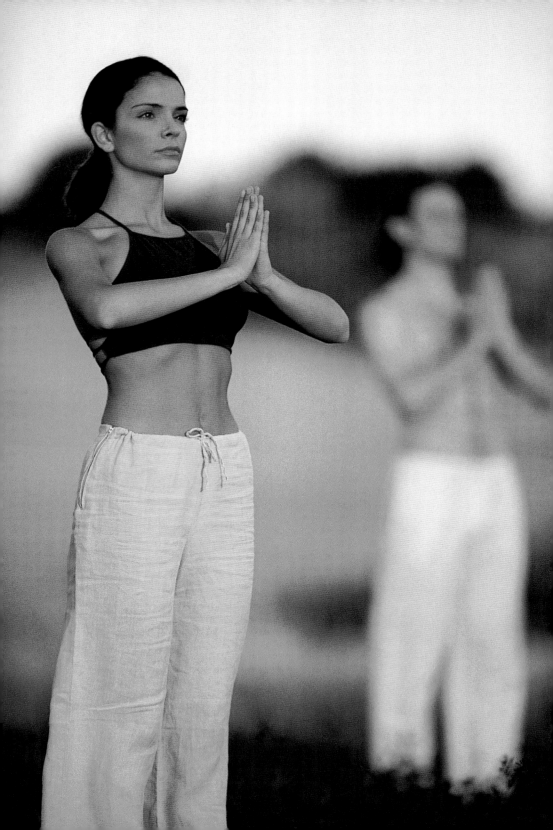

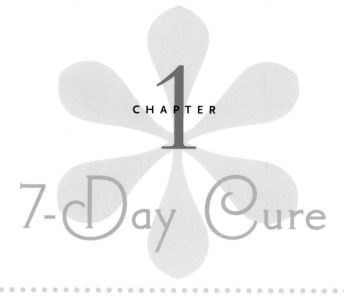

7-Day Cure

All of us take in toxic substances with our food, with the water we drink, with the air we breathe, or by means of skin contact. The human body has to process every poison it takes in. If this becomes impossible because the organs of detoxification (the intestines, kidneys, liver and gallbladder, lungs, and skin) are overburdened, then diseases and even death will occur. Thus, it is necessary to practice "inner" environmental protection.

Inner environmental protection means reducing our intake of toxins, which we can do, for example, by consciously selecting the foods we eat. Because, in the long run, none of us can totally avoid environmental toxins, it is even more important to use measures of detoxification to help the body cleanse itself.

Toxins that are produced internally are called "deposits." They consist of waste and food products that have built up not only in the intestines but also in the blood, muscles, joints, and tissues. The buildup of both deposits and toxins is a compounding problem and makes it difficult for the detoxification organs to eliminate both types of poisons. Since the process presented in Week 1 of the *30-Day Revitalization Plan* will purge both types, for our purposes, deposits produced internally and toxins that have entered the body from the outside environment are collectively called "toxins."

Because the fluid that delivers nutrients and oxygen to all the cells is connected to the intestines, kidneys, liver and gallbladder, lungs, and skin—the organs responsible for purging the body of waste—it is essential to target all five areas in this detoxification plan to eliminate blockage. Excess protein, sweets, and alcohol create acid that causes the fluid to thicken. This fluid will become an area of blockage for materials that should have been

7 · DAY CURE   13

eliminated a long time ago. Because the fluid of the connective tissues surrounds every cell in the body, the whole organism will be affected, and organs, muscles, tissues, and so forth will be poorly provided for or might even be destroyed.

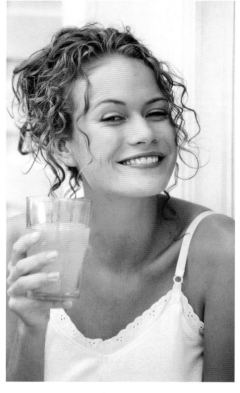

To keep the body running efficiently and properly disposing of toxins, the week-long program will not bring in new toxins unnecessarily while the body works on purging the old ones. This program will regularize bowel movements, essential to the process of detoxification; reduce the buildup of toxins on muscles and joints, which will improve flexibility and movement; clean up the liver, the body's internal purifier; improve the circulatory system; enhance the flow of oxygen throughout the body; and clear up your skin, which will instantly improve your appearance.

The interior cleansing of the body always takes place by means of the organs of elimination. With the aid of a measure of detoxification, first a specific organ of elimination, such as the liver or kidneys, will be cleansed. There are visible means of testing the effectiveness of cleansing, including a change in bowel movements, dark, strong-smelling urine, profuse perspiration, and bad breath. After the cleansing of the organ has been completed and it can function properly once more, then waste products and toxins that are found deeper inside the tissues will be dissolved and excreted.

The doses of a means of detoxification are critical in implementing a cure. If the doses are too low, then the treatment will be ineffective. If the doses are too high, then the body could be overburdened by the flood of freed toxins. Dosages cannot always be prescribed exactly, however, because every organism reacts differently. Therefore, the dosages given in this book are meant to serve only as guidelines. You yourself must find out which dose of a means of detoxification yields the best results for you. It is best to start with small amounts and increase them gradually.

Hunger Fades

This is what takes place during a fast:

- On the first day, the body still has carbohydrate reserves that it can draw upon for energy.
- As soon as these reserves have been depleted, the body switches over to a secondary source of energy, the fat cells. This process is known as "nourishing from within."
- Once the system of internal nourishment has been activated, the early pangs of hunger disappear.
- Because of this change in the metabolic process, most people find it easier to eat nothing than to eat small amounts. The reintroduction of new carbohydrates disturbs the system of internal nourishment.
- Each fast makes the change from external to internal systems easier, causing fasting to become less arduous over time.

Extreme Fasts

In a healthy person, the body's energy reserves can last up to 60 to 80 days. After that, the person can die. However, some exceptions have been reported, such as fasts of 200 days after which no serious damage was found, barring radical losses in weight and energy. A member of the Sikh religion fasted 204 days for religious reasons; he subsisted on only water and broth. In January 1995, when he ended his fast, he had lost half his weight, but otherwise he was in good health.

Such exceptions should not, however, be viewed as endorsements for extreme fasting. For medical reasons, extended fasting must be strictly avoided, because it can deplete the body's vital reserves. Moreover, the body needs many years to fully recover from such an assault.

Keep Moving

In addition to the fat cells, the protein reserves play a role in the body's search for energy during a fast. A complex series of events in the liver and the kidneys leads to the transformation of protein into carbohydrates that can be used by the body for energy. Alanine, an amino acid, is just one of the chemicals produced in the liver during this process.

Alanine is found in the body's muscles, but only during exercise. Sports, light physical labor, or even a brisk walk help to maintain energy during a fast.

Outdoor activity can also be good for our moods and can distract us from our hunger. Too little activity during a fast, on the other hand, can lead to poor circulation, which can create further problems.

Fasts from the Past

Fasting as a method for treating or preventing illness is probably as old as humankind. The Germanic tribes regularly set aside days on which to fast. According to Herodotus, a Greek historian from the fifth century BC, the ancient Egyptians fasted once a month because they recognized that too much food is damaging.

The famous physicians Hippocrates (c. 460—375 BC) and Paracelsus (1493–1541) prescribed fasts for all kinds of ailments. It is also well known that the Spartans kept strict fasting periods, thereby training their bodies to be especially productive.

Fast Trends

Up until the end of the eighteenth century, fasting was a popular medical therapy. According to the notes of Alfons Ferrus, who practiced medicine in the eighteenth century, slow and impassive people find fasting easiest, whereas those people readily irritated and quick to become angry find fasting more difficult. Around 1840, Osbeck, a Swedish professor, popularized his undernourishment diet for treating illness. The Swedish government commended him for his efforts.

During the nineteenth century, the age of the Industrial Revolution, technology and science moved into the foreground, and fasting went the way of so many ancient things in the modern world. Doctors forgot about fasting. New, chemically produced medicines and modern machines made it appear old-fashioned.

Modern Cures

Henry Tanner (1831-1919) and Edward Hooker Dewey (1840–1904), both American doctors, re-popularized fasting in the United States in the second half of the nineteenth century. They count as among the pathfinders of modern methods of fasting. Dr. Dewey, from Meadville, Pennsylvania, sought out alternative methods of treatment that were focused on the whole human being and not on isolated symptoms. He discovered that through fasting he could achieve the best results for healing various disorders. He especially recommended the morning fast for slightly overweight patients and patients with metabolic problems.

In the German-speaking world, patients have been medically treated with fasts since the beginning of the twentieth century. Dr. F. X. Mayr (1875–1965) and Dr. Otto Buchinger Sr. (1878–1966), were the first to study the effects of fasting scientifically and worked for its validation among their colleagues.

The Buchinger Cure

Dr. Otto Buchinger, Sr., is a pioneer in the field of medical fasting. He developed one of the most tried-and-true methods of fasting: the tea–juice fast.

In 1935, Buchinger wrote *Curative Fasting and Its Helpful Methods*, a book in which he established the principles of fasting therapy and made them accessible to his medical colleagues. In addition, he developed guidelines for healthy people who wished to fast at home.

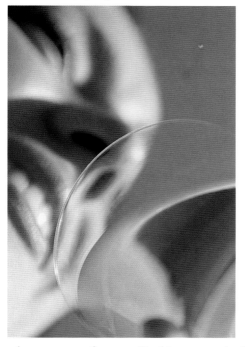

The idea of curing various disorders through the elimination of nutriments came to him after his own experience with a serious illness.

A case of recurring tonsillitis led to Buchinger's entire body being attacked by the infection, including the colon, the liver, the gallbladder, and the joints. The medical community was unable to help. Buchinger's condition worsened considerably and finally became life-threatening. Eventually, he could no longer perform his duties as general physician of the marines and was discharged as an invalid in 1918 at the age of 40.

In this difficult time and with his last reserves of energy, Buchinger searched through medical books for a solution. He came upon a report by an American doctor who had treated a similar hopeless case some 40 years before.

The patient was a young girl who was suffering from an infection that had spread to her entire body. Her condition finally improved when the attending physician stopped all food and medicine and administered only water to her. After about a month, this terminally ill patient, for whom all other doctors had given up hope, recovered fully.

Healing Success

Buchinger immediately underwent a three-month fast treatment under Dr. Gustav Riedlin in Freiburg. After that, his condition improved considerably, and soon he could work again. Following further treatments, he was cured completely.

After this experience, he prescribed fasts on an increasing basis for his patients, and in 1920, he opened up his own fasting clinic in Bad Pyrmont in Central Germany.

Religious Fasts

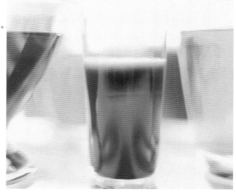

Since ancient times, fasting has been an important dictate in all the major religions. Because fasting requires an act of willpower, it is viewed as a victory of mind and spirit over body. Anyone who fasts overcomes physical needs and the desire for worldly pleasures, which is the declared aim of many faiths.

In addition, most religions attribute great significance to the mystical search for inner knowledge. Believers who practice meditation also often fast to purify both body and spirit. This can lead to mental highs and profound spiritual experiences that would otherwise be unattainable.

Islamic Customs

The Arab prophet and founder of the Islamic faith, Muhammad (570–632), taught: "Prayer brings us halfway to God, fasting takes us to the gateway of heaven." Muslims today still go without food or drink from dawn to dusk during the month of Ramadan in the spring. Smoking is banned as well.

According to the Koran, the holy book of the Muslims, the faithful should make a pilgrimage at least once in their lives to Mecca, the birthplace of Muhammad. The trip is undertaken while fasting. The pilgrims must travel without food for three days on their way to the holy site and for seven days on their way back.

Asceticism in Hinduism and Buddhism

In the Vedas, the religious texts of Hinduism, which were written many centuries ago, is the injunction for Indian ascetics to take in their nourishment as if they were consuming medicine. Siddhartha Gautama, the Buddha, or "the awakened one" (560–480 BC), following this decree, lived for six years on only grass and seeds.

Judaic and Christian Fasts

In the Old and New Testaments of the Bible, fasting often comes up as a means of purification. Moses, the prophet of the Old Testament, fasted for forty days on Mount Horeb. Jesus also fasted for forty days in the desert. One of the early founders of the Christian Church, St. John Chrysostom, wrote: "Fasting is the soul's nourishment, it reins in language and seals one's lips, it tames desire and calms the choleric temperament. It awakens consciousness, renders the body docile, dispels nightly dreams, cures headaches, and strengthens the eyes."

Days of fasting were found regularly on the Christian calendar. People fasted before Easter as an act of humility and contrition and in preparation for the coming celebration. Fridays were also days of fasting, on which meat or alcohol, for example, were forbidden under the law of abstinence.

Today, among Catholics, there are just two days of fasting: Ash Wednesday and Good Friday. On these days, Catholics between the ages of 21 and 60 who are healthy are supposed to fast. They are, however, permitted to eat one main meal and two snacks (without meat) during this time. Protestants, on the other hand, do not set aside specific days for fasting.

Jews still fast traditionally on the holiday of Yom Kippur, also called the Day of Atonement.

"Primitive" Fasts

In one of his books, Dr. Max Bircher, a physician, reported on the situation faced by the Hunzas, a tribe of some ten thousand people living in a Himalayan valley cut off from the rest of the world.

As with many so-called primitive peoples, the Hunzas had no way of storing food, and their agriculture wasn't sufficient to tide them over through an entire year. As a result, they had to fast in early spring until the first barley was ready to be harvested in early summer. Sometimes this fasting period lasted two months. The Hunzas didn't become sick or weak during this period, as might be expected, but continued to work vigorously in the harsh climate. These people normally had no need for doctors—or for police, for that matter, because they coexisted peacefully.

"Civilized" Fasts

With the encroachment of so-called civilization, the Hunzas lost the need to fast. Now that they could store flour, sugar, and canned goods, there was enough to eat year-round. Unexpectedly, the Hunzas began to suffer from a wide range of ailments: cavities, diabetes, obesity, digestive problems, stomach ailments, and gallbladder diseases—in other words, disorders caused by a poor diet. Struck by the epidemic scale of these ailments, the Hunzas soon began to develop asocial behavior, and outside help was required to maintain order. Suddenly these once healthy and peaceful people needed doctors and police in their isolated valley.

Animal Fasts

We cannot speak properly of animals fasting, because fasting requires the voluntary decision to abstain from food. Animals do, however, go through periods in which for different reasons they get by without sustenance.

Animals abstain from food instinctively when they are sick. Their bodies need all their energy to fight the disease, and digestion places a high demand for energy on the body.

Many animals have to go without food when its availability is limited, which is often the case in the winter. The bear, the hedgehog, and the marmot hibernate during the winter, living from the fat reserves gained over the summer and the fall. When they wake up in the spring, they have lost half of their body weight. Other animals, such as mountain goats, chamois, deer, and wolves, all of which do not hibernate, are also forced to eat less depending on the season.

For deer and chamois, the period of fighting between males for the female occurs during the time of food shortage. Although they eat nothing over the entire period, the bucks are still in top shape.

Fish and birds also seem most active when they have the least amount to eat. Salmon do not eat while heading upstream. And some migratory birds can fly for thousands of miles without pecking even the smallest grain.

This week-long program is appropriate for all people who are healthy and would like to undertake some preventive measures for the upkeep of their health, as well as generally to purify and regenerate their body. But a week of purification also has proven to be very effective in treating a number of ailments, such as skin problems, muscle tension, depression, digestive problems (acid indigestion, constipation), obesity, and high uric-acid or cholesterol counts. However, anyone who is seriously ill and under the care of a physician, takes medication regularly, or has any kind of misgivings should consult a physician beforehand.

CHAPTER 2

Meditation

In order to revitalize yourself fully, it is essential to adapt a healthy attitude. Meditation is a way of helping us see the outer world—and ourselves—more clearly. Meditation has been called "mindful awareness," a consciousness of both the world around us as well as our own inner world, with its drama, conflicts, and fears. It is also an awareness of the calmer, intelligent, inner essence that some religions call the soul.

Mental and psychological benefits of meditation include the following:

- increased ability to be calm
- improved mental focus
- expanded perspectives
- greater empathy and compassion for others
- enhanced creativity
- improved memory
- improved sleep
- deeper contact with one's spiritual essence
- reduced use/interest in drugs and alcohol
- greater feelings of optimism
- greater efficiency at work and school
- a clearer sense of one's personal goals

Over the past few years, an increasing amount of research has been done revealing the many benefits of meditation. On a purely physical level, regular meditation practice has been found to:

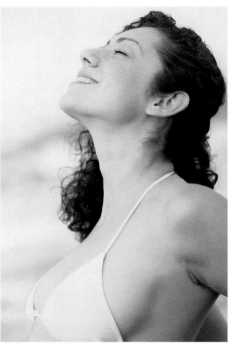

- lower blood pressure
- reduce anxiety and stress
- improve immune system function
- increase energy and stamina
- help manage asthma flare-ups and other allergic reactions
- help manage pain

Every human action is the result of some inner activity. All too often it is our desires and uncontrolled thoughts that drive us, and this can bring about all sorts of difficulties and even have harmful consequences, both for the individual and for humankind in general. This is why it is essential that we become the masters of our own inner realm, creating in this subjective world only what we consider to be right and constructive, and contributing to the common good on these inner planes as much as we would in the outer world.

 ## The Process

Since our attitudes, feelings, and beliefs are constantly manifesting themselves every single day, our most important task is to become aware of what we think, how we feel, and what we believe.

Though it's not always comfortable, we especially need to become aware of those negative thoughts and feelings that are hidden from view, because their power is greatest when we don't know (or merely suspect) that they are there.

At the same time, we need to acknowledge and honor our positive thoughts and feelings and allow them fuller expression. Like a gardener who nurtures a tiny acorn until it is able to grow into a powerful oak tree, we need to nurture our positive thoughts and feelings until they become a dominant aspect of our nature.

Whenever we focus on what is going on inside and observe our inner landscape in greater detail, our awareness of who we really are is strengthened. We also contact what teachers call "the infinite self," which helps us to become more integrated and whole. It allows us to transform negative attitudes, destructive emotions, and limiting beliefs into positive qualities that bring more excitement, fulfillment, and happiness into our lives.

Thus meditation must be handled as a part of our daily life. In all our activities, expressions, and relationships, meditation has to be present, not as an object by itself, but as a vital factor in all our undertakings.

As with any other skill, meditation works best when practiced daily. In time, we become more able to tap into the wellspring of unlimited love and wisdom that promotes inner healing as well as harmony in all of our relationships and activities. Simply stated, meditation can help us create a new life.

Just as water is essential for our physical well-being, meditation is essential for our mental and spiritual well-being. Yet if we drink water too quickly, or if we consume water in excess, it can be harmful to our health. By the same token, we can only derive maximum benefit from meditation if it is practiced appropriately and with care. The following are some "rules of the road" for prospective meditators:

- The desire to meditate should be based on good intentions as opposed to developing mental, emotional, or psychic power to wield over others. Psychic power, especially, needs to evolve naturally through self-awareness and selfless service.

- Because meditation challenges old emotional and mental patterns, an open-minded attitude is essential from the start. Otherwise, meditation can actually reinforce negative habits.

- If meditation practice is too intense over a long period of time, insomnia, irritability, and emotional instability can result. This can be due to excessive breathing exercises, meditation sessions that are too long, or the overuse of mantras.

- The insights gained through meditation need to be real. Ask yourself: How can this truth be expressed in my everyday life?

- Meditation can make us more aware of our faults. We need to avoid indulging in negative self-judgments and focus instead on acknowledgment of faults and transformation.

Do not meditate (or stop meditating) if:

- you feel tired
- you feel nervous
- you are having digestive problems
- you have a headache
- you have taken drugs or alcohol
- you feel aggressive or critical toward others
- you are becoming forgetful
- you feel that you are being forced to meditate

The Essentials

By paying attention to four elements—space, posture, relaxation, and breathing—we can greatly enhance our meditation experience.

Sacred Space

Although one can meditate anywhere, at any time of the day or night, those of us who have the opportunity to meditate at home can create an environment that will help us get the most out of this practice.

Quiet

First, find a place that is quiet. Those with lots of space can devote an entire room to meditation, using it exclusively for that purpose. Decorating the

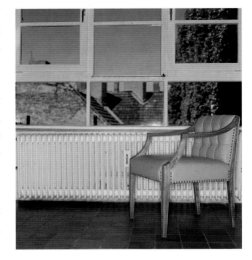

room with a thick carpet, white or light-colored walls, and ensuring good ventilation, along with a simple chair or meditation cushions or mats to sit on, will help create a comfortable environment conducive to meditation. The idea is to create a space that will uplift your spirits— a personal sanctuary apart from the workaday world.

If you do not have the space to create a meditation room, the next best choice is to use a space in a

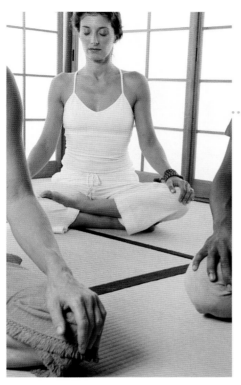

study, a den, or another room where you can be apart from the rest of the household for thirty minutes at a time.

Home Altars

Creating an altar in your home is a very personal undertaking. The altar exists to remind you of your inner life. It also can serve as a centerpiece for your meditation practice or where you recite your daily prayers.

You can create your altar on a small table, or even on a shelf in the den, but it should be located where you can visit frequently and in private, away from the most frequented areas of your home. Decorating the altar depends on your personal taste, and should reflect what you want rather than what you think is appropriate for an altar. Some people create an altar from empty space in a cluttered room, which sets it apart from the rest of the home. Whatever type of altar you choose to create, include only elements that are personally important to you.

As a sacred place in your home and a focal point to help you commune with the spiritual realm, your altar should always be kept clean and free from dirt, dust, or anything else that is not intended to be part of the altar.

In time, your altar can become a veritable "power spot" in your home. Like an electrical generator, it can be a repository of all of your feelings of devotion, compassion, and positive intent—a continual source of positive energy in your home for the benefit of all who reside or visit there.

Incense

Incense has been traditionally used not only to eliminate odors but also to clean the subtle energies of a room. It is also believed to uplift the spirit. Many different types of incense are available, and you need to choose the type that is most compatible with your needs. If you are studying meditation with a teacher, he or she will be able to recommend a particular type that is best for you. If you are choosing your own incense, the following guide may be helpful.

- Rose opens your heart and awakens love.

- Lavender stimulates the yin and yang balance and steadies and calms the emotions.

- Jasmine enhances self-image and promotes confidence.

- Lotus inspires the desire to meditate; it also helps develop trust and receptivity in relationships.

- Patchouli awakens the desire for transformation and helps increase your energy level.

- Sandalwood stimulates the intuitive senses and awakens the desire to merge with the Divine within.

- Frankincense inspires spiritual recognition and elevates the mind and the emotions.

- Myrrh strengthens endurance and helps preserve youthful innocence.

- Musk stimulates your primal instincts and helps draw a sexual partner. This incense may not be suitable for spiritually oriented meditation.

- Saffron awakens us to the Joy of the Gods; it is sometimes used in tantric yoga and other forms of sexual ritual and devotion.

- Gardenia is believed to assist in opening the energy centers or chakras.

- Olive arouses passion and bonding; it develops grounded sensuality.

- Almond helps to rekindle an awareness of sexual mysteries.

- Coconut arouses desire for the exotic and opens you up to new horizons; it is said to help bring out deep inner feeling.

As an alternative to incense, you can use aromatic oils to eliminate room odors and cleanse the subtle atmosphere of a room. Place several drops of mint, pine, or eucalyptus oil into a glass of water, and place the water near the place where you practice meditation.

Outdoor Altars

For those who have a quiet backyard, an outdoor altar can be a source of serenity and strength during the warmer months of the year, or all year-round if you live in a warm or temperate climate.

The creation of an altar will, of course, vary according to your personal taste. Some people erect a small religious statue surrounded by a protective structure, while others prefer the statue or religious object to be exposed to

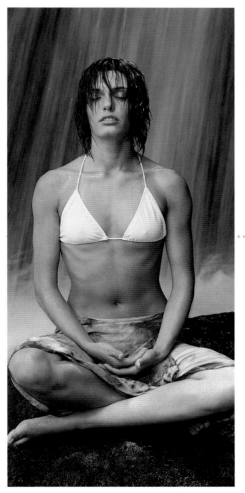

the elements. The altar is often surrounded by flowers and decorative shrubbery, such as ornamental conifers or flowering plants such as roses.

Like the altar in a room in your home, an outdoor altar should be kept clean and well maintained and should not be used for purposes other than those related to your spiritual practice.

The "Living Bridge"

The place inside or outside your home that becomes your sacred meditation space will be the primary space (or one of the primary places) in which you will engage in meditation. After you meditate, do not immediately get up and begin your daily tasks. Linger for a few moments in receptive silence in the sacred space you have created. Follow this by quietly doing some simple tasks around the home or garden in a meditative spirit, which will serve as a "living bridge" between your meditation practice and more mundane responsibilities and tasks.

Postures

There are numerous postures that people use when they meditate. Some are better designed for Westerners than others are. While a full lotus posture may be appropriate for an Indian saddhu, or holy man, it may be extremely difficult (let alone uncomfortable) for a stressed-out middle-aged executive who is exploring meditation for the first time. Some postures involve sitting on the floor or on a meditation mat, while others call for sitting in a chair or lying on a mat or on the floor.

No matter what posture you choose, some general guidelines may be useful:

- Your back and neck need to be reasonably straight, resulting in what some meditators call a "dignified" posture.

- The inner organs (especially the stomach, lungs, and intestines) should be free from pressure. If you feel that your shirt and pants are tight, loosen or unbutton them until you are comfortable. Some people meditate in comfortable Indian-style clothing that fits the body loosely and does not bind the internal organs in any way. Others prefer to wear a jogging suit or sweatpants and a T-shirt.

- During meditation, your blood should circulate unimpeded. If your legs fall asleep during meditation, the discomfort will disrupt your practice. It may also make it impossible to get up when you are finished!

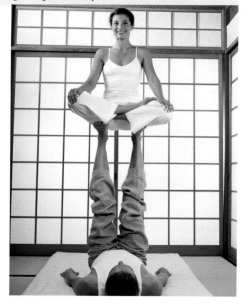

You may feel comfortable sitting cross-legged on a cushion or a mat. Many Westerners prefer to meditate in a simple, straight-backed chair that is neither too Spartan nor too comfortable. Attempting to meditate in an overstuffed lounge chair or on a comfortable sofa often leads to drowsiness or sleep. Whatever posture you choose, be aware if your body or head leans forward or to the side. Gently correct your posture so that your spine is comfortably straight, head resting naturally atop your spine.

Chair

Sit in a comfortable chair, feet placed firmly on the floor, with knees comfortably straight. This helps balance your body and keeps it free from tension.

Then, place your hands on your knees facing either up or down. You could also place your left hand on your lap facing up, and your right hand, also palm up, on top of it. With the palms facing up, you may also intertwine your fingers and place them on your lap; another recommended hand position is to place your hands on your thighs, palms facing up. Gently place your thumb between the tips of your index and middle fingers.

Half Lotus

The half-lotus posture involves sitting cross–legged on the floor or on a mat or cushion. Place your right foot gently on your left thigh. Be sure to keep your left foot on the floor under your right thigh. Reposition yourself until you're comfortable. Place your hands, palms up, on your thighs, either open or with your thumb between the tips of your index and middle fingers.

Full Lotus

As in the half lotus, sit on the floor, preferably on a meditation mat or thin cushion. Gently place your right foot on your left thigh and your left foot on your right thigh. Like the half lotus, place your hands, palms up, on your thighs, either open or with your thumb between the tips of your index and middle fingers. Newcomers to meditation often find this position impossible to achieve, so don't feel badly if you have trouble with it, especially at first. One of the goals in meditation is to feel comfortable. While your ability to achieve the full-lotus posture may well be an indicator of a flexible body, it is not necessarily a sign of advanced spirituality!

Squatting

Kneel on the meditation cushion with feet together, and place your weight on your knees and feet.

Extras

Many people choose to close their eyes during meditation. You can also close your mouth and breathe through your nose, if you want. Place the tip of your tongue gently on the roof of your mouth behind the front teeth.

There is no magic period of time for meditation. Begin meditating for five to ten minutes, and gradually increase the length of your meditation sessions over time to twenty or thirty minutes. Experienced meditators are able to remain in a posture for three hours or more.

When you are ready to rise after concluding your meditation, do so gently. If you feel stiffness or pain anywhere in your body, massage that area gently until it feels better. Get up slowly and gently, with dignity.

Basic Relaxation Exercises

The following exercises help you to relax. Before you begin any of the meditations described in this book, you may want to try one or more of these simple methods, or take elements from them that you feel work for you.

Tension/Release Exercise

This simple technique can lay the groundwork for many of the meditations that follow. It can also serve as a complete meditation in itself.

1. Sit in a comfortable position, either in a half-lotus posture on a cushion or upright on a comfortable, straight-backed chair.

2. Become aware of your breathing. Gradually, slow down your breathing rate, taking deeper, more rhythmic breaths.

3. When you exhale, say the word "peace" aloud, or use another word with peaceful connotations, such as "shanti" or "shalom." Try to slow your breathing so you can count slowly to six as you inhale, and slowly to six as you exhale.

4. Be aware of any tension in your body. Silently scan your face, neck, shoulders, chest, arms, hands, stomach, pelvis, legs, and feet to perceive any areas of tension.

5. If you come upon an area that is tense, direct your calming breath to that area.

6. When you inhale, visualize the breath moving toward the tense area and bathing it with warmth and calming energy. As you exhale, visualize the tension leaving that part of your body. Continue this process until your body is completely relaxed.

Progressive Relaxation Exercise I

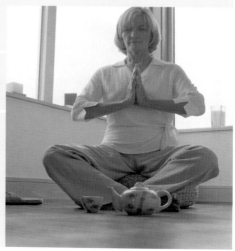

1. Sit comfortably in a chair or cross-legged on a bed or floor. First, tense the muscles in your face, and hold this tension for a few seconds. Then completely relax.

2. Now gradually move to your neck and tense the muscles there. Then completely relax.

3. Repeat this exercise in different sections of the body by working down through the shoulders, arms, chest, stomach, buttocks, anus, thighs, calves, and feet. By the time you reach your feet, you will almost surely be in a relaxed state.

As a variation, you can tense all the muscles of your body and then relax them all at the same time. You could also tense a particular muscle and then relax and gently massage it.

4. When you release tension, you can let your breath out, accompanied by a long "aaahh" or a sigh. This will help you get in touch with your deeper feelings and help you release them.

5. Quiet, deep breathing can follow this exercise.

Progressive Relaxation Exercise II

1. Sit in a comfortable position, either in a straight-backed chair or on a meditation cushion.

2. Close your eyes and focus on your breath. Take full and easy breaths. As you inhale, feel life-giving oxygen flow into your lungs. As you exhale, feel your body relax. With each exhalation, feel your body relax more and more. Feel your shoulders relax, your buttocks relax, your legs and feet relax, your belly relax, your arms and hands relax, your head, face, and jaw relax. Tension is progressively leaving your body and will continue to do so throughout this exercise.

3. Feel your mind release as well. As it relaxes, imagine that your mind is becoming more open, more alert, and more free.

4. Slowly let go of any anxieties, emotional tension, and fears with each exhalation of your breath. Feel yourself becoming emotionally relaxed as you exhale. Say to yourself, "I am relaxing." Continue this process for five minutes, or until you reach a level of deep relaxation.

Breathing

Although all of us breathe, we usually view the rhythm of our breathing as automatic. We are seldom aware of the quality of our breathing and tend to take partial, shallow breaths using only the upper part of our lungs. We often hold our breath or take light, quick breaths, especially when we are tense, fearful, or nervous, without being conscious of it.

Try the following simple breathing exercise: Consciously, take a few short, shallow, and irregular breaths. Be aware of how you feel. Chances are you will feel anxious, uneasy, and ungrounded.

Now take a few deep, full breaths, counting slowly to six at each inhalation and slowly to six as you exhale. Chances are that this deeper, slower breathing will help you feel more calm and comfortable.

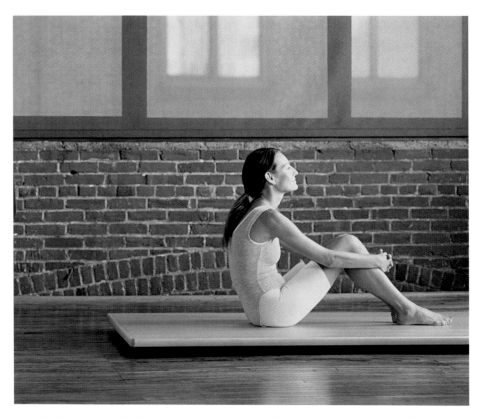

When rapid, shallow breathing becomes habitual or chronic, we limit the amount of air that we take into our body. This not only impairs our body's ability to oxygenate the blood and other vital tissues, but it often makes us feel nervous, mentally sluggish, and tired. In contrast, deep, rhythmic breathing is essential for proper oxygenation and can have a positive impact on how we feel mentally and emotionally. Here are a number of simple breathing techniques that promote both relaxation and vitality.

Awareness Breath

Sit in a comfortable position. Gently inhale while you do a slow count to four (approximately 4 seconds). Hold your breath quietly for a count of two, and then slowly exhale for a count of four.

As you breathe, your mind will probably begin to wander. Simply be aware of this, and gently bring yourself back to paying attention to your breath. By constantly directing your thoughts back to your breath, you are building a "muscle" of attentiveness and one-pointedness that will help you in your daily activities.

Counting Breath

With practice, the following breathing method will enable you to relax whenever you feel nervous or anxious. You can perform it at any place and at any time. Moreover, it can also lay the foundation for meditation practice.

1. Sit in a comfortable position. Gently inhale while you do a slow count to four (approximately 4 seconds), hold your breath quietly for a count of two, and then slowly exhale for a count of four. You can easily extend this breathing for a longer period, counting to six or even eight, while holding your breath for a count of four. Remember that such breaths should never be forced or uncomfortable. Breathe with awareness, and feel the life-giving oxygen being drawn into your body. As you exhale, imagine your body being cleansed.

2. Sitting comfortably, as you inhale, count "One, one, one, one . . ." and count "Two, two, two, two . . . " as you exhale slowly. Then count "Three, three, three, three . . ." as you slowly fill your lungs again with air. Continue this process up to the count of ten, and then begin from "one" once more.

3. As you inhale, count slowly up to ten, and then count from one to ten as you exhale. Repeat this process as many times as you need to in order to fully concentrate on your breathing.

4. Another method involves counting "one" while you inhale and while you exhale, so that each complete breath counts as one number. After a complete inhalation and exhalation, you begin again and count "two," until you complete your second full breath. Continue to count your breaths up to the number "ten," and then begin again from "one."

Standing Breath

Stand comfortably with your spine straight and your knees slightly bent, inhaling slowly and deeply through your nose. Make sure that you are breathing into your abdomen rather than your chest; place your hand on your belly to feel the air expand it as you inhale; gently pull in your stomach muscles as you exhale.

As you inhale, see in your mind's eye that you are surrounded by a brilliant golden light that is flowing into your body toward your abdomen and onward through the rest of your body, including your hands and feet. After inhaling, hold your breath and count slowly to three—with each count representing one second. (With practice, you can hold your breath for up to ten seconds.) Slowly exhale through your mouth, feeling any tension in your body melt away. Yawn and stretch. Repeat this exercise three times.

Learning how to breathe in a way that involves both the upper and lower parts of the lungs has been viewed as vital by yogis for centuries. Perhaps the most important breath to learn is known as the Yogi Complete Breath, first introduced to the West by Yogi Ramacharaka in the early part of the twentieth century. He described performing this breath as follows.

Stand or sit erect. Breathing through the nostrils, inhale steadily, first fill-

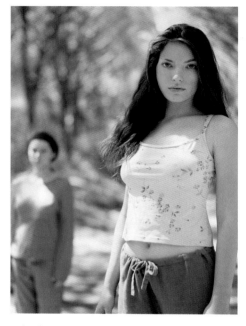

ing the lower part of the lungs, which simultaneously brings the diaphragm into play and exerts a gentle pressure on the abdominal organs by pushing forward the front walls of the abdomen. Then fill the middle part of the lungs, pushing out the lower ribs, breastbone, and chest. Then fill the higher portion of the lungs, protruding the upper chest, thus lifting the chest, including the upper six or seven pairs of ribs. In the final movement, the lower part of the abdomen will be slightly drawn in, which gives the lungs support and also helps to fill the highest part of the lungs.

In *The Science of Breath*, Yogi Ramacharaka reminds us that this breath does not consist of three distinct movements, but is rather one continuous, fluid movement. He recommends that we retain the breath for a couple of seconds and then exhale slowly, drawing in the abdomen slightly as the air leaves the lungs, and relaxing the chest and abdomen after releasing the air.

You can do the Yogi Complete Breath whenever you feel like it, though at first you may want to do it during a period of quiet contemplation, or just before beginning your daily meditation. Gradually, you can begin consciously breathing fully and deeply in more and more of your daily activities, until deep, rhythmic breathing becomes a normal part of your life.

Only living people breathe. The more we breathe, the more alive we are. And the more we practice deep, rhythmic breathing, the more we partake of oxygen—the essence of life itself.

Methods

Alignment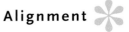

One of the goals of meditation is to align our thoughts and emotions with our deepest essence, or "core." There are many ways to do this. The following method is but one of many possibilities and can easily be modified according to your personal needs and goals.

1. Find a comfortable place where you can be quiet and alone.

2. Select a comfortable position—sitting in a chair (see page 28) or cross-legged on a cushion or rug. If you are outdoors, you may wish to lean against a tree or lie on the ground.

3. Practice one of the Basic Relaxation Exercises described earlier.

4. If you prefer to meditate with your eyes open, select something simple to focus your eyes upon, like a candle, a flower, a religious symbol, or another beautiful object. This will keep your mind from wandering. If you keep your eyes closed, try to visualize a field of white light.

5. Begin to breathe slowly and deeply, becoming aware of your breath as it enters and leaves your body. Each time your mind wanders to other thoughts or is disturbed by outside noises, gently bring your attention back to the easy, natural rhythm of your breathing. If you have trouble focusing on your breathing, count each inhalation and exhalation up to ten, and then start over again.

6. As you relax physically, various feelings may come and go. Don't repress them. Calmly observing them may cause them to gradually lose their intensity.

7. Gradually intuit and then visualize the concept of oneness with all beings. Express your desire to experience the reality of oneness as an integral part of your life today, either in silence or aloud: "I pray to realize my oneness with nature today." Repeat this visualization slowly several times. You can also express other desires or yearnings that you want to integrate into your life during the day. This process is akin to "sending a letter of intent to the universe."

8. After having expressed your keynote visualization, relax and be receptive once more. Continue your relaxed, deep breathing for at least three minutes and feel the sense of oneness living inside your body, near your heart. Feel it streaming out into the room, into the neighborhood, and further out into the world. End your meditation gradually and in silence.

Basic Zazen

Zazen, or "sitting meditation," places emphasis on direct seeing through sitting quietly and not thinking. A practice of Zen Buddhism, zazen is known as Chan meditation in China. The following meditation method is based on the teachings of the Japanese Zen master Dogen Zenji.

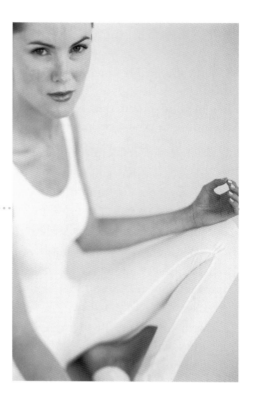

Place

As with other meditation practices, zazen should be done in a quiet place where you can meditate without disturbances. The room should be neither too dark nor too bright, it should be warm in winter and cool in summer, and it should be kept clean. Ideally, this space should contain a picture or statue of the Buddha. Fresh flowers and incense should be placed in front of the image.

Zazen *Tips*

When doing *zazen*, consider the following guidelines:

- Do not meditate if you haven't had sufficient sleep or when you are very tired.
- Avoid overeating and excessive alcohol before sitting.
- Wash your hands and face before sitting.
- Wear clean, loose-fitting garments.
- Place a thick mat (known in Japan as a *zanbuton*) in front of the wall and place a cushion (*zafu*) on top of it. Sit cross-legged on the zafu, placing the base of your spine at the center so that half the zafu is behind you. Rest your knees firmly on the zanbuton.

Body Position

If possible, sit in the full-lotus position described earlier, known in Japan as *kekkafuza*. If this is too difficult, sit in the half-lotus position, known as *hankafuza*. In either of these positions, you can rest both knees on the zanbuton.

Posture

Straighten the lower part of your back, push your buttocks outward, and push your hips forward. Straighten your spine, but not so that you feel uncomfortable.

Pull in your chin and extend your neck as though reaching the crown of your head to the ceiling. Your ears should be parallel to your shoulders. Your nose should be in line with your navel. After straightening your back, relax your shoulders, back, and abdomen without changing your posture. Sit up straight, leaning neither to the right nor to the left, neither forward nor backward.

Hands

Moving your hands near your lap, place your right hand (palm up) on your left foot, and your left hand on your right palm. The tips of your thumbs should touch each other lightly. This position is called *cosmic mudra* or *hokkai-join*. Place the tips of your thumbs in front of your navel, holding your arms slightly apart from your body.

Mouth

In zazen, the mouth is kept closed. Place your tongue lightly against the roof of your mouth.

Eyes

Zen masters recommend that you keep your eyes slightly open, with your vision cast down at about a forty-five degree angle in front of you. Without focusing on anything in particular, allow your field of vision to encompass everything in front of you. If your eyes are closed, it is easier to daydream or become drowsy.

Breathing

Begin your breathing by quietly making a deep exhalation and inhalation. Then open your mouth slightly and exhale slowly and smoothly. In order to expel all the air from your lungs, exhale from your abdomen, pulling the abdomen in slowly. Then close your mouth and inhale through your nose naturally. This form of breathing is known in Japanese as *kanki-issoku*.

Generally speaking, continue doing abdominal breathing through your nose during meditation. Do not try to control your breathing, but allow it to happen naturally. Allow your long breaths to be even and long, and short breaths to be short; strive to become aware of the difference. Your breathing should be so quiet that others cannot hear you. Beginners may wish to count their breaths, which increases awareness and helps regulate breathing.

Swaying

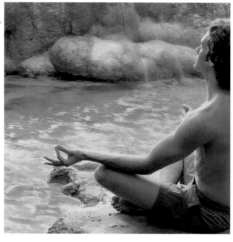

When you feel the need, swaying the body can be a part of zazen meditation. Place your hands with palms up on your knees, and gently sway the upper part of your body from side to side. You can do this several times. Without moving your hips, move your trunk as though it were a long, flexible pole leaning to the right and to the left, so that you stretch your hip muscles. You may also sway forward and backward.

As you sway, let each movement become smaller and smaller until it ceases with your body in an upright position. This exercise should take several minutes. At this point, assume the cosmic mudra position with your hands once more.

Awareness

During meditation, do not concentrate on any particular subject or attempt to control your thinking. When you maintain the proper posture, and as your breathing settles down, your mind will become quiet as well.

If thoughts come up, don't struggle with them or try to escape from them. Simply leave them alone and allow them to come and go freely. Your goal when this happens is to awaken from distraction or drowsiness and return to the correct posture and breathing moment by moment.

Completing Zazen

When you finish zazen, bow, place your hands palms up on your thighs, and gently sway your body (left to right, right to left, and forward and backward) a few times. Then sway a bit more extensively, so that you actually feel your muscles stretching. Take a deep breath. Slowly unfold your legs. Stand up slowly and carefully, especially if your legs are asleep.

Thought

One of the primary purposes of meditation is to make us more aware of our thought processes. The following meditation is designed to assist in this process of self-awareness.

1. Do one of the Basic Relaxation Exercises (see page 29).

2. As you breathe, be aware of each thought as it comes up, without censoring it, resisting it, or judging it in any way. Try to observe the connection (if any) of one thought to another. Watch each thought as it departs, and be aware of the next thought that comes up. Continue this process of active observation for three to five minutes.

3. You will probably find a combination of present-day concerns, old memories, odd associations, and projections for the future. After you have completed your exercise, record these thoughts in a notebook, describing them as you saw them. Write down everything you can remember.

4. If you continue this meditation for several days or weeks, review your notes from time to time, comparing the thoughts that come up each day during your practice.

Mind Expansion

1. Sit in a quiet place. Devote several minutes to any of the relaxation techniques described earlier.

2. When you feel sufficiently relaxed and centered, read a spiritual or other thought-provoking statement. Some possible statements include:

> Let the kingdom of your heart be so wide that no one is excluded.
> — *N. Sri Ram*

> He who does not attempt to make peace when small discords arise, is like a bee's hive which leaks drops of honey. Soon, the whole hive collapses.
> — *Nagarjuna*

> People ought not to consider so much what they are to do as what they are; let them be good and their ways and deeds will shine brightly.
> — *Meister Eckhart*

> The key to humanity's trouble . . . has been to take and not give, to accept and not share, to grasp and not distribute.
> — *Alice A. Bailey*

> It is in the heart center that our inner nature grows to fullness. Once the heart center opens, all blockages dissolve, and a spirit of intuition spreads throughout our entire body so that our whole being comes alive.
>
> — *Tarthang Tulku*

3. Devote several minutes to thinking about the idea and exploring its meanings.

4. At the same time, open yourself to inspiration and understanding regarding this idea. At this point, your mind is more alive and expansive, opening itself to new possibilities and ways of perception.

5. Close your eyes and continue to observe your thoughts, being aware of any wandering or unrelated thinking. Gently bring your consciousness back to the concept at hand.

6. After a few minutes, take several deep breaths and conclude your meditation.

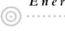 Energy

The following meditations are designed to enable you to safely access the energy of the universe, known in the East as *chi* or *prana*. Although best done in the morning, they can be performed whenever you feel the need for more energy during the course of the day.

Contacting Universal Energy

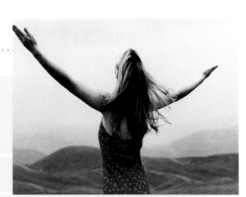

1. Seated comfortably in a straight-backed chair or on a cushion or mat, do one of the Basic Relaxation Exercises (see page 29).

2. Continue to pay attention to your breathing. Close your eyes.

3. Visualize yourself flying upward like a soaring bird. Light is shining all around you. Feel the radiance and warmth of this dazzling, bright light. Feel this light flowing through you, bathing you with energy. This energy brings with it a sense of inner peace and well-being. Acknowledge that this light not only invigorates you but guides you in making the correct choices in your life as well. Continue to be aware of your breathing.

4. After several minutes, visualize yourself descending to earth again, yet continue to feel some of this bright light within you.

5. Open your eyes and slowly come out of your meditation.

Illumination

1. Sit comfortably in a straight-backed chair or on a cushion or mat. Perform one of the Basic Relaxation Exercises, being especially aware of your breathing.

2. Visualize your body and mind as being a dark gray mass, totally devoid of light. Feel the heaviness, the emptiness, the lack of energy and inspiration. Allow this feeling to continue for a minute or two.

3. Now imagine a tiny source of pure, white light beginning to shine within you. It can originate in the heart, at the base of your spine, in your brain, or in any other part of your body.

4. Imagine this light growing in both size and brightness. Feel its warmth and its healing. See this light expand while it permeates your entire body with light—your arms and legs, fingers, and toes. As you breathe, see this light radiating outward, filling the atmosphere with its energy and warmth.

5. Now, mentally reduce the force until you feel the core of light and its radiance filling your entire body.

6. Quietly conclude your meditation while retaining the feeling of being filled with light. Take a few deep breaths and stretch before getting up from your seated position.

Eightfold Path

According to traditional Buddhist teachings, the way of liberation is The Noble Eightfold Path. Less a religious doctrine than a form of moral psychology, the eight factors of the path include:

1. Right understanding, or a knowledge of the true nature of existence.

2. Right thought, or thought that is free from negativity, sensuality, ill will, and cruelty. Right thought also involves being aware of our inaccurate, separative, or destructive beliefs.

3. Right speech, calling for speech that is not only true, kind, and helpful, but also without gossip, harshness, or idle chitchat.

4. Right action, involving not just the avoidance of killing, stealing, and adultery, but involvement in personal, political, and social activities that heal, nourish, and alleviate pain in the world.

5. Right livelihood, involving an occupation that does no harm to conscious living beings, but also a vocation or avocation that does good for society and benefits the earth.

6. Right effort, which involves not only cultivating wholesome qualities in ourselves, but getting involved in activities that benefit other living beings.

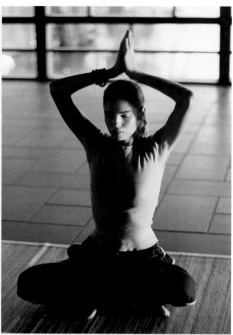

7. Right mindfulness, which involves developing mental awareness and clarity; it also calls upon us to focus on ideas and concepts that are important in life, as opposed to devoting our thoughts to worry, trivia, or celebrity gossip.

8. Right concentration, calling for the cultivation of a mind that is both collected and focused through meditation.

Eight-Day Plan

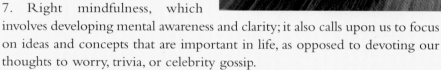

The following meditation plan is designed to be used over a period of eight days. Each day is devoted to meditating on one aspect of the Noble Eightfold Path. For this meditation, you will need a notebook and a picture or other image of the Buddha. You may also wish to write down each aspect of the Eightfold Path on an index card to refer to during meditation.

1. Seat yourself comfortably in a chair or on a cushion on the floor. Perform one of the Basic Relaxation Exercises, or another relaxation method of your choice (see page 29). Be aware of your breathing, which should be deep, slow, and even.

2. With the Buddha image before you, pray for clarity and enlightenment. This can be a short prayer such as, "I pray to open myself to the wisdom of the Noble Eightfold Path and learn to follow it in my daily life."

3. Choose an aspect of the Noble Eightfold Path and read the card that you wrote the words on. Ponder the meaning and ramifications of this aspect carefully. Ask about its meaning. To what extent do you manifest it in your life? In what areas is your understanding and practice lacking? Be totally honest with yourself, allowing your thoughts to flow freely, writing them down in your notebook. At the same time, strive to be objective, being aware of feelings of pride, remorse, or guilt that may come up. Devote five to ten minutes to this exercise.

4. When you are ready to conclude your meditation, take a few deep breaths. Express gratitude for your insights. Gently stretch your body as you slowly rise from your meditation posture.

Mantras

We live in a world of sound. Sound is essentially a form of energy that is transmitted through air and other conductors. Sounds can be soothing—the movement of the wind through the trees, the gurgling of a stream, or the breaking of waves on a rocky shore. Other pleasant sounds include the quiet ringing of bells. Discordant sounds such as rap music, the screeching of brakes, or the incessant barking of a dog tend to inhibit our ability to think clearly. Noise pollution affects us physically, emotionally, and mentally, often producing stress and feelings of ungroundedness.

By the same token, human speech can also have a powerful impact in our daily life; we really know very little about how it affects us. Speech tones and volume, as well as certain words, are types of energy that make us react in different ways. In some cases, a hateful word or a careless phrase can hurt us even more than a punch in the stomach.

The human voice has long played a role in religious practices through-out the world. Chanting, praying, and singing are all powerful methods of using voice vibration and the power of sound to elevate our consciousness and make us more receptive to spiritual forces. Singing spiritual hymns and chanting heartfelt prayers and the holy names of God have always been viewed as an essential part of daily spiritual practice. Serious devotees of the spiritual life, from Catholic monks to Hindu yogis, Jewish kabbalists to Tibetan Buddhist monks, have a powerful tradition of chanting that has survived to this day.

The word "mantra" comes from the Sanskrit language, meaning "the thought that liberates and protects." A mantra has been defined as a combination of sacred syllables which forms a nucleus of spiritual energy or a sacred syllable or word or set of words through the repetition and reflection of which one attains perfection or realization of the Self. Using a mantra in spiritual practice involves chanting, singing, or even humming a sacred sound that can either help prepare the foundation for meditation or elevate our consciousness during meditation itself. A mantra involves the repetition of the name of God, such as "Yahweh" by the Christians or "Elohim" by the Jews. Chanting the name of Jesus has been a vital aspect of Christian meditation, while chanting the name of the goddess Oshoun or the god Oshala has been practiced by adherents to African religions such as Macumba and the Brazilian Candomble. It can also involve repeating a sacred word such as "shanti" or "peace."

Aside from the vibration of the actual names or sacred words, a mantra can have powerful personal associations. For Muslims, there is no word more meaningful than "Allah," while the word "aum," or "om" is viewed by the Hindus as symbolizing the essence of spiritual reality. Yet we must beware of mechanically reciting a mantra or any sacred sound. The power of a mantra is proportionate to the feeling that we put into its expression. For this reason, our personal choice of a mantra is extremely important; it should ideally be a sacred word or name that we can personally relate to.

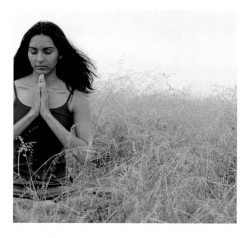

Having said this, we can acknowledge that many mantras are universal in scope. Based on the idea that there is no such thing as a "Jewish soul" or a "Christian soul," but rather a "divine soul," the actual mantra is unimportant; any sacred word or name can impart a powerful spiritual vibration and uplift the consciousness of any receptive individual.

Reciting a mantra produces the following benefits:

- It calms the mind and the emotions.
- It elevates the consciousness.
- The breath becomes more regular and controlled.
- It provides us with a vehicle for expressing our deepest emotions and yearnings.
- It "feeds" the Higher Self and allows it to play a larger role in our daily life.

Advice on Chanting

When you recite a mantra, gently pull in your abdominal muscles, allowing the chest to widen as you vocalize. Breathe through your nose. Exhale evenly while paying attention to your breath. The "melody" of the mantra needs to be consistent and should not change with each vocalization.

Vocalizing a sacred word in a low, gentle tone increases its power. However, if you find yourself in a place where chanting a mantra is not appropriate (such as on a bus or in any public place), you can recite the sound mentally and envision it totally enveloping your being as if you were making the sound with your voice.

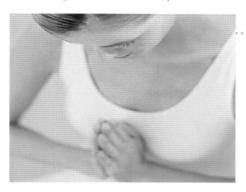

Christian Mantras

Ave Maria is considered an expression of love and devotion towards the Cosmic Mother, who is often personified by the Virgin Mary. Often used as a blessing for others, it is a powerful mantra that can be vocalized either aloud or silently.

Holy Mary Mother of God

Nonsectarian English Mantras

Oh God Beautiful
Peace
One
I Am

Arabic Mantras

La Illaha Illa Allah (There is no God but Allah)
Allah Akbar (There is no one greater than Allah)
Allah

Hebrew Mantras

Elohim (Great Living One)
Kodosh (Holy One)
Adonai (Lord)
Ahavah (Love)
Shalom (Peace)
Ribbono shel Olem (Master of the Universe or Source and Substance of
    All Reality)

Om is a most sacred mantra; it means "the divine energy." It represents the trinity of the physical, mental, and spiritual aspects of our being, as well as an individual, universal, and transcendental consciousness.

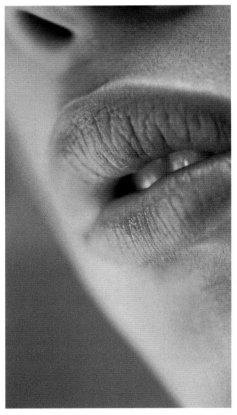

The "o" and the "m" should be sounded for fifteen seconds each, making a total of thirty seconds (be sure to inhale deeply before beginning the mantra!). H. Saraydarian suggests that we vocalize "om" three times before beginning meditation and three times after we complete meditation. He recommends that the first "om" be vocalized softly, the second "om" be louder, and the third still louder. After the three "oms" are sounded solemnly, we should visualize their effects during a period of silence. "Om" can also be sounded silently. If you have heard others recite this mantra (especially a guru or yoga teacher), recall how it sounds and reproduce the sound in your mind.

"Om" is considered the mantra for healing, one that will preserve the body and mind in a state of health so that we can attain spiritual realization. In Hindu mythology, "Hari" is the name for the god Vishnu, the "preserver" of the spirit. Chanting "hari" is also viewed as a sign of repentance for our disharmonious actions and attitudes. This mantra can be chanted once per breath, or in two sequences per breath to strengthen concentration.

"Om shanti" combines the sacred "om" with the Sanskrit word for "peace," not unlike the Hebrew word "shalom." The words can also be reversed, recited as "shanti om."

"Om mani padmi hum" means "The Jewel of the Lotus" and symbolizes completion and integration. A very powerful mantra, it should be recited slowly, but in one complete breath.

"Om nama sivaya" is believed to help destroy ignorance. It asks God to help us transform our negative qualities and destroy the obstacles to living a spiritual life. Like the previous mantra, it should be vocalized slowly in one breath.

"Om krishna guru" is recommended when you are seeing a spiritual teacher, either on the concrete level or as a spirit guide. In addition to "om," meaning the Supreme Energy, "Krishna" is said to represent the supreme energy manifested in a form that becomes personal to us. "Guru" is the Sanskrit term for spiritual teacher.

"Om ah hung" is a mantra used primarily by Tibetan Buddhists. In Buddhism, "ah" is the source of all speech and sound; it is also a sound of purification, warmth, and healing. It represents the energy of expansion and empowerment. "Hung" (pronounced "hoong" with a soft h) is a sound of infinity, enlightenment, and oneness. When "om," "ah," and "hung" are recited together, the Tibetan monk Tulku Thondup suggests that the length of each sacred word may be varied.

"Om sri rama yaya rama" is an appeal to the soul to live according to Divine Will. In the Hindu religion, the god Rama represents the King or Pillar. As a "call to victory" of the Higher Self, this mantra is ideal for a person seeking transformation and self-realization. A related mantra is the "hare Rama."

"Aum" is closely related to "om." Swami Sivananda taught that the cosmic "aum" is traditionally chanted in three parts, with equal time devoted to each part. When you chant this sacred sound, visualize the "ah" being chanted in the area of your body near the navel, the "oo," just above the diaphragm, and the "mm" at the base of the throat. Like the "om," this mantra should be done slowly and clearly in one long complete breath.

"Aum nama bhagavate gajananaya namah" is a mantra to invoke the presence of the god Ganesha, whose power is believed to remove obstacles and to provide clarity and wisdom when we need to make an important decision.

"Radha govinda" is a mantra used to discover the Divine within. It is to be chanted with intense feelings of love and devotion, as if the mantra is the key that will open a buried treasure. In Hindu mythology, Radha was the lover of Lord Krishna and is seen as a symbol of unceasing love for God.

Judeo-Christian Mantras

"Shalom" is one of the most important and beautiful words in the Hebrew language. When you use it as a mantra, you can elongate the syllables so it is expressed as:

"shhhhaaa . . . looooo . . . mmmmm," not unlike the "om" described above. The syllables can be pronounced in equal lengths, or in varying lengths. The mantra can be chanted in one long breath if desired.

Basic Mantra Meditation Technique

As with any other form of mediation, take a few moments to relax. You can use one of the Basic Relaxation Exercises (see page 29) or select another of your choice.

Choose a mantra that has significance to you. While sitting or standing in a comfortable position (see page 27), recite it aloud clearly and with awareness of your outgoing breath. Remember that different mantras may require a specific form of expression, so refer to the guidelines for the specific mantras offered above. Allow the sound to both permeate the surrounding atmosphere and vibrate deep within your body and mind, so that you feel the power of the manta completely envelop your being.

Continue to recite the mantra for several minutes at first; with practice, you may want to extend your chanting to a half hour or more.

When you wish to stop chanting, make your final recitation and devote several minutes to quiet, rhythmic breathing. You may wish to say a short prayer before you conclude the meditation.

Namo Amitabha

The repeated intoning of the name of a Buddha is a powerful method of focusing the mind and calming the emotions. The phrase "namo amitabha," means "taking refuge in boundless life and enlightenment." The following mantra meditation was inspired by the technique taught by the Won school of Buddhism in Korea. It is intended to help us to discover the amitabha of our own minds and return to the paradise of our own original nature.

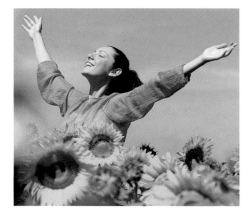

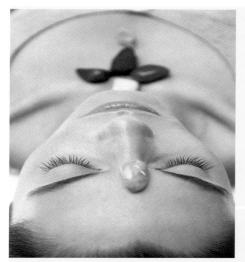

1. Sit on a chair or on a comfortable cushion placed on the floor. Maintain an upright posture and relax your body and mind. Do not swing or shake your body. You may wish to do the Basic Relaxation Exercises (see page 29) or another form of relaxation before you begin chanting. You may also want to use sacred beads for counting each chant as you recite it.

2. Speaking in your normal voice, concentrate your mind, body, and spirit on intoning the name of a Buddha, linking your entire being with the phrase "namo amitabha." Recite the phrase slowly and clearly with each exhalation. Merely verbally intoning "namo amitabha" without concentration of thought is said to be of little effect, but the silent repetition of the name of a Buddha can be very powerful if you do it consciously.

3. Allow your mind to relax completely as you chant. Do not imagine the figure of Buddha as something you seek from outside, but allow the words to surround you totally, bringing life to your own innate Buddha nature.

4. Continue this chanting meditation for five minutes at first. With practice, you can extend your meditation to ten minutes or longer.

5. When you are finished, take several deep breaths and slowly rise from your seated position.

Teachers of Won Buddhism suggest that you intone the name of the Buddha whenever you are annoyed by "delusive thoughts," involving emotions such as greed, envy, or fear, or while you are walking, standing, sitting, or reclining; however, you should not chant the Buddha's name if it will distract you from what you are doing, such as driving a car or operating machinery.

Goodness

Many of us underestimate our gifts and do not acknowledge our good deeds and other accomplishments. While not intended as an ego trip, the following meditation helps us to take stock of the good things we have done in our lives.

1. Sit comfortably in a straight-backed chair or on a meditation mat. Perform one of the Basic Relaxation Exercises (see page 29). Be aware of your breathing and take deep yet gentle breaths.

2. As you watch your breathing, pray, "I ask to acknowledge the good I have done in my life."

3. With pen in hand, begin to write down all the beautiful, loving things you have done in your life. These may include acts of compassion and generosity, right attitudes, or acts of courage—anything that you feel particularly good about (even if you might have forgotten it up to now). Be aware of any period in your life that was especially rich in good deeds and loving actions.

4. After several minutes of brainstorming, read the list over. Say to yourself, "I acknowledge the goodness within me." At this point, you may wish to express gratitude for your life and your innate gift of goodness. Ask the Great Spirit for more opportunities to express goodness in your life.

✳ Gratitude

Many of us experience feelings of melancholy from time to time. We sometimes focus on our failings and highlight what is missing, rather than acknowledging the positive aspects of ourselves and what is good in our lives. While not encouraging us to seek an escape from our problems, the following meditations are designed to help us come in contact with the many positive aspects of our life at present and to feel gratitude for what we have.

Gratitude 1

1. Do one of the Basic Relaxation Exercises (see page 29).

2. Say a simple prayer such as, "I pray to be aware of what I am grateful for."

3. Pen and journal in hand, begin writing a list of what you have to be grateful for. This list can include aspects of your personality you are happy with, the presence of certain people in your life, your pet, certain possessions you have, your job, knowledge or insights you may have gained, your health, your favorite tree in your front yard, and whatever else may come into your mind.

4. Do not censor the flow of ideas; simply allow your active mind to brainstorm as you record your impressions in your journal. Allow several minutes for this exercise. When you are finished, read over each impression either silently or aloud.

5. When you have finished reading your list, devote a minute or so to quiet breathing. Conclude your meditation with a prayer of thanks.

1. Perform one of the Basic Relaxation Exercises (see page 29).

2. On a piece of paper, write the name of every person who has been kind to you, either today or during your lifetime. This may include people who have done you a special favor, listened to your troubles, helped you with a problem, given you a hug when you needed it, or performed an especially caring act that you have never been able to forget.

3. When you have finished, read their names, either singly or as a group, and say, "May [name] receive God's grace," "I thank God for having [name] in my life," or another expression of your choosing.

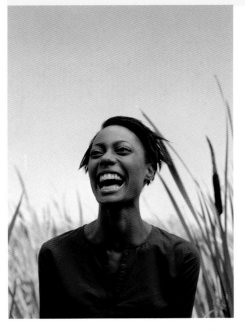

Healing Meditations

Meditation can be a powerful tool for healing because it allows us to explore the deeper issues of health and disease. As opposed to curing, healing is a process rather than a goal. It encompasses the entire spectrum of the human being— physical, emotional, mental, and spiritual.

Healing implies viewing our situation with a wider perspective that goes beyond the treatment of symptoms, to embrace all aspects of our lives. Rather than becoming fixated on symptoms (which often distracts us from the healing process), healing means learning from the crisis (or from the symptom), not trying to control or eliminate it. It involves developing the flexibility we need to change the attitudes that keep us out of touch with our innate intelligence, respect, and love.

Healing also involves enduring pain or discomfort while expanding our perspective to learn what our suffering has to teach us. Rather than trying to compete with symptoms or pain from the outside (through therapeutic means, natural or otherwise), healing implies taking responsibility for growth and change from the inside. When viewed from this perspective, meditation can be a powerful tool to facilitate self-healing and inner growth.

Visualization

Creative visualization is often used in a healing meditation. Louise L. Hay, author of *You Can Heal Your Life* and other books, outlines the three basic parts of a positive healing visualization, which we can adapt to our individual needs:

1. An image of the problem or pain or disease, or the diseased part of the body.

2. An image of a positive force eliminating this problem.

3. An image of the body being rebuilt to perfect health, and then the image of the body moving through life with ease and energy.

Remember that positive visualization can incorporate literal images, symbolic images related to treatment, or abstract images. One universal image you can use is a bright, white healing light. Imagine it shining around (and through) every aspect of your being.

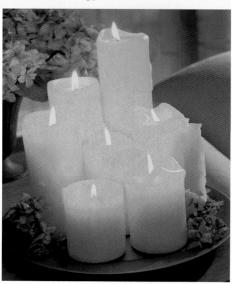

A powerful tool for this type of visualization meditation is the "Divine Light Invocation" mantra taught by Swami Sivananda Radha:

> *I am created by Divine Light*
> *I am sustained by Divine Light*
> *I am protected by Divine Light*
> *I am surrounded by Divine Light*
> *I am ever growing into Divine Light.*

Guidance

Many of us are taught to believe that healing has to do with our physician's level of expertise or the medication we are given. We often overlook the fact that it is our own body that is doing the work: healing is essentially an inside job. We may call on a health professional to help us initiate and maintain the healing process, but we ourselves are doing the healing.

This simple meditation is designed to help us take greater responsibility for our healing and access inner wisdom regarding our health.

1. Sit comfortably in a chair or on a meditation mat. Do one of the Basic Relaxation Exercises (see page 29), or use another relaxation method of your choice.

2. After you feel comfortable and relaxed, say clearly, slowly, and purposefully: "I am a self-healing being. I have an unlimited capacity to heal myself. I pray to access my body's innate healing power to the fullest." You may want to repeat this prayer several times so that it becomes more integrated into your consciousness.

3. Devote several minutes to receptive silence. Chances are that many thoughts and feelings will come, including fear, anger, frustration, doubt, and judgments; you may have feelings of resistance to healing or even a desire to remain sick. By the same token, you may experience inspiration and lightness, along with a feeling that you are open to new ideas and possibilities; some may involve practical guidance that can facilitate your healing and assist your health practitioner in helping you. Allow these thoughts and feelings to surface, without judging or censoring them. Write your impressions in a notebook. Some of these ideas or impressions may be subjects of meditation themselves.

4. When you feel ready to end your meditation, take several deep breaths before slowly getting up.

Repeat this daily meditation as often as you need to. Since self-healing may involve many personal issues, such as childhood hurts, poor self-image, negative attitudes, wrong assumptions, and anger toward oneself, family, or friends, this meditation serves as a vehicle for self-exploration and self-discovery as we embark on our personal healing journey.

Deeper Wisdom

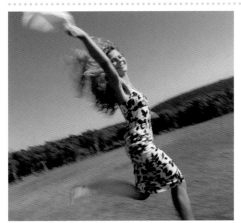

This meditation is similar to the previous one, but it is intended to be used by those who have already done some exploration with the previous method.

Many of us feel victimized when we are ill, or have suffered an accident and are eager to have unpleasant symptoms relieved as soon as possible. Yet we can also use our pain and suffering as a springboard to learn more about ourselves and to develop new goals and areas of interest. This meditation allows us to move deeper into the healing process and to work with specific issues that may have come to our attention.

1. Sit comfortably in a chair or on a meditation mat. Do one of the Basic Relaxation Exercises (see page 29) or use another relaxation method of your choice.

2. After you feel comfortable and relaxed, say clearly, slowly, and purposefully: "I pray to discover the inner meanings of my health problem." You may want to repeat this prayer several times so that it becomes more integrated into your consciousness.

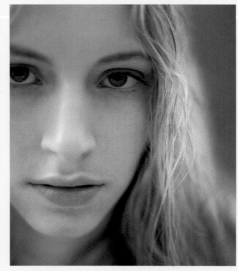

3. As you breathe quietly and evenly, allow yourself to ponder your prayer request. Rather than feel victimized by your health problem, ask if there might be a pattern or rhythm to your symptoms, especially if you have suffered a similar health problem previously. Is your health problem offering you any opportunities for personal growth? Are there any positive components to your health problem, such as time off from work, greater self-nurturing, or changes in your thinking and goals? What new insights have you gained about your life and relationships? What would you like to change about your life if you could? Are there any areas of interest you would like to pursue? Allow your responses to surface, without judging or censoring them. Write down your impressions in a notebook.

4. When you feel ready to end your meditation, take several deep breaths before slowly getting up.

As with the previous exercise, repeat this daily meditation as often as you need to.

Healing Light

This powerful meditation is designed to enable you to access the powers of healing in the universe.

1. Sit comfortably either in a straight-backed chair or on a cushion or mat. Once in a comfortable posture, do one of the Basic Relaxation Exercises (see page 29).

2. As you sit quietly with your hands folded on your lap, visualize a tiny point of pure, white light located about six inches above your head.

3. Visualize this light getting brighter. As it brightens, it sends out strong beams of light just in front of you, to your right, to your left, and behind you. See yourself surrounded by brilliant white light on all sides. That makes you feel secure and blessed.

4. As you continue to be aware of your breathing, inhale this light through your nose. Feel the light entering your lungs and penetrating every part of your body. Feel its healing power. Feel its wisdom.

5. Now visualize a blue light beginning to move through your body, exiting through the soles of your feet. This is a cleansing light, and it is sweeping away any negative thoughts, inner disharmony, pain, and tension that you may have been holding. Breathe in the white light, and exhale the blue light, knowing that you are being healed by the incoming "white" breath and cleansed by the outgoing "blue" breath.

6. Continue this exercise for several minutes. As you slowly come out of your meditation, visualize the light fading until it again becomes the tiny point of light above your head. Express gratitude to the light, and ask that it remain with you throughout the day. Know, too, that you can access its power at any time.

Healing Hand

The following meditation is similar to the previous one, except that it involves the use of your own hand for channeling additional healing energy to a specific area of your body that is ill or in pain.

1. Sit comfortably either in a straight-backed chair or on a cushion or mat. Once in a comfortable posture, do one of the Basic Relaxation Exercises (see page 29).

2. As you sit quietly, visualize a tiny point of pure, white light located about six inches above your head.

3. Visualize this light getting brighter. As it brightens, it sends out strong beams of light just in front of you, to your right, to your left, and behind you. You see yourself surrounded by brilliant white light on all sides of you. It makes you feel both secure and blessed.

4. As you continue to be aware of your breathing, inhale this light through your nose. Feel the light entering your lungs and penetrating every part of your body. Feel its healing power. Feel its wisdom.

5. Imagine that your right hand is receiving an extra abundance of healing energy; it is almost as though the healing light is radiating out of your hand.

6. Gently place your hand on an area of your body or mind that needs healing, and envision this light penetrating that area, bathing it with healing energy. If you have been feeling pain in that area, imagine the pain being dissipated by the energy from your hand. Remember that the light may make you feel either warm or cool.

7. Continue this exercise for several minutes. As you slowly come out of your meditation, visualize the light fading until it again becomes the tiny point of light above your head.

Managing Pain

1. Sit comfortably either in a straight-backed chair or on a cushion or mat. Once in a comfortable posture, do one of the Basic Relaxation Exercises (see page 29).

2. Remember an event or experience that you thoroughly enjoyed. It may be a time that made you happy, a special meal, or an experience with a special person you remember with fondness. Recall the details of that experience, including sights, sounds, colors, and tastes. Recall the feelings that you had, and savor the memories.

3. Now move your visualization to another event, such as a celebration. Recall the laughter, the play, the feelings of happiness you had. Savor your memory of the experience, and bring it into the present moment.

4. Visualize some of your accomplishments in life, or aspects of your life that are special sources of pride and happiness for you. Allow yourself to feel good about yourself and your accomplishments.

5. Continue to be aware of your breathing. Visualize these good feelings flowing into the area of your body that is in pain. Feel their warmth and healing power. Know that these memories and experiences are parts of your total being—your living history.

6. Slowly conclude your meditation. Take several deep breaths, stretch, and slowly rise from your meditation posture.

Inner Wisdom

This meditation helps us to come in contact with our body's inner wisdom; the ultimate source of healing.

1. Sit comfortably either in a straight-backed chair or on a cushion or mat. Once comfortable, do one of the Basic Relaxation Exercises (see page 29).

2. As you take full, deep, and easy breaths, feel your body relaxing totally. At the same time, feel the aliveness of your body: your energy is flowing, your emotions are stable, your mind is alert.

3. Perform a "mental scan" of your body. Be aware of circulation, digestion, elimination, temperature regulation, and protection, which your brain, nervous system, immune system, muscles, and organs do on their own, without you having to think about them. Feel your body to maintain and heal itself.

4. Allow yourself to experience a sense of gratitude and wonder. Tell your body that you are grateful.

5. Now ask your body what it needs at this time to facilitate healing. You may need to ask more than once. Be open to receiving any answer that may come up; it may involve proper nutrition, rest, exercise, therapeutic procedures, herbs, or something else. Write your impressions in a journal.

6. Slowly conclude your meditation. Take several deep breaths, stretch, and slowly rise from your meditation posture.

Trauma and Shock

Life involves constant change. However, major changes, such as sudden traumas, unexpected loss, or surprising news, can be difficult to deal with.

1. When faced with sudden or traumatic change, find a quiet place and perform one or more of the Basic Relaxation Exercises (see page 29).

2. At the same time, strive to focus your attention on the present moment, being especially aware of your thoughts and feelings. Allow them to surface and record them in your journal.

3. After several minutes (or for as long as this process lasts), offer these feelings to God or the Great Spirit. Ask for assistance in dealing with your situation (you may wish to say, simply, "Lord, please help me!")

4. Continue your breathing for several minutes before concluding.

5. Repeat as necessary.

The following meditation is based on a sacred exercise taught by Sun Bear, a Native American shaman and founder of the Bear tribe. It is designed to help us release negative feelings (often involving pain, anger, and frustration) and send them to the Earth Mother for healing and transformation.

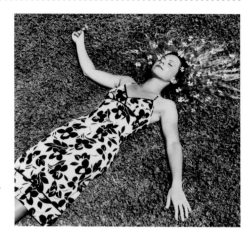

Go to an isolated place in the forest, preferably out of earshot of surrounding homes and businesses. Ideally, the area would be a place where you could use a blanket to lie comfortably on your stomach or back.

While standing or sitting in a cross-legged position, spend several minutes doing one of the Basic Relaxation Exercises (see page 29). Try to feel your connection with the Earth Mother. After several minutes, say, "Earth Mother, I pray to release my feelings and give them to You for healing and transformation."

Lying on the ground, feel free to scream, cry, or yell, in order to empty your being of anger, fear, hurt, frustration, or resentment. Pound your fists on the ground, if you wish (this is not a "dignified" exercise!). Express your feelings directly into the earth, and at the same time, observe your train of thought and feelings without censoring or judging them.

When you are finished, return to a sitting or standing position. Breathe deeply and feel your connection to the earth. Be aware of the healing power of the Earth Mother, your source of life and nurturing. Conclude your meditation with a prayer of thanks.

Kabbalah

Among the early Jews, the date palm represented the symbolic tree of life in the Kabbalah, the ancient system of Jewish mysticism. The mystical tree of life, known as Sephiroth, is made up of the ten emanations of the infinite God, or the "qualities of God's infinity made manifest in a finite world."

Like the cosmic Asvatha tree of the Buddhists, the Sephirothic tree is inverted, symbolizing the manifestation of the cosmos from a single transcendent source. Each of the ten Sephira represents a group of exalted ideas, titles, and attributes, which are listed opposite.

First Sephira: Kether (the crown or the primordial point)

Second Sephira: Chokmah (wisdom or the primordial idea)

Third Sephira: Binah (intelligence and understanding)

Fourth Sephira: Chesed or Gedula (mercy or love)

Fifth Sephira: Geburah (The "power" of God, chiefly manifested as severity, strength, fortitude, and justice)

Sixth Sephira: Tipereth (compassion, beauty, the heart and center of the Sephirothic tree)

Seventh Sephira: Netzach (firmness, victory, or lasting endurance)

Eighth Sephira: Hod (glory or majesty)

Ninth Sephira: Yesod (formation, or the foundation or basis of all active forces in God)

Tenth Sephira: Malkuth (the kingdom of earth, action, and all nature)

The Sephiroth are considered by kabbalists to be a bridge connecting the finite universe with the infinite God. In the Zohar, a compendium of kabbalistic teachings, it is said that the Torah is the Sephirothic tree of life and that all who occupy themselves with it are assured of life in the world to come.

Nature

Nature is a powerful source of beauty and inspiration, and meditating in a natural setting can be an unforgettable experience. However, even if we cannot meditate in a natural setting, we can visualize nature in our minds. The following meditations are devoted to exploring our connection with the natural world and using its magic to facilitate inner healing and transformation.

Outdoors

Being in nature helps mobilize our five basic senses and stimulates our sixth sense—intuition. When you go into nature to meditate, choose a natural form that attracts you, such as a lake, a stream, or some other body of water; a tree; a flower; a cliff; a meadow; or a mountain. Using your senses of sight, hearing, smell, touch, and (if appropriate) taste, "observe" the natural form. Breathe fully, but without forcing your breath.

Close your eyes, but continue to visualize the natural form in your mind's eye. As you breathe, be aware of any thoughts, feelings, memories, or personal associations that come up. Be especially aware of your feelings, without judging them one way or the other.

Slowly open your eyes and come out of your meditation. Devote several minutes to recording your impressions in a journal. Conclude by giving thanks to the natural form that assisted you in your meditation practice.

The following meditations can be done indoors.

In Apple Orchards

1. Sit comfortably in a chair or on a meditation mat on the floor. Do one of the Basic Relaxation Exercises (see page 29) or use another relaxation method of your choice. Be aware of your breathing.

2. After you have relaxed your body and mind, imagine yourself walking down a path toward an apple orchard.

3. Visualize the trees in the orchard bearing the ripest of fruit. Bees, butterflies, and songbirds are everywhere. In the distance, you hear a rushing stream. Pause for a moment and listen to it.

4. Feel yourself being welcomed into the orchard by the bees, the birds, and the trees themselves. It's a magical feeling. Pause and reflect.

5. Imagine yourself bowing in honor of the tree, and express the greeting, "Your life is one with mine." Pause and reflect.

6. Picture yourself picking an apple from the tree. Bring it to your chest and hold it up in front of you. Pause and reflect.

7. Imagine yourself biting into the apple. It is the most delicious and juicy apple you have ever tasted. Imagine the apple's essence awakening your taste buds and then permeating your entire being, bringing you nourishment, cleansing, and inner healing.

8. After several minutes, respectfully take leave of the orchard and return to your normal state of consciousness. Take several deep breaths and stretch, if you like. Slowly leave your sitting position.

By Rivers

1. As in the previous meditation, sit comfortably in a chair or on a meditation mat on the floor. Do one of the Basic Relaxation Exercises (see page 29) or another relaxation method of your choice. Be aware of your breathing.

2. After you have relaxed your body and mind, place your focus on your heart. It is constantly pumping blood throughout your body and is also the abode of your love.

3. Visualize your heart as a river of pure, clean water. On the shore of the river is an altar made up entirely of precious stones, including amethysts, emeralds, rubies, and diamonds. Behind the altar are lush tropical trees in full blossom. The blossoms are beautiful to behold, and their aroma permeates all of your senses.

4. Visualize yourself seated within this beautiful scene, feeling as one with it. Your heart feels rich and expansive. It is the center of your life. Enjoy your visit here. Express gratitude to be able to enjoy such richness in your life.

5. After several minutes, respectfully take your leave and return to your normal state of consciousness. Take several deep breaths and stretch, if you like. Slowly leave your sitting position.

Four Elements

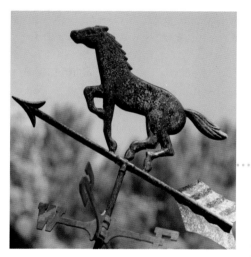

The purpose of these meditations is to allow us to deepen our connection with the four elements: earth, fire, water, and air. These meditations are most successful when done outdoors in a natural setting, but that is not essential.

Earth

As you sit comfortably or lie down on your back using a mat or blanket, devote several minutes to relaxation, using one of the Basic Relaxation Exercises (see page 29). Pay special attention to your breathing. Visualize all the tension leaving your body until you feel completely relaxed.

Feel your physical and energetic connection to the earth. Imagine that the earth's strength not only is supporting you, but is giving you vital energy. Remember that the earth contains minerals, such as iron, calcium, silica, and magnesium that are also found in your body, so you have both an energetic and a biochemical connection to the earth. Feel this connection and your gratitude toward the earth elements as you continue to breathe deeply. After several minutes, respectfully take your leave and return to your normal state of consciousness. Take several deep breaths and stretch, if you like. Slowly leave your sitting position.

Fire

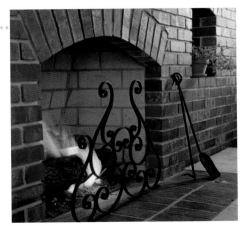

This meditation is best done on a sunny day (wear a hat or sunscreen as needed).

Sit comfortably or lie down on your back using a mat or blanket. As in the previous meditation, devote several minutes to progressive relaxation. Take full, deep breaths, knowing that you are bringing the life force into your body with each incoming breath.

Feel the warmth and light of the sun on your body. The fire of the sun can destroy, but it is essential for life and creation. As you breathe, focus on the essential qualities of life: heat, passion, purification. Feel the heat within your body, filling you with passion and inspiration. Know too that the fire element in your body allows your immune system to function, killing viruses, bacteria, and germs with its purifying heat. Feel the fire within fill you with the energy to develop creative visions and achieve new goals. Feel your gratitude for the fire element in your life. After several minutes, respectfully take your leave and return to your normal state of consciousness. Take several deep breaths and stretch, if you like. Slowly leave your sitting position.

Water

Sit or lie down using a mat or blanket near a river, a lake, or some other body of water. If this is not possible, sit near a fountain. A glass of water will do also!

As in previous exercises, devote several minutes to relaxation and deep breathing until you feel completely relaxed.

Visualize the element of water and the importance it has in your life. Ponder its nourishing and purifying qualities. Think about the spiritual essence of water and about flowing water as symbolizing the movement of life. Remind yourself that more than 75 percent of your body is made up of water, and imagine how water functions in your organs, tissues, and body processes, including circulation, locomotion, elimination, and digestion. Visualize the water element bringing you cleansing and healing, and feel your gratitude toward it. After several minutes, respectfully take your leave and return to your normal state of consciousness. Take several deep breaths and stretch, if you like. Slowly leave your sitting position.

Air

This meditation is best done outdoors. Sit comfortably on a chair or on the ground. Devote several minutes to deep, rhythmic breathing, as described in one of the breathing exercises earlier in this book. Continue to practice deep breathing until you feel completely relaxed.

Focus your attention on the all-pervading qualities of air: the air that you breathe and that gives you the gift of life, the gentle breezes that caress your face, and the winds that bring new ideas and fresh perspectives. Feel your connection with the air element within—the oxygen that energizes and nourishes every cell of your body. As you breathe deeply of the life-giving air, feel your gratitude toward it. After several minutes, respectfully take your leave and return to your normal state of consciousness. Take several deep breaths and stretch, if you like. Slowly leave your sitting position.

Flowers Meditations

In addition to their beauty, flowers can provide us with a potent source of inspiration and wisdom. They possess the ability to elevate our spirits and bring us hope and comfort during times of difficulty. Many feel that the presence of flowers in a hospital room can help speed the patient's recovery considerably.

Meditating with flowers can be a powerful experience that is both gentle and transformational. The following four meditations utilize the power of flowers in different ways. You can vary the first three meditations endlessly with different species of flowers, which will impart a different keynote quality to each meditative experience.

Flowers

1. Sitting, place a single flower in a vase and set it before you. If you do not have access to a fresh flower, a color photograph of a flower will do.

2. Perform one of the Basic Relaxation Exercises (see page 29).

3. Observe the flower carefully: its colors, textures, aroma, and form.

4. After a few minutes of observation, gently close your eyes, seeing the flower in your mind's eye.

5. Think about what the flower means to you, both as a symbol and as a friend. As you observe your thoughts about the flower, be aware of other associations that come to mind.

6. As the mental images of the flower begin to fade, open your eyes again.

7. After a few minutes of observation, gently conclude your meditation.

1. Go to a garden or to some wildflowers in a field. It is important that you allow yourself to be drawn to the specific flowers you wish to work with. Sit comfortably on the ground with a mat or blanket if desired. Devote several minutes to one of the Basic Relaxation Exercises (see page 29) or another one that works for you, until you feel comfortable and relaxed.

2. Silently observe the flowers. As you contemplate them, visualize their beginning from a tiny seed deep in the earth. Imagine them breaking through the soil. Observe the flower's color, form, and overall beauty. Feel its strength and vitality, its utter joy to be alive, and its ability to express itself to the fullest, even in a difficult environment. Allow yourself to connect with the energy of the flower.

3. Take several deep breaths. Turn your focus back to yourself and your own physical and emotional condition. Note that both you and the flowers share the same life force that comes from the earth, which assures your survival, growth, and healing, and that the possibilities for healing are tremendous.

4. Offer a prayer such as, "I pray for the power of nature to help me heal my life," or create one that applies more to your specific health situation. And allow yourself to feel inspiration and appreciation for the beauty around you. Devote at least ten minutes to this meditation, but end it if you feel tired.

5. Before concluding your meditation, take several deep breaths and stretch. Repeat the meditation as often as you wish.

Red Roses

The red rose is a powerful symbol of human love. Among the most valued of garden flowers, the rose is an enduring symbol of unfolding love.

1. Sit comfortably in a straight-backed chair or on a meditation cushion or mat.

2. Be aware of your breathing. Take slow, deep, and even breaths. At each exhalation, feel the tension drain out of your body and mind.

3. When you feel fully relaxed, visualize your heart chakra as a pure, fresh rosebud ready to open.

4. Continue your breathing. Visualize the rosebud opening slowly. As it unfolds, pay attention to each individual petal as representing a quality of love. These may include compassion, caring, devotion, protection, passion, kindness, selflessness, service, caring, and nurturing.

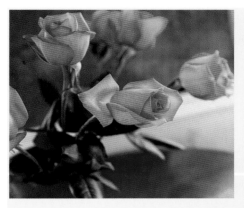

5. As your heart center continues to open, think of those you love and send them love at this time. As the rose opens, imagine these feelings of love radiating outward into the world. Don't forget to include yourself as well. Allow at least several minutes for this part of the meditation.

6. As you continue to breathe, allow your heart feelings to expand their range so that you are radiating love to the larger community. See your heart as full and healthy, radiating love and light.

7. As you conclude your meditation, take several deep breaths, holding your hands to your heart center. After a few stretches, slowly get up from your meditation position.

Trees

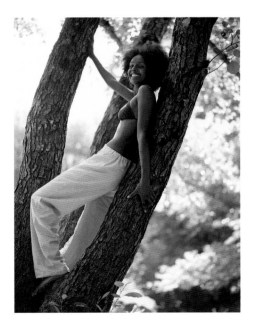

Trees have always played a central role in the survival of humanity and in the flowering of myriad cultures, including the ancient Egyptian, Hebrew, Greek, Roman, Indian, Japanese, Chinese, and Native American. Although many of us consider trees to be inanimate objects, native peoples have long considered them sacred beings offering wisdom, guidance, inspiration, and healing. Many believe that because humans and trees both live in the vertical dimension (although trees remain in one place throughout their lives while humans are constantly moving), we share a special bond of friendship. The following meditations are designed to help us create a deeper connection with trees and open ourselves to their life-giving and life-affirming nature.

Individual Trees

Repeat these first five steps for all the individual tree species meditations.

1. Stand near a tree, or imagine yourself standing near a tree.

2. Stand comfortably erect, bending your knees slightly, making sure they are not locked. Feel your feet on the ground and the ground supporting your body.

3. Imagine a vertical line in the center of your being, moving down from the sky through your spine and continuing through both feet, penetrating the earth.

4. Breathe normally, with an awareness of your breath.

5. Try to "feel" what it is like to be a tree (devote at least two minutes to each of the following exercises):

Oak Trees

6. Feel your body strong and straight.

7. Hold your arms open, palms turned upward.

8. Feel yourself stable against the winds of life; while flexible and able to adapt to meet the challenges, affirm your groundedness in truth.

9. Visualize yourself as providing others with nourishment, strength, and protection.

10. Feel your connection to both the earth and the sky, drawing both wisdom from the earth and nourishment from the sky and sun.

Pine Trees

6. Feel your body strong and straight. Imagine your head to be higher than it actually is.

7. Hold your arms open at a 45-degree angle to your body, palms facing downward.

8. Feel your connection to the earth.

9. Feel yourself solid yet flexible, with your boughs offering a blessing to those around you.

10. Meditate on the concept of compassion and see yourself as a source of understanding and compassion for others.

Gingko Trees

6. Feel yourself as ancient as the earth itself, going back to the time of the dinosaurs, unique and unconventional.

7. As an aged being from the East, acknowledge your ability to adapt and thrive, even in difficult circumstances.

8. Specifically acknowledge how you have succeeded in your life up to now, and how you have persevered. What innate talents and abilities did you use to accomplish this?

9. See yourself as having succeeded while keeping your beauty and maintaining your individuality.

10. Finally, acknowledge that your challenges in life are gifts from the Earth Mother that have strengthened you and increased your power and resourcefulness.

Maple Trees

6. Feel yourself as abundant and receptive, with your branches opening in all directions, reaching out to others.

7. Imagine your branches as a form of antennae, receiving information from the world around you.

8. At the same time, be conscious of how you affect others around you through your thoughts, feelings, and actions.

9. Visualize yourself receiving the best from others and giving your best in return.

10. Finally, experience the joy of the maple tree—strong, bright, and intimately involved with life around it.

Weeping Willow Trees

6. Stand erect, with your shoulders relaxed and your arms at your sides.

7. Visualize yourself as a tree of calm and grace, even when you are experiencing difficulty in your life. You are grounded in reality and acknowledge the truth of your situation at the moment.

8. Now feel your strong connection to the water element with its inherent fluidity and nourishing properties, giving life to every cell of your body.

9. Acknowledge the water element as a part of you that is ever present; at the same time, see yourself as part of this eternal movement of life.

Acorns

1. After performing one of the Basic Relaxation Exercises (see page 29), take an actual acorn and hold it in your hand; if an acorn is not available, use a photograph or hold a mental image of an acorn in your mind's eye.

2. As you hold or imagine it, allow your mind to explore any associations the acorn has for you. Continue to be aware of your breathing.

3. If your mind moves too far afield from your subject, gently move your focus back to the image of the acorn.

4. After several minutes, conclude your meditation.

Healing with Trees

Choose a large, healthy tree to which you feel drawn. Sit down on a mat or blanket either facing the tree or with your spine resting against the tree, or lie down with your feet touching (or almost touching) the tree. If you feel especially needful of support or of a physical connection to the tree, embrace the tree with your body pressed against it.

1. Devote several minutes to one of the Basic Relaxation Exercises (see page 29) until you feel comfortable and relaxed.

2. As you breathe evenly and fully, feel your energetic connection with the tree. Like the tree, imagine yourself to be in total alignment in your body, mind, and emotions. Feel the energy of the tree intermingling with yours. Feel the vital power of the tree strengthen your energy field and your feeling of being "grounded" in the earth.

3. Ask the tree for healing. You can say something such as "Brother/sister tree, my life force is one with yours. Please help me to heal." Say this with feeling and sincerity, as though the tree is a dear friend who can truly assist you in the healing process.

4. Devote several minutes to receptive silence and contemplation. Allow yourself to be open to new (and possibly unexpected) ideas, impressions, and insights about your health situation and how you might improve it. Continue to breathe, taking slow, natural breaths, and feeling your connection to the tree and its indwelling spirit of intelligence, love, and power. Record your experiences in a journal, if you wish.

5. After ten minutes, you are ready to conclude your meditation. Express your gratitude to the tree and slowly take your leave. If you feel that you have benefited from this meditation, return to the tree again for additional healing sessions.

Sit near a lake, stream, river, or ocean. As you breathe quietly and evenly, observe the light reflecting on the water, and see how it is constantly changing. Observe the changing light. As you do, see your mind alive and changing as well.

Alternatively, place a glass of water in front of you.

1. As you breathe, observe the water as essential to your life. Observe your mind as you explore the meaning that water has for you.

2. If your mind wanders, gently and patiently bring your focus back to the water. This part of the meditation can take several minutes.

3. As you continue your meditation, gently lift the glass and slowly drink the water, taking small sips. Devote several minutes to ingesting the water. Be aware of any feelings as you do this.

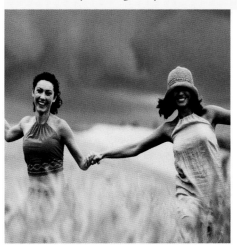

Walking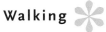

Most people believe that meditation is best practiced sitting on a cushion or mat. Yet walking meditation can trace its roots back hundreds of years to the Zen tradition. Like sitting meditations, walking meditations help the meditator to be aware. Yet unlike sitting, walking offers us a constant stream of images and experience that require constant observation.

Walking Indoors

For this meditation, you'll want to create a clear path at least twelve feet long. It is best to remove your shoes for this exercise so you can be in better contact with the floor.

1. Begin by standing, devoting several minutes to one of the Basic Relaxation Exercises (see page 29) or another form of relaxation. With your body relaxed, bend your knees slightly and feel your feet connected to the floor. Place your hands gently at your sides, or clasp your hands behind you. Remain conscious of your breathing.

2. Begin walking slowly, looking down at the floor several feet ahead of you. Be aware of the forward movement of your body, as well as the connection as each foot touches the floor. Your mind will continually shift its focus as you apply one foot to the floor, place your weight on that foot, bend your knee, and move your other foot. Simply stay aware of your movement, which should be gradual, fluid, and easy.

3. When you reach the end of your indoor path, gently turn around. Be aware of your movements as you do this. Continue to observe your breathing, and be aware of any thoughts that come up. If you find yourself daydreaming or being otherwise distracted, gently bring your focus back to your movement.

4. When you return to your starting point, conclude your walking meditation. Stand still for several minutes. Bend your knees slightly and be aware of your breathing, noting your inner calm and dignity.

Walking Outdoors

For this walking meditation, you will want to either go barefoot or wear light shoes or sandals. Choose a predetermined route that will be approximately 12 to 27 feet in length.

1. As you stand comfortably with your knees slightly bent, take a few moments to relax. As you watch your breathing, feel your feet firmly planted on the earth.

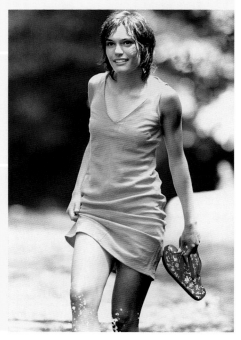

2. Begin walking slowly, looking down at the earth several feet ahead of you. Be aware of each foot as it touches the ground. Feel the living earth supporting your body as it moves.

3. When you reach the end of your path, stop and then turn around slowly. Remain mindful of your movement, as well as your connection to the earth. Slowly return to your starting point, being mindful of your breathing, your movement, and your connection to the earth.

4. When you return to your starting point, stand still for several minutes, knees slightly bent. Continue to be aware of your breathing as well as the supporting earth beneath your feet. As in the indoor walking meditation, note your feelings of inner calm and dignity.

Walking Outdoors with a Partner

This walking meditation requires a partner and a blindfold. Your partner will gently lead you, blindfolded, for a short walk on a route that you have both determined is safe.

1. Before you begin, devote several minutes to one of the Basic Relaxation Exercises (see page 29). As in the previous walking meditation, bend your knees slightly and feel your connection to the earth, which is supporting you totally.

2. Put on the blindfold and have your partner to turn you around several times so that you lose your sense of direction. Take your partner by the arm and have him or her silently lead you on a slow yet steady walk.

3. As the two of you walk in silence, be aware of your feelings and sensations, without censoring them in any way. If you feel fear, observe it and breathe into the areas of your body where you experience the fear as you walk. Be aware, too, of feelings of enjoyment, trust, and surrender.

4. Devote several minutes to this walking meditation. After you return to your starting point, stand quietly for several minutes, being aware of your breathing as well as any feelings that come up.

5. After concluding your meditation, write your impressions in a journal or share your experience with your partner. Allow your partner to share his or her experience with you as well.

Seeing and Listening

We often go through life in a state of inattention. In order to function more efficiently in today's modern world, we often block out sights and sounds we don't wish to deal with. As a result, we may isolate ourselves from the rhythms of life and limit our life experiences.

Seeing.

This simple meditation helps us cultivate the art of seeing. Leave your home for a walk through your neighborhood; devote from thirty to sixty minutes to this meditation so that you don't feel rushed. You may decide to choose the same route as you might take on an ordinary day, but this time you will walk slowly (at about half your normal speed) while paying close attention to everything in your range of vision.

In this walking meditation, you may wish to stop and observe a neighborhood tree, gaze at a flower by the roadside, or examine the shingles on the roof of a nearby house. You may pause to watch children playing, or silently observe shoppers as they enter and leave the supermarket. Simply allow these sights to enter your consciousness without censoring or judging them in any way.

Continue walking. Chances are that you will see many familiar things but will view them from a refreshingly new perspective.

Listening.

As in the previous meditation, walk in silence for thirty minutes to an hour. This may involve a walk in your neighborhood, in the park, or by the seashore. In this exercise, you are not to speak, but merely to listen, so you may want to limit your interaction with others. Listen to the sounds of nature, traffic, music, people talking, construction, and 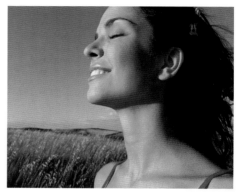 airplanes flying overhead. Try not to censor or block out any sounds. If any sounds distress you, breathe deeply to regain your composure.

Silently Walking in a Group

Walking in nature as a group can be a highly rewarding experience. There are many types of walking meditations, and your natural environment will often determine them. A moonlight meditation on a path through the forest or a walking meditation along the shore at dawn will be very different experiences. Yet there are some general guidelines to help maximize your experience. This meditation is often conducted by a facilitator who can gently lead the group in the meditation process.

1. Before starting, the group should come together in a circle, joining hands. After the facilitator offers a brief description of the program, members quietly focus their consciousness on the unique experience they will have both as individuals and as a group.

2. With the facilitator leading the group, members walk in single file at a slow to moderate pace.

3. Silence is observed as they walk. In this silence, the participants are invited to use all of their senses, especially sight, hearing, and smell. Be aware of the trees, animals, and sky, and feel your connection to them all.

4. Ideally, the group should have a predetermined destination, such as a stream, a lake, or a large tree or clearing. Participants maintain their silence as they arrive at their destination.

5. The facilitator can lead a small ceremony at this site. Members of the group join hands while sitting in a circle. Prayer, chanting, or other forms of ritual can be done here, or silence can be maintained throughout. The type of ceremony may vary according to the destination. For example, a tree meditation can be especially powerful under a large oak or redwood tree, while a meditation exploring the mysteries of moving water is appropriate when you are visiting a lake or ocean shore. However, some people may prefer to be alone at this time, finding a personal spot for meditation, prayer, or silent reflection.

6. After a predetermined period of time (which might last from fifteen minutes to an hour), the group can assemble once more. The participants return to their starting place, walking in single file and in silence.

7. Upon their return to the starting place, members again join hands and have the opportunity to share their experiences and feelings about the meditation walk. A closing prayer by the facilitator or other members of the group may conclude the meditation.

Seeking Wisdom

In traditional cultures, community members often have access to a wise elder who is a source of instruction and advice. Often a shaman or medicine person, the elder is regarded as a type of community treasure, whose advice is highly valued by tribal members. In many cases, this person helps us to access our own innate wisdom by telling stories or asking questions. However, most of us today do not have access to a wise and trusted older adult who can offer us clarity and vision when we are facing a difficult problem.

The following exercise is designed to help us access wisdom in our life by contacting "the sage within" through meditation.

1. Perform one of the Basic Relaxation Exercises (see page 29).

2. Close your eyes. Imagine that you are in the presence of a sage—a wise person of limitless knowledge and compassion. Know also that this person is very concerned about your welfare and is eager to help you in any way

possible. Imagine yourself making respectful contact with this elder.

3. Ask this person a question about an issue that has been troubling you: it may concern a problem in your relationship, an important career decision you have to make, or a question about how you can improve your health. Continue to be aware of your breathing as you ask this question.

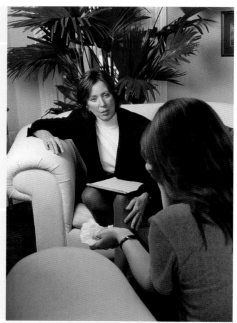

4. Allow yourself to be receptive to whatever response comes up. You may receive a direct answer, or you may be asked another question in return. Allow yourself to be open to whatever response you receive.

5. After several minutes, express gratitude to this person and take leave of him or her. Conclude your meditation.

6. Write down your experiences in a journal. You may not receive a final answer to your question in one session. It is possible that the information you receive during your meditation may lead to additional questions to ponder before you arrive at a satisfactory solution. With practice, this meditation can become an important learning tool.

Daily Reviews

We human beings are made up of a variety of often contradictory currents. We have qualities that we view as positive, such as compassion, humor, courage, and openness to new ideas. We also have qualities we call negative, such as jealousy, possessiveness, fearfulness, and dishonesty. Very often, we tend to ignore the negative currents or downplay their significance in our lives.

This process is not unlike having to deal with noisy children who constantly demand our attention. We want them to leave us in peace, and we may either ignore them or send them to their rooms. We often ignore our negative feelings or simply pretend that they do not exist. Unfortunately, like children who feel that they are being ignored by their parents, the negative feelings demand our attention with greater and greater intensity. When unresolved feelings are not dealt with directly, they often create situations in our life that force us to deal with them anyway. Very often these situations form a pattern. Though we often judge them to be "bad," our difficulties can provide us with the stepping stones to enable us to make positive changes in our ways of thinking and feeling.

Spiritual teachers have told us that one of the goals of meditation is to explore what are known as "lower self issues" in order to transform them into positive qualities. Like digging through a layer of mud and dirt to uncover a buried treasure, so must we dig through the "dirt" of our lower nature to discover our universal soul.

Evening Reviews

The best time to do this meditation is when you are ready for bed. You may also wish to do it whenever you are having trouble sleeping due to worry or another form of emotional disturbance. To do this meditation, have a notebook or journal at hand, as well as a quiet place where you can be alone.

1. Sit quietly for several minutes at the end of your day. Take several deep, gentle breaths and affirm that you wish to explore areas of your being that have caused you difficulty during the day. You may make a prayer of your own, or simply say, "I pray to explore areas of my being that have caused me difficulty today."

2. After several minutes of receptive silence, write down keywords or sentences describing situations or feelings that caused disharmony in your life during the day. Be completely honest and candid in your statements, which are intended to be only between you and God. "I lost my temper with my wife today," or "I spread gossip about my co-worker today," are two examples.

Such statements may reveal resentment, jealousy, anger, sadness, feelings of low self-esteem, or acts of deception. Though you may feel ashamed about these feelings or actions, write them down anyway. They are all part of you and make up part of your internal "family."

Be careful not to judge yourself or make the feelings or actions worse than they really are. Remember that even the most uncomfortable or shameful situation can be a stepping stone to spiritual fulfillment.

3. Continue to write for seven to ten minutes. Be mindful of how your thoughts, feelings, and actions caused disharmony during the day. When you've finished writing, say, "I ask God [or the Great Spirit] to help me transform areas of disharmony within my being."

4. Over the days and weeks that you will do this meditation, you will notice that clear patterns often reveal themselves. Ask yourself:

- "How do they appear?"
- "When do they come up and with whom?"
- "How do they cause disharmony in my life?"
- "What role do I have in creating this inner disharmony?"
- "How can I change these negative currents?"

5. Over weeks and months of regular meditation, you will become more aware of the geography of your lower nature. You will also become aware of many of the subtle tricks that you have used to avoid recognizing and dealing with difficult issues. By bringing disharmonious issues to light, you will find that you can work with them more effectively and transform negative currents into positive qualities that bring inner peace and greater awareness. Continue to ask God (or your Higher Self) for help with any area in your life that continues to cause you difficulty.

Morning Reviews

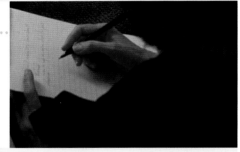

As in the evening review, many people who enjoy writing can practice a simple morning meditation that can help them achieve greater harmony and awareness during the day.

1. Sit quietly for a few minutes, taking regular breaths.

2. Ask God or your Higher Self for help in exploring areas that are of concern to you as you begin your day.

3. While in a receptive state, simply write down phrases or keywords that describe feelings of disharmony or concern. These may have to do with your feeling anger toward another person, anxiety about an interview at work, or fears about money or health. As in the evening review, simply write down whatever comes up without making judgments about it. Write for seven to ten minutes.

4. Read what you have written. Ask God or your Higher Self to help you be aware of these issues during the day, and ask for help in transforming them and dealing with them from a place of intelligence and higher understanding.

As you explore these issues at the beginning of every day, you can relate to them with greater clarity and purpose. Over time, you will see that this morning meditation will allow you to understand the inner meaning of troublesome issues and how they can be a catalyst for spiritual growth and inner peace.

Knowing Your Potential Self

Sit in a straight-backed chair. Adjust your body so it is comfortable, with your spine straight, your palms on your thighs facing up, and your feet flat on the floor.

Slowly close your eyes and start to breathe slowly, deeply, and rhythmically.

Continue to breathe deeply as you count from one to ten. The higher the number, the more deeply relaxed you become.

"One . . . two . . . three . . . four . . ."

Feel the energy pulsate through your body as you watch your breath.

"Five . . . six . . . seven . . ."

You feel that the boundaries of your body are gently disappearing.

"Eight . . . nine . . . ten."

Your mind is awake while your physical body is at rest.

Now imagine that your mind has expanded beyond the boundaries of your body. It is free from physical tension and bodily limitations. You can now experience profound insights and life-transforming breakthroughs.

Using all your senses, including sight, smell, hearing, touch, and taste, imagine that you are standing in a meadow near a flowing stream. You feel very comfortable here. There are flowers everywhere. An apple orchard is in

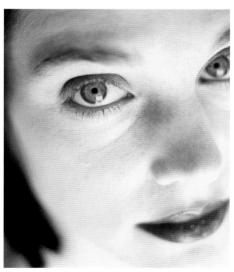

the background, and the trees are all in full bloom. Birds are singing. Bees and other insects are humming. You can hear the sound of water splashing on the rocks, and you can smell the spring flowers. The sky is blue, the air is crisp, and you feel a slight breeze on your face.

What do you see? What colors are there? What do you smell? What sounds do you hear? What do you feel touching you? What emotions do you feel? Feel the peace that is here.

While you are in this place of peace and beauty, imagine that you see a friendly figure approaching you. As you observe, imagine that the person coming toward you is you at your fullest potential. What qualities do you have within that are manifested in your life now? What do you look like? What qualities does that person have that you have not yet expressed in your life? Feel the kindness, the strength, and the enthusiasm that this person has as he or she walks towards you.

What is the chosen life path of that individual? What qualities has he or she developed? Breathe gently and continue to observe this person.

Now imagine that this person has a message to share with you. What is the message? Can you open your ears to hear it? Hear it now.

Finally, imagine this person walking up to you and making eye contact. See the love and understanding in the eyes of your realized self. Acknowledge your connectedness and love for each other.

Now slowly begin counting down from ten to one.

"Ten . . . nine . . . eight . . . seven . . ."

You feel both an inner calm and a deep connection to your true self.

"Six . . . five . . . four . . . three . . . two . . . one."

You are wide awake and alert, both physically and mentally. You feel rested and relaxed, with an inner calm and a deep connection to your true self. You will retain an inner knowing of who you are as you live your daily life.

Remember that through this meditation, you can return any time you want to enjoy the peace of this place and commune with your full potential self.

 ## Rainbow Colors

Color is a form of vibrational energy that can affect the way we think and feel: colors can depress us or enable us to feel more optimistic; they can even help stimulate the immune system by their subtle influence on the human mind. We all know that walking into a room painted robin's-egg blue, for example, will produce a different feeling from walking into a room painted bright red. By using color consciously, we can help bring about major changes in all areas of our lives.

The following meditations help us to access the hidden powers of color and the power that they can bring to our lives on physical, psychological, and spiritual levels.

After performing one of the Basic Relaxation Exercises (see page 29), visualize a field of color. You may also see the color as a flower, a light, a cloth, or a flame, such as a red rose, a blue sky, or a bright yellow sun.

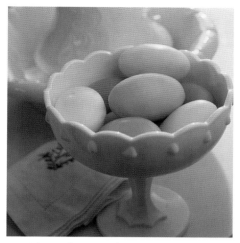

Visualize the color penetrating your entire being. In your mind's eye, feel the power that the particular color brings to your life, and how it can enhance your present-day reality.

Red arouses passion and desire. It is a color that is helpful to visualize when your energy level is low, or when you're lacking courage or motivation. Red can help you to feel your connection to nature. It also helps stimulate masculine energy and enables you to connect with qualities such as strength, activity, assertiveness, protection, stability, realism, and objectivity.

Orange mobilizes your courage to try something new. It enhances your desire for forward movement and overcoming obstacles. Orange also helps you to become more open to your feelings and energizes psychic vision.

Yellow has long been linked with stimulating intellectual activity and increasing mental capacity, and for this reason it is a good color to meditate on when you have research to do or an important decision to make. The color yellow rekindles dormant creativity and helps you feel more open to joy and humor. Drawing upon yellow also facilitates communication and helps you to become aware of new ideas.

Green is the color of healing and renewal. It enhances the desire for self-development and personal expansion and facilitates getting in touch with your innate optimism and enthusiasm. Meditate on the color green when you feel that your health needs improvement or that you need to find a new direction in life.

Blue is viewed as a "quiet" color, which facilitates receptivity and relaxation. It helps you to surrender and access inner peace. The color blue also allows you to better feel your connection to celestial realms and stimulates your feminine qualities, such as sensitivity and intuitive recognition.

Indigo arouses the life force within and helps you to integrate your sexuality with your spirituality. Long connected to helping people become committed to a spiritual path (as well as embrace spiritual values in general), the color indigo inspires you to realize your inner divinity. Meditate on indigo if you want to find your spiritual direction in life.

Violet awakens inner devotion and enhances your perceptions of universality and universal consciousness. It inspires soul-mate recognition and helps you develop deeper psychic and spiritual connections with loved ones. Violet is a healing color. It also helps you to learn the value of forgiveness, so it is a good color to meditate on if you are angry or annoyed with yourself or anyone else.

White is not technically a color, but it is composed of all seven colors of the rainbow. Meditating on white helps you to perceive the universality of people and things and enables you to view life from a perspective of wholeness. At the same time, white awakens innocence and purity.

Rainbows

You can also meditate on all the colors of the rainbow together. When you perform a Rainbow Meditation, imagine yourself sitting underneath a rainbow's shining bands of color. Focus on each color one by one, and ponder the meaning it has in your life.

Three Points

This meditation technique, based on the teachings of H. Saraydarian, involves gathering together diverse ideas, opinions, and inventions and creating something new. It is not unlike dealing with an outdated, messy house. By cleaning it, repairing the cracked walls, repainting it, installing better lighting, and adding new furniture, we have created a completely different living space.

The Three Points meditation involves choosing a subject or an object you will think about from three viewpoints: form, quality, and purpose.

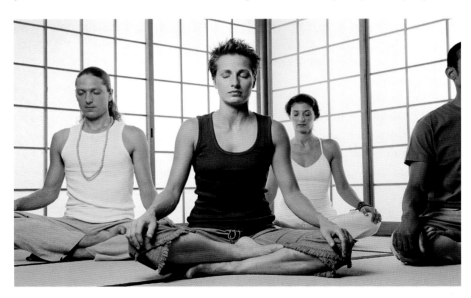

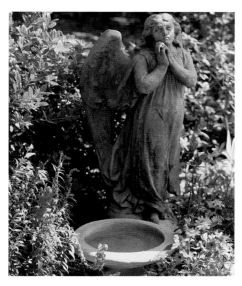

Possible choices for a meditation subject include:

- God
- God is Love
- Angel
- Telling the truth
- Education
- Justice
- Kindness
- Responsibility
- Open-mindedness
- Enlightenment
- Energy
- The goal of life
- Health

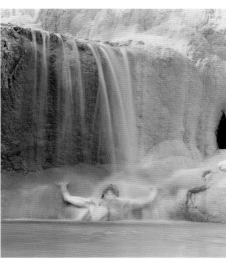

Possible choices for a meditation object include:

- Tree
- Leaf
- Candle flame
- Shell
- Illuminated bulb
- Waterfall
- Flower
- Mandala
- Open circle
- Image of a religious leader
- Cross
- Square in the circle

After you have chosen the subject or object of your meditation, think about it from the following three points of view, allowing your mind to expand and deepen its natural curiosity.

Form:

This involves not only the outer appearance of the physical form itself, but your feelings about the form; it also has to do with mental images that you associate with a concept such as "justice" or "God."

Quality:

This has to do with the aspects of the subject or object that set it apart from others. In this part of the meditation, you find the differences in quality as opposed to form.

Purpose:

Here you discern the purpose of the concept or image, including its life task, inner direction, higher calling, or destiny.

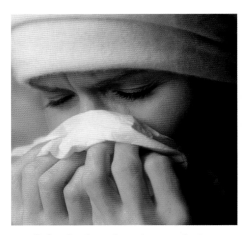

After devoting several minutes to any of the basic relaxation techniques described earlier, think about your chosen subject or object for three or four minutes as it pertains to form, quality, and purpose. As you become more comfortable with this meditation, you can devote more time to each point of view—up to a total of nine to twelve minutes.

You may also wish to record your impressions in a journal for future reference.

 Twenty Yamas

According to traditional Hindu teachings, the way to lead a virtuous life is to cultivate high moral values and manifest them in daily life. The term "yama" comes from the Sanskrit and means roughly "a way of self-restraint" or "a way of self-control." Less a religious doctrine than a form of moral psychology, the twenty basic yamas include:

1. **Ahimsa:** Nonviolence or noninjury; not harming others through hurtful thoughts, words, or deeds.

2. **Satya:** Truthfulness; speaking out for truth; keeping your promises.

3. **Asteya:** Not stealing; not coveting the property of others; prudence in your financial affairs.

4. **Brahmacharya:** Restraint in sex, including celibacy when single and faithfulness in marriage.

5. **Kshama:** Forgiveness, including sending goodwill to others.

6. **Dhriti:** Firmness; overcoming indecision and fear.

7. **Daya:** Compassion towards all beings.

8. **Arjava:** Honesty in all personal and business situations.

9. **Mitahara:** Control over your appetite; abstention from eating meat.

10. **Saucha:** Purity in body, mind, and emotion.

11. **Hri:** Feeling remorse for your personal misconduct.

12. **Santosha:** Contentment; being happy with what you have; seeking fulfillment in yourself rather than in the accumulation of wealth and outer recognition.

13. **Dana:** Tithing; giving generously to help others.

14. **Astikya:** Having deep faith in the grace of the Divine.

15. **Pujana:** Performing daily meditation or some other spiritual practice.

16. **Shravana:** Studying holy scriptures and listening to the teachings of the wise ones.

17. **Mati:** Sharpening your intellect through spiritual practice. In India, this is often done with the help of a guru or spiritual guide.

18. **Vrata:** Observing your sacred vows faithfully.

19. **Japa:** Chanting God's names and other sacred mantras daily.

20. **Tapas:** Austerity; in India, this often involves following a spiritual discipline as outlined by your guru.

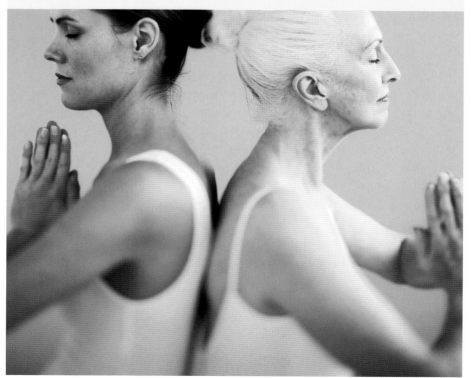

The following meditation plan is designed to be used over a period of twenty days. Each day will be devoted to meditating on one of the twenty yamas. For this meditation, you will need a journal. You may also wish to write each yama on an index card to refer to during meditation.

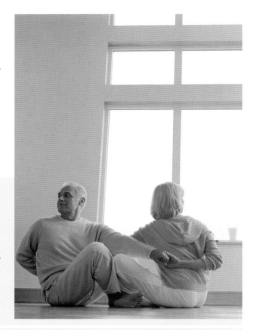

1. Seat yourself comfortably in a chair or on a cushion on the floor. Perform one or more of the Basic Relaxation Exercises (see page 29), or another relaxation method of your choice. Be aware of your breathing, which should be deep, slow, and even.

2. Pray for clarity and enlightenment. This can be a short prayer such as "I pray to open myself to the wisdom of the sacred yama and learn to follow it in my daily life."

3. Choose a yama and read the card that this aspect is written upon. Ponder the meaning and ramifications of the yama carefully. Ask about its meaning. To what extent do you manifest this yama in your life? In what areas is your understanding and practice lacking? Be totally honest with yourself, allowing your thoughts to flow freely, writing them down in your journal. At the same time, strive to be objective, being aware of feelings of annoyance, pride, remorse, or guilt that may come up. You will relate to some of them more strongly than others: for example, you may have more personal issues connected with *satya* (truth) than you have about *dana* (tithing). Devote five to ten minutes to this exercise.

4. When you are ready to conclude your meditation, take a few deep breaths. Express gratitude for your insights. Gently stretch your body as you slowly rise from your meditation posture.

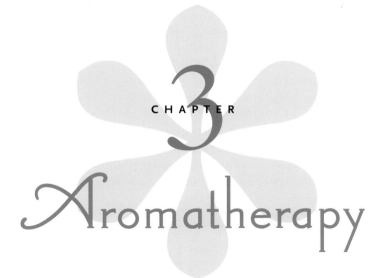

CHAPTER

3

Aromatherapy

· ·

Aromatherapy is the use of pure essential oils, which are extracted from trees, shrubs, flowers, herbs, and grasses. These precious oils can be used as an extension of the natural atmosphere. Indulge in as many formulas as you wish. Don't deny yourself pleasure, take advantage of the benefits awaiting you, and make every day a special one from now on!

Essential oils are fragrant components extracted from petals of flowers, leaves, roots, seeds, fruits, woods, grasses, and resins. Some plants yield oil from only one part, while others contain oil in several parts. Orange trees yield oil from the flowers, twigs, leaves, and rind of the fruit. The leaves, buds, and stems from the clove tree contain oil, while only the fruits from the tree of *Litsea cubeba* are used to produce an essential oil.

The quality and quantity of essential oil produced depends on various factors: location where the plant is grown, including altitude, moisture, climate; condition of soil; and even the season or time of day or night the plant material is harvested. The extraction process also plays a key role in the quality of an oil. Oils extracted by steam distillation, carbon dioxide extraction, and cold-pressing are preferable, while solvent extracted oil should be avoided, since harmful chemicals are used in the extraction process.

Essential oils, sometimes referred to as ethereal substances, are certainly more than just nice smelling. The oils can be used simply and effectively to scent and beautify the body, create a wonderful environment, and help promote inner peace and thus a happier mental state.

The Essentials

✳ Methods

Application

In this self-application method, apply the oil on the skin, rubbing it in until it is fully absorbed. Application is used when a massage is not absolutely necessary.

Diffusers

Diffusers disperse a mist of microparticles of essential oil, which creates an aromatic atmosphere indoors. Different types of diffusers are available on the market. Choose a smaller or larger unit, depending on the size of the area to be fragranced. The formulas given for diffuser use are in percentages rather than drops due to the different types of units. In one type, essential oils are added to a pad and are vaporized by an electric fan. A second type has a small glass bottle into which essential oils are placed. The oil is then propelled into a nebulizer and vaporized into the air. A third type requires that the essential oils be placed on a pad and releases the vapors though a warming process.

Massage

An aromatherapy massage can provide a means of counteracting the pressures of daily life. Only after receiving a massage do we realize how tight our muscles have been and recognize the high amounts of tension stored in our body. Some people think of massage as a luxury and utilize it only in times of severe distress. But living under the strains of modern society, we should recognize massage as an extraordinarily beneficial measure for stressed individuals to receive on a regular basis.

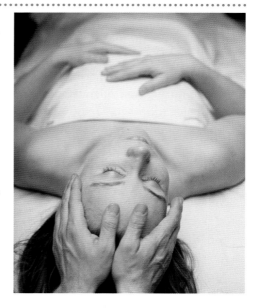

For the best possible massage, follow these guidelines:

- Choose a room that is quiet, warm, and comfortable.
- Play soft music to promote relaxation.
- Mist a blissful essential oil fragrance in the room before the treatment.
- Be in a calm state before giving the massage. Tension can be easily transferred from one person to another.
- Make sure your fingernails are short before giving a massage, to avoid scratching the recipient's skin.
- Remove all jewelry.
- Use a firm cushion if a massage table is unavailable. The recipient should be covered with a sheet or blanket for warmth.
- Choose the appropriate aromatherapy massage formula, and place all oils nearby to avoid searching for them during the massage.
- Wash hands with warm or hot water before and after giving the massage.
- Wear comfortable clothing.
- Warm the carrier, or base, oil by placing the small container in warm water. Pour an ample amount into the palm of your hand, rub your hands together, and apply the oil to the recipient's skin.

Mist Sprays

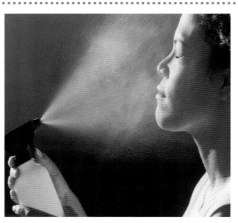

A convenient and effective way to disperse aromatic vapors into the air is through the use of a mist spray. As the aromas mature in the bottle, the fragrance improves and becomes more pleasant.

Directions: Fill a four-ounce fine-mist spray bottle with purified water and add the essential oils. Tighten the cap and shake well.

To use: Shake the bottle well. Sit comfortably in a chair, close your eyes, spray the mist above your head approximately 10 times (2 to 3 sprays at a time), and take slow, deep breaths, breathing the vapors deeply. Use indoors to receive the full benefit.

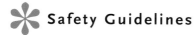
Safety Guidelines

To ensure safe use of essential oils, please adhere to the following guidelines:

- Essential oils are highly concentrated substances and should be diluted in a carrier oil before applied to the skin. Common carrier oils are almond (sweet), apricot kernel, avocado, borage, flaxseed, grape seed, hazelnut, jojoba, kukui nut, sesame, sunflower, and walnut.

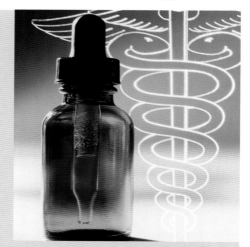

- Only pure essential oils and pure unrefined carrier oils should be used. Never purchase oils that are solvent extracted, synthetic, or refined. The refining process removes valuable nutrients, and chemical preservatives are added to extend the shelf life of the product.

- The oils of basil (sweet), bergamot, cinnamon leaf, clove, grapefruit, lemon, lemongrass, lime, mandarin, orange, pepper (black), peppermint, spearmint, and tangerine can irritate the skin, especially dry skin. If any skin irritation should occur as a result of the essential oils, immediately apply lavender oil neat or a carrier oil to the area. This will quickly soothe the skin.

- If a person is sensitive, the number of drops of essential oils in the massage and bath oil formulas can be reduced to make the formulas half-strength.

- When applying essential oils to the skin using a spray mist, or when taking a scented bath, be careful not to get essential oil vapors into the eyes. If the oils have already irritated the eyes, flush with cool water.

- Care should be taken when using carrier and essential oils during pregnancy. Many of the oils have a stimulating effect on the uterus that can be very helpful at the appropriate time to facilitate childbirth. However, if those oils are used prior to the time of childbirth, they can bring on premature labor. Even certain common foods, spices, and vegetable oils—celery, carrots, parsley, basil, bay leaves, marjoram, and safflower oil, for example—can stimulate uterine contractions.

- Small amounts (2 to 3 drops at a time) of the following essential oils are safe during pregnancy: bergamot, coriander, cypress, frankincense, geranium, ginger, grapefruit, lavender, lemon, lime, mandarin, neroli, orange, patchouli, petitgrain, sandalwood, spearmint, tangerine, tea tree, and ylang-ylang. Sesame oil can be used as a carrier oil.

- If a person is highly allergic, a simple test can determine if there is any sensitivity to a particular oil. Rub a drop of carrier oil on the upper chest area, and in 12 hours check for redness or any other skin reaction. If the skin is clear, place one drop of an essential oil, diluted in 15 drops of the same carrier oil, and again rub on the upper chest area. If there is no skin reaction after 12 hours, both carrier and essential oil can be used.

- Do not consume alcohol, except a small glass of wine with a meal, in the time period when using essential oils.

- Do not use essential oils while on medication; the oils might interfere with the medicine.

- After an application of citrus oils on the skin, avoid sunbathing, saunas, and hot baths, to prevent skin damage.

Oils

- Essential oils spilled on furniture will remove the finish; therefore, be careful when handling the bottles.

- Store essential oils in brown-colored glass bottles and keep them in a dark, cool place.

- Always use a glass dropper when measuring drops of essential oil.

- Keep all bottles tightly closed to prevent the oils from evaporating and oxidizing.

- Always store essential oils out of reach and out of sight of children.

Measurements

100 drops = 1 teaspoon = 5 milliliters
300 drops = 1 tablespoon = 15 milliliters
600 drops = 1 ounce = 30 milliliters
4 ounces = 120 milliliters
4 ounces (dry) = 100 grams

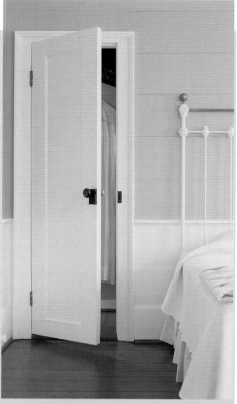

- Find a peaceful and comfortable place to relax.

- Make sure you will not be disturbed by the telephone, doorbell, people entering the room, or noisy pets.

- Be sure that the room temperature is comfortably warm.

- Play soft music in the background, if desired, to enhance relaxation.

- Determine the easiest and most natural method to relax:

  1. Listening to a relaxation tape.

  2. Guiding yourself with images.

  3. Using thoughts to create a state of mind.

- Choose an appropriate relaxation position: sitting comfortably in a well-supported chair with your back straight and feet flat on the floor, or lying in a supine position.

Relaxation Exercise

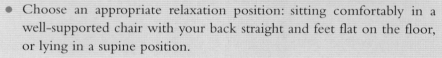

Take a deep breath. As you exhale, close your eyes. Continue breathing slowly and fully. Pause and reflect. Scan your body and pinpoint tense areas. Focus on sending deep relaxation to each individual area. Pause and reflect. With each inhalation, you relax further. As you exhale, the tension releases and exits your body, enabling you to feel peaceful and serene. Let go of any extraneous thoughts, and give yourself permission to experience inner peace and stillness. Pause and reflect. Focus on your breathing. Begin to count down slowly from 20 to 1, taking a full breath with each number. Allow yourself to enter a deeper level of tranquility. Detach yourself from the outside world until you cease to be aware of it.

$\mathcal{S}$cents

❋ Allspice (Pimento Berry)

Botanical name: *Pimenta officinalis*

Allspice is an evergreen tree that grows to 30 to 70 feet and has leathery leaves and small white flowers that are succeeded by aromatic berries. The berries turn black when ripe.

Scent: Clove-like

Effects on the mind and emotions: calms, uplifts mood, improves mental clarity and memory, promotes restful sleep, reduces stress

Effects on the body: warms, relaxes tight muscles, lessens pain, helps breathing, improves digestion, helps reduce cellulite deposits, purifies

Other use: disinfectant

Precaution: Essential oil of allspice can irritate the skin.

❋ Amyris

Botanical name: *Amyris balsamifera*

Amyris is an evergreen tree growing to about 60 feet with clusters of white flowers and edible bluish black fruit.

Scent: Smoky sweet

Effects on the mind and emotions: calms, promotes a peaceful state of mind, releases anxiety

Effects on the body: cools, purifies

Other use: fixative for fragrances

❋ Anise

Botanical name: *Pimpinella anisum*

Anise reaches a height of about 2 feet and has small white flowers.

Scent: Licorice-like

Effects on the mind and emotions: calms, promotes restful sleep

Effects on the body: lessens pain, helps breathing, improves digestion, stimulates lactation in nursing mothers

Precaution: Essential oil of anise is stupefying in large amounts.

☀ Basil (Sweet)

Botanical name: *Ocimum Basilicum*
Basil is a bushy plant that grows to 2 feet and has white, blue, or purple flowers. About 150 varieties of basil exist.

Scent: Licorice

Effects on the mind and emotions: calms, uplifts mood, helps relieve mental fatigue in small amounts, improves mental clarity and memory, promotes restful sleep, sharpens the senses, reduces stress, helps in meditation

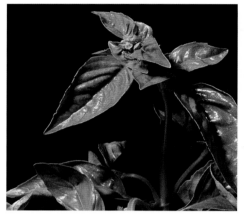

Effects on the body: cools, lessens pain, improves digestion, stimulates lactation in nursing mothers, helps reduce cellulite deposits, purifies

Other use: soothing aid to the skin after insect bites

Precaution: Essential oil of basil can irritate the skin. In large amounts, the oil can be toxic.

☀ Bay (West Indian)

Botanical name: *Pimenta racemosa or Pimenta acris*
Bay is a tropical evergreen tree that grows to about 30 to 50 feet. The tree has aromatic leathery leaves, clusters of white or pink flowers, and black or purple oval berries.

Scent: Spicy

Effects on the mind and emotions: calms; improves mental clarity, alertness, and memory; sharpens the senses; promotes restful sleep; reduces stress

Effects on the body: warms, relaxes tight muscles, soothes sprains, lessens pain, helps breathing, improves digestion, promotes perspiration, helps reduce cellulite deposits, purifies

Other uses: disinfectant, insect repellant

Precaution: Essential oil of bay can irritate the skin.

☀ Benzoin

Botanical name: *Styrax benzoin or Styrax tonkinensis*
The benzoin tree grows to about 115 feet and has fragrant white flowers.

The trunk secretes an aromatic resin when injured. The resin is also known as gum benjamin.

Scent: Cinnamon–vanilla

Effects on the mind and emotions: calms, uplifts mood, promotes restful sleep, reduces stress, helps in meditation

Effects on the body: warms, relaxes tight muscles, breaks up congestion, reduces inflammation, improves the breathing, helps reduce cellulite deposits, purifies, aids in healing of the skin

Other uses: preservative in cosmetics, fixative for fragrances

❋ Bergamot

Botanical name: *Citrus bergamia*
Bergamot is an evergreen citrus tree that grows to a height of about 15 feet and bears green to yellow fruit.

Scent: Citrus

Effects on the mind and emotions: calms; promotes restful sleep; uplifts mood; relieves anxiety, nervous tension, and stress; helps relieve mental fatigue; improves mental clarity and alertness; sharpens the senses; refreshes; balances the nervous system

Effects on the body: cools, helps reduce cellulite deposits, purifies

Other use: disinfectant

Precaution: Essential oil of bergamot can irritate dry skin. Skin can burn if exposed to sunlight after topical application.

❋ Bois de Rose (Rosewood)

Botanical name: *Aniba rosaeodora*
Bois de rose is a large evergreen tree with yellow flowers.

Scent: Slightly rosy

Effects on the mind and emotions: calms, uplifts mood, relieves nervousness and stress

Effects on the body: lessens pain, regenerates and moisturizes the skin

❋ Cajeput

Botanical name: *Melaleuca Leucadendron* or *Melalleuca cajuputi*
Cajeput is an evergreen tree that grows to a height of 50 to 100 feet. The

tree is cultivated in many areas as an ornamental for its outstanding white, pink, or purple flowers. It belongs to a family of more than 150 trees.

Scent: Camphor-like

Effects on the mind and emotions: calms, promotes restful sleep, reduces stress

Effects on the body: warms slightly, relieves muscle aches and pains, breaks up congestion, helps breathing

Other uses: disinfectant, insect repellant

✳ Cardamom

Botanical name: *Elettaria Cardamomum*
Cardamom grows to a height of about 10 feet and has small yellow flowers and fruit with seeds inside.

Scent: Spicy

Effects on the mind and emotions: uplifts mood, improves mental clarity and memory, energizes

Effects on the body: warms, relieves pain, improves physical strength, improves digestion

✳ Cedarwood (Atlas)

Botanical name: *Cedrus atlantica*
Cedarwood is an evergreen tree that grows to a height of about 130 feet and has needle-like leaves. These trees can reach an age of one thousand to two thousand years if undisturbed.

Scent: Woody

Effects on the mind and emotions: calms, promotes restful sleep, relieves anxiety and tension, helps in meditation

Effects on the body: cools, relaxes tight muscles, lessens pain, helps breathing, helps reduce cellulite deposits, purifies

Other use: insect repellant

✳ Celery

Botanical name: *Apium graveolens*
Celery grows to a height of 1 to 2 feet and has white flowers.

Scent: Strong celery

Effects on the mind and emotions: cools, calms, promotes restful sleep

Effects on the body: helps reduce cellulite deposits, purifies

Precaution: Essential oil of celery is very cleansing to the tissues; it is best used in small amounts due to its detoxifying properties.

❋ Chamomile (Roman)

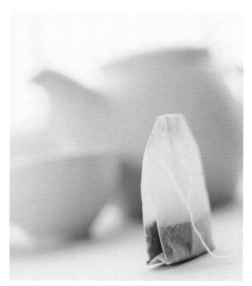

Botanical name: *Anthemis nobilis* Chamomile grows to a height of about one foot and has small, daisy-like flowerheads.

Scent: Apple-like

Effects on the mind and emotions: calms, uplifts mood, promotes restful sleep, reduces stress and tension

Effects on the body: lessens pain, reduces inflammation, improves digestion, helps heal the skin

Other use: soothing aid to the skin after insect bites

❋ Cinnamon Leaf

Botanical name: *Cinnamomum zeylanicum*
The cinnamon tree grows to a height of about 50 feet and has leathery leaves and small white flowers and light-blue berries.

Scent: Cinnamon

Effects on the mind and emotions: uplifts mood, helps relieve mental fatigue, reduces stress, revives

Effects on the body: warms, relaxes tight muscles, lessens pain, improves digestion, helps reduce cellulite deposits, purifies

Other uses: disinfectant, insect repellant

Precaution: Essential oil of cinnamon can irritate the skin.

❋ Citronella

Botanical name: *Cymbopogan Nardus*
Citronella is an aromatic tall grass.

Scent: Lemony

Effects on the mind and emotions: calms, uplifts mood, improves mental clarity and alertness, reduces stress, acts as a mental stimulant

Effect on the body: cools

Other use: insect repellant

❋ Clary Sage

Botanical name: *Salvia sclarea*
Clary sage grows to a height of about 3 feet. The flowers are pink, white, or blue, depending on the variety.

Scent: Sweet and spicy

Effects on the mind and emotions: calms, uplifts mood, promotes restful sleep, relieves stress and tension, acts as an aphrodisiac, encourages communication

Effects on the body: lessens pain, improves digestion, contains a hormone-like substance similar to estrogen

Precaution: Essential oil of clary sage can be stupefying in large amounts.

❋ Clove

Botanical name: *Eugenia caryophyllata*
Clove is an evergreen tree that grows to about 40 feet and has bright pink buds that develop into yellow flowers, then into purple berries.

Scent: Hot and spicy

Effects on the mind and emotions: uplifts mood, helps relieve mental fatigue, improves mental clarity and memory, revives, acts as an aphrodisiac

Effects on the body: warms, relieves pain, helps breathing, improves digestion

Other uses: disinfectant, insect repellant

Precaution: Essential oil of clove can irritate the skin.

❋ Copaiba

Botanical name: *Copaifera officinalis*
The copaiba tree grows to about 50 feet.

Scent: Woody

Effects on the mind and emotions: calms, promotes a peaceful state of mind, uplifts mood, improves mental clarity and alertness, promotes restful sleep, reduces stress and tension, helps in meditation

Effects on the body: warms, opens breathing passages, soothes the intestines, allows deeper breathing, helps heal the skin

Other use: fixative for fragrances

❉ Coriander

Botanical name: *Coriandrum sativum*

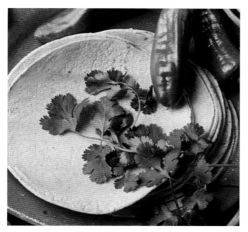

Coriander grows to a height of about 3 feet and has small white flowers that develop into green seeds. Coriander is also known as cilantro, or Chinese parsley.

Scent: Musky

Effects on the mind and emotions: helps relieve mental fatigue, improves mental clarity and memory, revives, energizes

Effects on the body: relieves pain, improves digestion

❉ Cubeb

Botanical name: *Piper Cubeba*
Cubeb is an evergreen climbing woody shrub that grows to a height of about 20 feet and has clusters of flowers that develop into small berries resembling peppers.

Scent: Peppery

Effects on the mind and emotions: refreshes, uplifts, and stimulates

Effects on the body: relieves pain, breaks up congestion, reduces inflammation, helps breathing, improves digestion

❉ Cumin

Botanical name: *Cuminum cyminum*
Cumin grows to a height of about 1 foot, has thread–like leaves, small white or pink flowers, and aromatic seeds.

Scent: Strong, spicy

Effects on the mind and emotions: calms, uplifts mood, helps relieve mental fatigue, reduces stress, revives, helps in meditation

Effects on the body: warms, relieves pain, improves digestion, helps reduce cellulite deposits, purifies

✳ Cypress

Botanical name: *Cupressus sempervirens*

Cypress is an evergreen tree that grows to a height of about 160 feet. Some trees are believed to be older than three thousand years.

Scent: Woody

Effects on the mind and emotions: calms, uplifts mood, improves

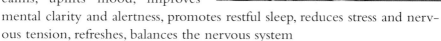

mental clarity and alertness, promotes restful sleep, reduces stress and nervous tension, refreshes, balances the nervous system

Effects on the body: relaxes the muscles, reduces perspiration, contains a hormone-like substance similar to estrogen, helps reduce cellulite deposits, purifies, contracts weak connective tissue, tones the skin

✳ Dill

Botanical name: *Anethum graveolens*

Dill grows to a height of about 3 feet and has small yellow flowers.

Scent: Spicy

Effects on the mind and emotions: calms, promotes restful sleep

Effects on the body: relieves pain, improves digestion

Other use: insect repellant

✳ Elemi

Botanical name: *Canarium luzonicum*

Elemi is an evergreen tree that grows to a height of about 100 feet and has yellow fragrant flowers and green fruits with nuts inside called pili nuts. These nuts are a valuable food for millions of people.

Scent: Lemon-like, balsamic

Effects on the mind and emotions: calms, uplifts mood, promotes restful sleep, reduces stress, helps to communicate feelings, helps in meditation

Effects on the body: warms, opens the breathing passages, helps heal the skin

✳ Eucalyptus

Botanical name: *Eucalyptus globulus*
The eucalyptus tree is one of the tallest trees, reaching over 300 feet and as high as 480 feet. The leaves are fragrant and leathery, the flowers are white, and the fruit is contained in a capsule. There are approximately seven hundred different species of eucalyptus.

Scent: Fresh, camphor-like

Effects on the mind and emotions: helps relieve mental fatigue, improves mental clarity and alertness, refreshes, revives, energizes, stimulates

Effects on the body: cools, relieves pain and aching sore muscles, breaks up congestion, reduces inflammation, helps breathing

Other uses: disinfectant, insect repellant

Precaution: Essential oil of eucalyptus can be toxic in large amounts.

✳ Fennel

Botanical name: *Foeniculum vulgare*
Fennel grows to a height of 3 to 7 feet and has green feathery leaves and clusters of small yellow flowers.

Scent: Strong licorice

Effects on the mind and emotions: calms, promotes restful sleep, reduces stress

Effects on the body: warms, relieves pain, improves digestion, contains a hormone-like substance similar to estrogen, stimulates lactation in nursing mothers, helps reduce cellulite deposits, purifies

Other uses: disinfectant, insect repellant

Precaution: Essential oil of fennel can be stupefying in large amounts.

✳ Fir Needles

Botanical name: *Abies balsamea*
Fir needles is an evergreen tree that grows to a height of about 40 to 80 feet and has needle-like leaves. There are approximately forty species of the tree.

Scent: Pine-like

Effects on the mind and emotions: calms, uplifts mood, improves mental clarity, refreshes, revives, encourages communication

Effects on the body: lessens pain, helps breathing, helps reduce cellulite, purifies

✳ Frankincense

Botanical name: *Boswellia thurifera*
Frankincense is a small tree that grows to about 20 feet and has white flowers.

Scent: Woody and camphor-like

Effects on the mind and emotions: calms, uplifts mood, promotes restful sleep, encourages communication, brings out feelings, helps in meditation

Effects on the body: reduces inflammation, helps heal the skin, reduces wrinkles

✳ Geranium

Botanical name: *Pelargonium graveolens*
Geranium grows to a height of about 3 feet. There are more than seven hundred species of the plant.

Scent: Rose-like

Effects on the mind and emotions: calms in small amounts, stimulates in large amounts, uplifts mood, reduces stress and tension, encourages communication

Effects on the body: cools, lessens pain, reduces inflammation, helps reduce cellulite deposits, purifies, soothes itching skin

Other uses: disinfectant, soothing aid to the skin after insect bites, insect repellant

✳ Ginger

Botanical name: *Zingiber officinale*
Ginger grows to a height of about 3 feet and has white or yellow flowers.

Scent: Spicy

Effects on the mind and emotions: uplifts mood, helps relieve mental fatigue, improves mental clarity and memory, stimulates

Effects on the body: warms, relaxes tight muscles, relieves aches and pains, improves digestion, relieves travel dizziness and nausea

Other use: disinfectant

✳ Grapefruit

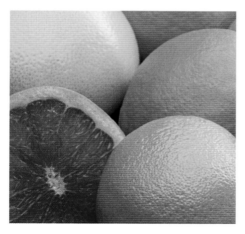

Botanical name: *Citrus paradisi*
Grapefruit is an evergreen citrus tree that grows to a height of about 30 to 50 feet and has fragrant white flowers and edible fruit.

Scent: Citrus

Effects on the mind and emotions: uplifts mood; helps relieve mental fatigue; improves mental clarity, alertness, and memory; sharpens the senses; reduces stress; refreshes; revives; energizes

Effects on the body: cools, increases physical strength and energy, helps reduce cellulite deposits, purifies

Precaution: Essential oil of grapefruit can irritate dry skin. Skin can burn if exposed to sunlight after topical application.

✳ Guaiacwood

Botanical name: *Guaiacum officinale*
Guaiacwood is an evergreen tree that grows to a height of about 40 feet and has leathery leaves and blue or purple flowers.

Scent: Sweet dried fruit

Effects on the mind and emotions: calms, helps in meditation

Effects on the body: reduces inflammation, purifies, helps heal the skin

✳ Helichrysum

Botanical name: *Helichrysum italicum* or *Helichrysum angustifolium*
Helichrysum is an evergreen plant that grows to a height of about 2 feet and has daisy-like yellow flowers.

Scent: Strong and sweet

Effects on the mind and emotions: calms, uplifts mood, improves mental clarity and alertness, reduces stress, revives, creates feelings of euphoria

Effects on the body: cools, helps breathing, increases muscle endurance

Other use: disinfectant

✴ Hyssop Decumbens

Botanical name: *Hyssopus officinalis, var. decumbens*
Hyssop decumbens is a semi-evergreen plant that grows to a height of about 1 to 4 feet and has aromatic leaves and spikes of white, pink, blue, or dark purple flowers.

Scent: Sweet, camphorous

Effects on the mind and emotions: calms, uplifts mood, improves mental clarity and alertness, revives

Effect on the body: helps breathing

✴ Juniper Berry

Botanical name: *Juniperus communis*
Juniper is an evergreen bush 2 to 6 feet high that sometimes reaches 25 feet, with silvery green, needle-like leaves. The green berries take three years to ripen to a blue color. The maximum lifespan of the bush is two thousand years.

Scent: Evergreen forest

Effects on the mind and emotions: relaxes, uplifts mood, improves mental clarity and memory, reduces stress, refreshes, revives

Effects on the body: lessens pain, reduces inflammation, cleanses the intestines, helps reduce cellulite deposits, purifies

Other uses: disinfectant, soothing aid to the skin after insect bites, insect repellant

Precaution: Essential oil of juniper, if used in large amounts, can cause the body to become dehydrated.

✴ Labdanum (Cistus)

Botanical name: *Cistus ladaniferus*
Labdanum is a small evergreen bush that grows to a height of about 10 feet and has large white flowers.

Scent: Sweet, prune-like

Effects on the mind and emotions: calms, uplifts mood, promotes restful sleep, reduces stress, encourages communication, brings out feelings, helps in meditation

Effects on the body: warms, loosens tight muscles

Other use: fixative for fragrances

❋ Lavender

Botanical name: *Lavandula officinalis or Lavandula augustifolia*

Lavender is an evergreen plant that grows to a height of about 3 feet and has

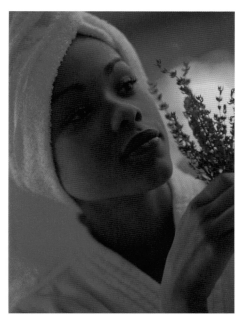

lilac-colored flowers. There are twenty-eight species of this plant.

Scent: Floral herbaceous

Effects on the mind and emotions: calms in small amounts, stimulates in large amounts, uplifts mood, promotes restful sleep, reduces stress and tension, soothes the nervous system, balances mood swings

Effects on the body: relaxes tight muscles, lessens aches and pains, breaks up congestion, reduces inflammation, helps breathing, improves digestion, soothes the intestines, helps reduce cellulite, purifies, helps heals the skin

Other uses: disinfectant, soothing aid to the skin after insect bites, insect repellant

❋ Lemon

Botanical name: *Citrus limonum*

Lemon is an evergreen citrus tree that grows to a height of 10 to 20 feet and has white, fragrant flowers and edible fruits.

Scent: Lemony

Effects on the mind and emotions: calms, uplifts mood, helps relieve mental fatigue; improves mental clarity, alertness, and memory; sharpens the senses; promotes restful sleep; reduces stress, refreshes, revives; calms or energizes; balances the nervous system

Effects on the body: cools, helps reduce cellulite deposits, purifies

Other uses: disinfectant, soothing aid to the skin after insect bites

Precaution: Essential oil of lemon can irritate dry skin. Skin can burn if exposed to sunlight after topical application.

✳ Lemongrass

Botanical name: *Cymbopogon citratus*
Lemongrass is a grass that grows to about 2 feet and has bulbous stems and sword-like leaves.

Scent: Strong lemon

Effects on the mind and emotions: uplifts mood, improves alertness, promotes restful sleep, reduces stress, refreshes, revives, balances the nervous system

Effects on the body: reduces inflammation, helps breathing, improves digestion, stimulates lactation in nursing mothers, contracts weak connective tissue, tones the skin

Other uses: disinfectant, insect repellant

Precaution: Essential oil of lemongrass can irritate dry skin.

✳ Lime

Botanical name: *Citrus limetta*
Lime is an evergreen citrus tree that grows to about 10 feet and has fragrant white flowers that develop into edible fruits.

Scent: Fresh citrus

Effects on the mind and emotions: uplifts mood; helps relieve mental fatigue; improves mental clarity, alertness, and memory; sharpens the senses; reduces stress; refreshes, revives, strengthens the nerves

Effects on the body: cools, helps reduce cellulite deposits, purifies

Other uses: disinfectant, soothing aid to the skin after insect bites

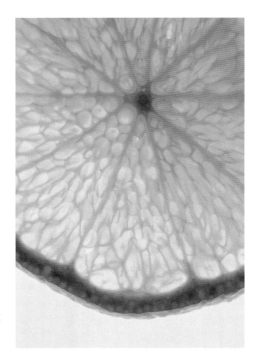

Precaution: Essential oil of lime can irritate dry skin. Skin can burn if exposed to sunlight after topical application.

❋ Litsea Cubeba

Botanical name: *Litsea cubeba*
Litsea cubeba is an evergreen tree that grows to about 30 feet and has white flowers that develop into small red or black berries.

Scent: Lemony

Effects on the mind and emotions: calms; uplifts mood; improves mental clarity, alertness, and memory; promotes restful sleep; refreshes; revives; creates feelings of euphoria; encourages communication

Effects on the body: cools, relieves pain, improves digestion

❋ Mandarin

Botanical name: *Citrus nobilis*
Mandarin is an evergreen tree that grows to a height of about 25 feet and has fragrant flowers and edible fruits.

Scent: Sweet citrus

Effects on the mind and emotions: calms, promotes restful sleep, uplifts mood, improves mental clarity and alertness, sharpens the senses, relieves stress and tension

Effects on the body: cools, helps reduce cellulite deposits, purifies

Precaution: Essential oil of mandarin can irritate dry skin. Skin can burn if exposed to sunlight after topical application.

❋ Marjoram

Botanical name: *Origanum majorana* or *Majorana hortensis*
Marjoram is a bushy plant that grows to a height of about 2 feet and has white or purple flowers and light-green leaves.

Scent: Spicy

Effects on the mind and emotions: calms, promotes restful sleep

Effects on the body: warms, relaxes tight muscles, relieves aches and pains, breaks up congestion, reduces inflammation, helps breathing, improves digestion

Other uses: disinfectant, soothing aid to the skin after insect bites

❋ Myrrh

Botanical name: *Commiphora myrrha*

Scent: Balsamic

Myrrh is a small tree growing to about 9 feet.

Effects on the mind and emotions: calms, uplifts mood, promotes restful sleep, helps in meditation

Effects on the body: cools, reduces inflammation, helps heal the skin

Other use: fixative for fragrances

❋ Myrtle

Botanical name: *Myrtus communis*

Myrtle is an evergreen shrub that grows to a height of 10 to 18 feet and has scented leaves and small aromatic white blossoms. The flowers are succeeded by bluish black berries that are edible, fresh or dried. There are about sixteen species of the myrtle shrub.

Scent: Fresh, camphor-like

Effects on the mind and emotions: calms, uplifts mood, refreshes, helps in meditation

Effects on the body: relieves pain, helps breathing

❋ Neroli

Botanical name: *Citrus aurantium*

Neroli is from the fragrant white blossoms of the bitter-orange tree.

Scent: Sweet floral

Effects on the mind and emotions: calms, uplifts mood, reduces nervous tension

Effects on the body: regulates the nervous system

❋ Nutmeg

Botanical name: *Myristica fragrans*

Nutmeg is an evergreen tree that grows to a height of 60 to 80 feet and has large, fragrant leaves, small yellow flowers, and yellow fruits. The female tree bears fruit after its flowers have been pollinated by the flowers of the male tree.

Scent: Spicy

Effects on the mind and emotions: calms and promotes restful sleep in small amounts, stimulates in large amounts, uplifts mood, improves mental clarity and alertness, revives

Effects on the body: warms slightly, relaxes tight muscles, relieves aches and pains, improves digestion

Precaution: Essential oil of nutmeg can be stupefying in large amounts.

✳ Orange

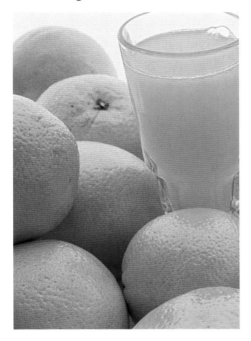

Botanical name: *Citrus aurantium* or *Citrus sinensis*
Orange is an evergreen citrus tree that grows to a height of about 25 feet and has fragrant white flowers and edible fruits.

Scent: Sweet citrus

Effects on the mind and emotions: calms, uplifts mood, promotes restful sleep, improves mental clarity, reduces stress

Effects on the body: cools, helps reduce cellulite deposits, purifies

Precaution: Essential oil of orange can irritate dry skin. Skin can burn if exposed to sunlight after topical application.

✳ Oregano

Botanical name: *Origanum vulgare*
Oregano grows to a height of 1 to 2 feet and has dark-green leaves and purple buds that blossom into white, pink, or lilac-colored flowers. The entire plant is aromatic. There are about twenty species of oregano.

Scent: Spicy

Effects on the mind and emotions: uplifts mood, improves mental clarity and alertness

Effects on the body: warms, loosens tight muscles, relieves muscle aches and pains, increases physical endurance and energy, helps breathing, improves digestion, promotes perspiration, helps reduce cellulite deposits, purifies

Other uses: disinfectant, insect repellant

Precaution: Essential oil of oregano can irritate the skin.

❋ Palmarosa

Botanical name: *Cymbopogon martini*
Palmarosa is a fragrant grass.

Scent: Sweet

Effects on the mind and emotions: calms, uplifts mood, reduces stress, refreshes

Effects on the body: warms; lessens aches and pains; reduces inflammation; regenerates, moisturizes, and heals the skin

❋ Patchouli

Botanical name: *Pogostemon patchouli* or *Pogostemon cablin*
Patchouli grows to about 3 feet and has whorls of light-purple or lavender flowers.

Scent: Musty

Effects on the mind and emotions: uplifts mood, acts as an aphrodisiac, creates feelings of euphoria, stimulates nerves, interferes with sleep

Effect on the body: helps heal the skin

Other use: insect repellant

❋ Pepper (Black)

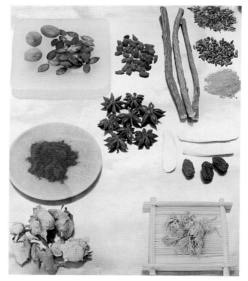

Botanical name: *Piper nigrum*
Black pepper is a tropical climbing vine that grows to a height of about 10 feet and has clusters of small white flowers.

Scent: Hot and spicy

Effects on the mind and emotions: improves mental clarity and memory, revives, stimulates

Effects on the body: warms, loosens tight muscles, improves digestion in small amounts, improves the benefits of other oils when combined

Precaution: Essential oil of black pepper can irritate the skin.

✳ Peppermint

Botanical name: *Mentha piperita*
Peppermint is a cross between mints and has been known of since the seventeenth century. It grows to a height of 1 to 3 feet and has a purplish stem and pale violet flowers.

Scent: Strong mint

Effects on the mind and emotions: uplifts mood; helps relieve mental fatigue; improves mental clarity, alertness, concentration, and memory; sharpens the senses; refreshes, revives, energizes; stimulates nerves; acts as an aphrodisiac; encourages communication

Effects on the body: cools, relieves pain, increases physical strength and endurance, reduces inflammation, helps breathing, improves digestion, increases the appetite, reduces lactation in nursing mothers, soothes itching skin

Other uses: disinfectant, insect repellant

✳ Peru Balsam

Botanical name: *Myroxylon pereirae*
Peru balsam is a slow-growing evergreen that grows to 60 to 120 feet and has fragrant flowers.

Scent: Vanilla

Effects on the mind and emotions: calms, uplifts mood, promotes restful sleep, reduces stress, helps in meditation

Effects on the body: warms, loosens tight muscles, purifies, helps heal the skin

Other use: fixative for fragrances

✳ Petitgrain

Botanical name: *Citrus biguarade*
Petitgrain is produced from the twigs and leaves of the orange, lemon, or tangerine tree.

Scent: Sweet floral, citrus

Effects on the mind and emotions: calms; uplifts mood; promotes restful sleep; reduces anxiety, tension, and stress; improves mental clarity, alertness, and memory; helps in meditation

Effects on the body: cools, helps heal the skin

❊ Pine

Botanical name: *Pinus sylvestris*
Pine is an evergreen tree that grows to a height of 115 to 130 feet and has greenish-blue, needle-like leaves. There are ninety species in the pine family. It is estimated that pine trees can live for twelve hundred years.

Scent: Fresh pine

Effects on the mind and emotions: uplifts mood; helps relieve mental fatigue; improves mental clarity, alertness, and memory; refreshes; revives

Effects on the body: lessens pain, helps breathing, helps reduce cellulite deposits, purifies

Other use: disinfectant

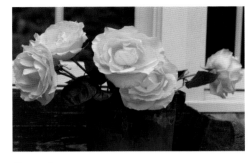

❊ Rose

Botanical name: *Rosa centifolia* or *Rosa damascena*
The rose bush grows to various heights and produces sweet, fragrant flowers.

Scent: Sweet floral

Effects on the mind and emotions: calms, uplifts mood, reduces stress, acts as an aphrodisiac

Effects on the body: cools, lessens aches and pains, reduces inflammation, balances the female hormonal and reproductive system, purifies, helps heal the skin

❊ Rosemary

Botanical name: *Rosmarinus officinalis*
Rosemary is an evergreen shrub that grows to 2 to 6 feet with needle-shaped leaves and blue flowers. The entire plant is aromatic.

Scent: Fresh, camphor-like

Effects on the mind and emotions: uplifts mood, helps relieve mental fatigue, improves mental clarity, alertness, and memory; sharpens the senses; refreshes; stimulates nerves

Effects on the body: warms, relaxes tight muscles, relieves aches and pains, helps breathing, improves digestion, helps reduce cellulite deposits, purifies

Other uses: disinfectant, insect repellant

✳ Sage (Spanish)

Botanical name: *Salvia lavendulafolia*
Sage is an evergreen plant that grows to a height of 2 to 3 feet and has small light-blue to purple flowers and aromatic, grayish green leaves. There are about five hundred different varieties of sage.

Scent: Spicy

Effects on the mind and emotions: improves mental clarity and alertness, reduces stress

Effects on the body: relaxes tight muscles, lessens aches and pains, improves digestion, reduces lactation in nursing mothers, reduces perspiration, helps reduce cellulite, purifies

Other use: disinfectant

Precaution: Some of the varieties of sage contain the toxic component of thujone. Essential oil of Spanish sage is relatively nontoxic.

✳ Sandalwood

Botanical name: *Santalum album*
Sandalwood is an evergreen tree that grows to a height of 30 feet and has small purple flowers and small fruits containing a seed. There are ten species of sandalwood.

Scent: Woody

Effects on the mind and emotions: calms, uplifts mood, promotes restful sleep, reduces stress, acts as an aphrodisiac, encourages communication, brings out emotions, helps in meditation

Effect on the body: helps heal the skin

Other uses: fixative for fragrances

✳ Sea Buckthorn

Botanical name: *Hippophae rhamnoides*
Sea buckthorn is a shrub that grows to a height of about 30 feet and has clusters of yellow flowers that develop into small orange berries.

Scent: Sweet, fruity

Effects on the mind and emotions: relaxes, uplifts mood

Effects on the body: warms, loosens tight muscles, softens the skin

Note: Sea buckthorn is considered a vegetal/carrier oil, not an essential oil, but has valuable properties similar to essential oils.

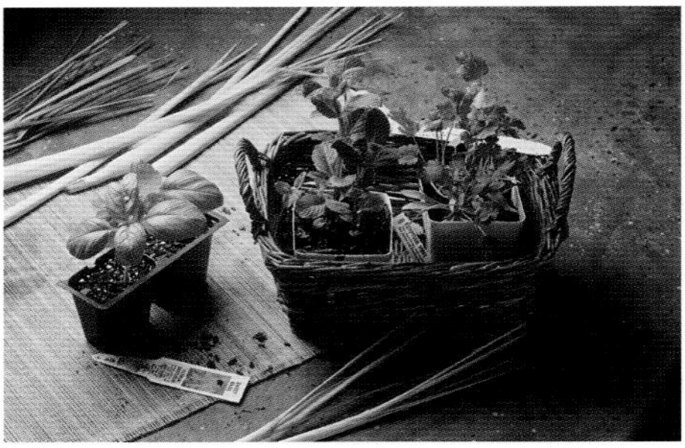

❋ Spearmint

Botanical name: *Mentha spicata*
Spearmint grows to a height of 1 to 3 feet and has small white or lilac flowers and shiny green leaves.

Scent: Minty

Effects on the mind and emotions: uplifts mood; helps relieve mental fatigue; improves mental clarity, alertness, and memory; sharpens the senses; refreshes; revives; energizing; stimulates nerves; acts as an aphrodisiac; encourages communication

Effects on the body: cools, relieves aches and pains, increases physical strength and endurance, reduces inflammation, helps breathing, improves digestion, increases the appetite, soothes itching skin

Other use: insect repellant

❋ Spikenard

Botanical name: *Nardostachys Jatamansi*
Spikenard is an aromatic plant that grows to a height of about 2 feet.

Scent: Sweet woody

Effects on the mind and emotions: calms, uplifts mood, promotes restful sleep, reduces stress

Effect on the body: reduces inflammation

❋ Spruce

Botanical name: *Picea mariana*
Spruce is an evergreen tree that grows to a height of 70 to 200 feet. There are about fifty species in the spruce family. It is estimated the tree can live for twelve hundred years.

Scent: Sweet, pine-like

Effects on the mind and emotions: calms, uplifts mood, improves mental clarity, encourages communication, brings out feelings

Effects on the body: breaks up congestion, helps breathing

Other use: disinfectant

✳ Tangerine

Botanical name: *Citrus reticulata*
Tangerine is an evergreen citrus tree that grows to about 20 feet and has fragrant white flowers and edible fruits.

Scent: Sweet citrus

Effects on the mind and emotions: calms, uplifts mood, promotes restful sleep, relieves stress and tension, improves mental clarity and alertness, sharpens the senses

Effects on the body: cools, helps reduce cellulite deposits, purifies

Precaution: Essential oil of tangerine can irritate dry skin. Skin can burn if exposed to sunlight after topical application.

✳ Tea Tree

Botanical name: *Melaleuca alternifolia*
Tea tree is an evergreen growing to 10 feet. It has needle-like leaves and purple or yellow flowers. It belongs to a family of more than 150 species of trees.

Scent: Camphor-like

Effects on the mind and emotions: uplifts mood, improves mental clarity, revives, stimulates

Effects on the body: relieves pain, helps breathing, helps heal the skin

Other uses: disinfectant, soothing aid to the skin after insect bites

✳ Thyme

Botanical name: *Thymus vulgaris*
Thyme is an evergreen plant that grows to 1 foot and has small leaves and pink or pale-lilac flowers.

Scent: Hot and spicy

Effects on the mind and emotions: uplifts mood; improves mental clarity, alertness, and memory; sharpens the senses; stimulates; relaxes the nerves

Effects on the body: warms, relaxes tight muscles, relieves aches and pains, increases physical strength and energy, breaks up congestion, reduces inflammation, helps breathing, improves digestion, promotes perspiration, helps reduce cellulite deposits, purifies

Other uses: disinfectant, insect repellant

Precaution: Essential oil of thyme can irritate the skin.

❋ Vanilla

Botanical name: *Vanilla planifolia*
Vanilla is a climbing plant that grows to about 12 feet with clusters of flowers.

Scent: Sweet vanilla

Effects on the mind and emotions: calms, promotes restful sleep, uplifts mood, reduces stress, acts as an aphrodisiac

Note: Vanilla extracted by the CO_2 method is recommended for use in aromatherapy formulas.

❋ Vetiver

Botanical name: *Vetiveria zizanoides*
Vetiver is a grass that grows to a height of 4 to 8 feet.

Scent: Earthy

Effects on the mind and emotions: calms, uplifts mood, promotes restful sleep, removes stress and tension

Effects on the body: relaxes tight muscles, relieves pain, improves digestion, helps heal the skin

Other use: insect repellant

❋ Ylang-Ylang

Botanical name: *Cananga odorata*
Ylang-ylang is an evergreen tree that grows to a height of about 100 feet and has large, fragrant yellow flowers and glossy leaves.

Scent: Sweet floral

Effects on the mind and emotions: calms, uplifts mood, promotes restful sleep, reduces stress, acts as an aphrodisiac, creates feelings of euphoria, encourages communication, brings out feelings

Effects on the body: relaxes tight muscles, lessens pain

Other use: disinfectant

Formulas

Appreciation

It is important to appreciate everything we have in life. It is unfortunate that too many people wait until they are on their deathbeds or for a tragedy to occur before experiencing feelings of contrition and regret at not having enjoyed the closeness of loved ones.

- Choose a method for your aromatherapy session: application, diffuser, mist spray. Select and use a formula (see below).

- Do Relaxation Exercise (see page 90). Allow yourself to reach a peaceful, quiet state. Think of the special people you know. Repeat this exercise whenever possible. Each session should last 20 to 30 minutes.

Application

Apply one of these formulas to the upper chest and back of the neck until the oil is fully absorbed into the skin. Breathe in the vapors deeply.

Ylang-ylang . . . . 4 drops Allspice . . . . 3 drops Vanilla . . . . 3 drops Carrier Oil . . . . 2 teaspoons	Sandalwood . . . . 4 drops Bergamot . . . . 3 drops Geranium . . . . 3 drops Carrier Oil . . . . 2 teaspoons
Litsea Cubeba . . . . . . 3 drops Palmarosa . . . . 3 drops Neroli . . . . 2 drops Labdanum . . . . 2 drops Carrier Oil . . . . 2 teaspoons	Bois de Rose . . . . 3 drops Anise . . . . 3 drops Ylang-Ylang . . . . 3 drops Cedarwood (Atlas) . . . 1 drop Carrier Oil . . . . 2 teaspoons
Frankincense . . . . 3 drop Vanilla . . . . 3 drops Orange . . . . 3 drops Sandalwood . . . . 1 drop Carrier Oil . . . . 2 teaspoons	Patchouli . . . . 3 drops Bois de Rose . . . . 3 drops Lime . . . . 2 drops Clove . . . . 2 drops Carrier Oil . . . . 2 teaspoons
Vanilla . . . . 3 drops Bergamot . . . . 3 drops Neroli . . . . 2 drops Cumin . . . . 2 drops Carrier Oil . . . . 2 teaspoons	Labdanum . . . . 5 drops Allspice . . . . 3 drops Peppermint . . . . 2 drops Carrier Oil . . . . 2 teaspoons

Diffusers

Depending on the type of diffuser you have, place the essential oils on the diffuser pad or in the glass bottle to disperse the aroma into the air. Breathe in the vapors deeply.

Ylang-Ylang 30%	Ylang-Ylang 25%
Bois de Rose 30%	Palmarosa 25%
Orange 20%	Citronella 25%
Clove 20%	Frankincense 25%

Lavender 50%	Allspice 30%
Petitgrain 20%	Citronella 30%
Allspice 20%	Geranium 30%
Bergamot 10%	Bergamot 10%

Mist Sprays

Fill a fine–mist spray bottle with purified water, then add the essential oils. Tighten the cap and shake well. Mist numerous times and breathe in the vapors deeply.

Lime . . . . 40 drops	Allspice . . . . 40 drops
Lavender . . . . 30 drops	Lavender . . . . 40 drops
Geranium . . . . 30 drops	Frankincense . . . . . . 40 drops
Ylang-Ylang . . . . 25 drops	Lemon . . . . 20 drops
Cedarwood (Atlas) . . . 25 drops	Palmarosa . . . . 10 drops
Pure Water . . . . 4 ounces	Pure Water . . . . 4 ounces

Bergamot . . . . 50 drops	Frankincense . . . . . . 40 drops
Geranium . . . . 40 drops	Petitgrain . . . . 40 drops
Bois de Rose . . . . 40 drops	Mandarin . . . . 40 drops
Sandalwood . . . . 20 drops	Anise . . . . 30 drops
Pure Water . . . . 4 ounces	Pure Water . . . . 4 ounces

Lavender . . . . 50 drops	Bergamot . . . . 40 drops
Ylang-Ylang . . . . 50 drops	Citronella . . . . 40 drops
Citronella . . . . 30 drops	Bay . . . . 40 drops
Sandalwood . . . . 20 drops	Sandalwood . . . . 30 drops
Pure Water . . . . 4 ounces	Pure Water . . . . 4 ounces

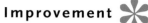

- Choose a method for your aromatherapy session: application, diffuser, or mist spray. Select and use a formula.

- Do the Relaxation Exercise (see page 90). Allow yourself to reach an inner peaceful and quiet state, then reflect on specific changes you have to make in your life so you can improve yourself. Repeat this exercise as many times as you feel necessary. Each session should last 20 to 30 minutes.

Application

Apply one of these formulas to the upper chest and back of the neck until the oil is fully absorbed into the skin. Breathe in the vapors deeply.

Elemi . . . . 3 drops Basil (Sweet) . . . . 3 drops Geranium . . . . 2 drops Palmarosa . . . . 2 drops Carrier Oil . . . . 2 teaspoons	Litsea Cubeba . . . . . . 4 drops Vanilla . . . . 3 drops Sandalwood . . . . 3 drops Carrier Oil . . . . 2 teaspoons
Sandalwood . . . . 5 drops Lemongrass . . . . 3 drops Pepper (Black) . . . . . . 2 drops Carrier Oil . . . . 2 teaspoons	Bois de Rose . . . . 4 drops Cedarwood (Atlas) . . . 3 drops Cardamom . . . . 3 drops Carrier Oil . . . . 2 teaspoons
Litsea Cubeba . . . . . . 4 drops Cardamom . . . . 3 drops Cedarwood (Atlas) . . . 3 drops Carrier Oil . . . . 2 teaspoons	Spruce . . . . 4 drops Vanilla . . . . 3 drops Grapefruit . . . . 3 drops Carrier Oil . . . . 2 teaspoons

Diffusers

Depending on the type of diffuser you have, place the essential oils on the diffuser pad or in the glass bottle to disperse the aroma into the air. Breathe in the vapors deeply.

Geranium . . . . 30% Frankincense . . . . 30% Orange . . . . 30% Pepper (Black) 10%	Bois de Rose . . . . 40% Litsea Cubeba . . . . . . 30% Geranium . . . . 20% Ginger 10%
Grapefruit . . . . 40% Lime . . . . 30% Frankincense 30%	Litsea Cubeba . . . . . . 50% Spruce . . . . 30% Basil (Sweet) 20%

Mist Sprays

Fill a fine-mist spray bottle with purified water, then add the essential oils. Tighten the cap and shake well. Mist numerous times and breathe in the vapors deeply.

Bois de Rose . . . . 50 drops	Lime . . . . 50 drops
Cardamom . . . . 40 drops	Geranium . . . . 30 drops
Lemongrass . . . . 40 drops	Orange . . . . 30 drops
Sandalwood . . . . 20 drops	Basil (Sweet) . . . . 20 drops
Pure Water . . . . 4 ounces	Ginger . . . . 20 drops
	Pure Water . . . . 4 ounces

Tangerine . . . . 50 drops	Frankincense . . . . . . 50 drops
Cedarwood (Atlas) . . . 50 drops	Spruce . . . . 50 drops
Spruce . . . . 50 drops	Palmarosa . . . . 50 drops
Pure Water . . . . 4 ounces	Pure Water . . . . 4 ounces

❋ Introspection

- Choose a method for your aromatherapy session: application, diffuser, or mist spray. Select and use a formula (see below).

- Do the Relaxation Exercises (see page 90). Allow yourself to reach a peaceful, quiet state. Then take a closer look at yourself. On a personal level, compare how your daily actions measure up to your moral values and the principles you stand for. On an interpersonal level, examine how you honor your promises, commitments, and responsibilities to the people in your life. Repeat this exercise as many times as you feel necessary. Each session should last 20 to 30 minutes.

Application

Apply one of these formulas to the upper chest and the back of the neck until the oil has been fully absorbed into the skin. Breathe in the vapors deeply.

Basil (Sweet) . . . . 3 drops	Elemi . . . . 3 drops
Sandalwood . . . . 3 drops	Frankincense . . . . 3 drops
Pepper (Black) . . . . . . 2 drops	Lemon . . . . 2 drops
Orange . . . . 2 drops	Tangerine . . . . 2 drops
Carrier Oil . . . . 2 teaspoons	Carrier Oil . . . . 2 teaspoons

Pepper (Black) ...... 3 drops	Myrrh .... 3 drops
Spruce .... 3 drops	Cypress .... 3 drops
Frankincense .... 2 drops	Labdanum .... 3 drops
Lemon .... 2 drops	Tangerine .... 1 drop
Carrier Oil .... 2 teaspoons	Carrier Oil .... 2 teaspoons

Petitgrain .... 3 drops	Cedarwood (Atlas) ... 3 drops
Sandalwood .... 3 drops	Basil (Sweet) .... 3 drops
Cajeput .... 2 drops	Spikenard .... 2 drops
Myrrh .... 2 drops	Rosemary .... 2 drops
Carrier Oil .... 2 teaspoons	Carrier Oil .... 2 teaspoons

Sandalwood .... 4 drops	Peru Balsam .... 3 drops
Bois de Rose .... 3 drops	Bois de Rose .... 3 drops
Nutmeg .... 2 drops	Myrrh .... 2 drops
Clove .... 1 drop	Rosemary .... 2 drops
Carrier Oil .... 2 teaspoons	Carrier Oil .... 2 teaspoons

Spruce .... 3 drops	Vetiver .... 4 drops
Bois de Rose .... 3 drops	Cypress .... 3 drops
Petitgrain .... 2 drops	Lemongrass .... 3 drops
Cedarwood (Atlas) ... 2 drops	Carrier Oil .... 2 teaspoons
Carrier Oil .... 2 teaspoons	

Diffusers

Depending on the type of diffuser you have, place the essential oils on the diffuser pad or in the glass bottle to disperse the aroma into the air.

Petitgrain 50%	Bois de Rose 40%
Basil (Sweet) 20%	Petitgrain 40%
Allspice 20%	Juniper Berry 20%
Rosemary 10%	

Frankincense 50%	Lime 40%
Spruce 50%	Tangerine 30%
	Cypress 30%

....

Fill a fine-mist spray bottle with purified water, then add the essential oils. Tighten the cap and shake well. Mist numerous times and breathe in the vapors deeply.

Frankincense . . . . 50 drops	Cedarwood (Atlas) . . . 45 drops
Vetiver . . . . 50 drops	Lime . . . . 45 drops
Orange . . . . 50 drops	Elemi . . . . 40 drops
Pure Water . . . . 4 ounces	Grapefruit . . . . 20 drops
	Pure Water . . . . 4 ounces

Bay . . . . 50 drops	Frankincense . . . . 40 drops
Sandalwood . . . . 50 drops	Nutmeg . . . . 40 drops
Cajeput . . . . 30 drops	Copaiba . . . . 30 drops
Mandarin . . . . 20 drops	Lime . . . . 30 drops
Pure Water . . . . 4 ounces	Pure Water . . . . 4 ounces

Loving Yourself

- Choose a method for your aromatherapy session: application, diffuser, or mist spray. Select and use a formula.

- Do the Relaxation Exercise (see page 90). Allow yourself to reach a peaceful and quiet state. Reflect on the things you enjoy doing that bring great satisfaction, make you feel good, and at the same time are beneficial to your well-being. Repeat this exercise as often as possible. Each session should last 20 to 30 minutes.

Application

....

Apply one of these formulas to the upper chest and the back of the neck until the oil is fully absorbed into the skin. Breathe in the vapors deeply.

Spruce . . . . 4 drops	Ylang-Ylang . . . . 4 drops
Sandalwood . . . . 3 drops	Orange . . . . 3 drops
Vanilla . . . . 3 drops	Sandalwood . . . . 3 drops
Carrier Oil . . . . 2 teaspoons	Carrier Oil . . . . 2 teaspoons

Sandalwood . . . . 4 drops	Bergamot . . . . 5 drops
Vanilla . . . . 3 drops	Copaiba . . . . 3 drops
Grapefruit . . . . 3 drops	Neroli . . . . 2 drops
Carrier Oil . . . . 2 teaspoons	Carrier Oil . . . . 2 teaspoons

Spruce	4 drops	Copaiba	5 drops
Frankincense	3 drops	Tangerine	3 drops
Ylang-Ylang	3 drops	Juniper Berry	2 drops
Carrier Oil	2 teaspoons	Carrier Oil	2 teaspoons

Vanilla	4 drops	Labdanum	5 drops
Ylang-Ylang	4 drops	Allspice	3 drops
Juniper Berry	2 drops	Lavender	2 drops
Carrier Oil	2 teaspoons	Carrier Oil	2 teaspoons

Vanilla	4 drops	Copaiba	8 drops
Labdanum	4 drops	Bergamot	8 drops
Rose	2 drops	Myrrh	4 drops
Carrier Oil	2 teaspoons	Carrier Oil	2 teaspoons

Spruce	8 drops	Ylang-Ylang	7 drops
Petitgrain	6 drops	Cumin	5 drops
Juniper Berry	6 drops	Orange	5 drops
Carrier Oil	2 teaspoons	Cedarwood (Atlas)	3 drops
		Carrier Oil	2 teaspoons

Cedarwood (Atlas)	3 drops	Sandalwood	8 drops
Clove	3 drops	Ginger	4 drops
Tangerine	3 drops	Grapefruit	4 drops
Myrrh	1 drop	Clove	4 drops
Carrier Oil	2 teaspoons	Carrier Oil	2 teaspoons

Diffusers

Depending on the type of diffuser you have, place the essential oils on the diffuser pad or in the glass bottle to disperse the aroma into the air. Breathe in the vapors deeply.

Ylang-Ylang	40%	Frankincense	40%
Juniper Berry	30%	Bergamot	40%
Clove	30%	Orange	20%

Bergamot	40%	Petitgrain	40%
Spruce	40%	Juniper Berry	30%
Ylang-Ylang	20%	Spruce	30%

```
Grapefruit . . . . . . . . . 50%        Ylang-Ylang . . . . . . . . 50%
Clove . . . . . . . . . . . . . 30%     Tangerine . . . . . . . . . 50%
Citronella . . . . . . . . . . 20%


Lime . . . . . . . . . . . . . . 50%    Grapefruit . . . . . . . . . 30%
Mandarin . . . . . . . . . . 30%        Petitgrain . . . . . . . . . . 30%
Ylang-Ylang . . . . . . . 20%           Ginger . . . . . . . . . . . . 20%
                                        Ylang-Ylang . . . . . . . 20%
```

Mist Sprays

Fill a fine-mist spray bottle with purified water, then add the essential oils. Tighten the cap and shake well. Mist numerous times and breathe in the vapors deeply.

```
Ylang-Ylang . . . . . . . . 50 drops      Cedarwood (Atlas) . . . 50 drops
Sandalwood . . . . . . . . 50 drops       Myrrh . . . . . . . . . . . . . 40 drops
Clove . . . . . . . . . . . . . 30 drops  Mandarin . . . . . . . . . . 40 drops
Citronella . . . . . . . . . . 20 drops   Clove . . . . . . . . . . . . . 20 drops
Pure Water . . . . . . . . 4 ounces       Pure Water . . . . . . . . 4 ounces


Grapefruit . . . . . . . . . 60 drops     Frankincense . . . . . . . 50 drops
Peru Balsam . . . . . . . . 60 drops      Cedarwood (Atlas) . . . 50 drops
Juniper Berry . . . . . . . 30 drops      Tangerine . . . . . . . . . . 50 drops
Pure Water . . . . . . . . 4 ounces       Pure Water . . . . . . . . 4 ounces


Bergamot . . . . . . . . . . 50 drops     Peru Balsam . . . . . . . . 50 drops
Copaiba . . . . . . . . . . . 50 drops    Citronella . . . . . . . . . . 50 drops
Peru Balsam . . . . . . . . 50 drops      Tangerine . . . . . . . . . . 50 drops
Pure Water . . . . . . . . 4 ounces       Pure Water . . . . . . . . 4 ounces


Allspice . . . . . . . . . . . 40 drops   Lemon . . . . . . . . . . . . 60 drops
Ylang-Ylang . . . . . . . . 30 drops      Peru Balsam . . . . . . . . 60 drops
Spruce . . . . . . . . . . . . 30 drops   Bois de Rose . . . . . . . 30 drops
Myrrh . . . . . . . . . . . . . 30 drops  Pure Water . . . . . . . . 4 ounces
Orange . . . . . . . . . . . . 20 drops
Pure Water . . . . . . . . 4 ounces
```

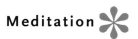
The meditative state not only relaxes the body, but rejuvenates the mind and nervous system.

- Choose a method for your aromatherapy session: application, diffuser, or mist spray; select and use a formula.

- Do Relaxation Exercise (see page 90). Allow yourself to reach a peaceful and quiet state of mind, and maintain this level of calmness for 20 to 30 minutes. Practice as often as you can.

Application

Apply one of these formulas to the upper chest and the back of the neck until the oil is fully absorbed into the skin. Breathe the vapors deeply.

Frankincense . . . . 5 drops Orange . . . . 5 drops Carrier Oil . . . . 2 teaspoons	Elemi . . . . 5 drops Litsea Cubeba . . . . . . 5 drops Carrier Oil . . . . 2 teaspoons
Copaiba . . . . 5 drops Lemon . . . . 3 drops Nutmeg . . . . 2 drops Carrier Oil . . . . 2 teaspoons	Sandalwood . . . . 4 drops Basil (Sweet) . . . . 4 drops Lavender . . . . 2 drops Carrier Oil . . . . 2 teaspoons
Cedarwood (Atlas) . . . 5 drops Spruce . . . . 5 drops Carrier Oil . . . . 2 teaspoons	Labdanum . . . . 6 drops Clary Sage . . . . 4 drops Carrier Oil . . . . 2 teaspoons
Peru Balsam . . . . 4 drops Nutmeg . . . . 3 drops Spikenard . . . . 3 drops Carrier Oil . . . . 2 teaspoons	Guaiacwood . . . . 5 drops Tangerine . . . . 5 drops Carrier Oil . . . . 2 teaspoons
Guaiacwood . . . . 5 drops Petitgrain . . . . 3 drops Frankincense . . . . 2 drops Carrier Oil . . . . 2 teaspoons	Peru Balsam . . . . 5 drops Orange . . . . 3 drops Cumin . . . . 2 drops Carrier Oil . . . . 2 teaspoons

Diffusers

Depending on the type of diffuser you have, place the essential oils on the diffuser pad or in the glass bottle to disperse the aroma into the air. Breathe in the vapors deeply.

Frankincense 50%			Lavender 50%	
Orange 30%			Basil (Sweet) 25%	
Petitgrain 20%			Anise 25%	

Litsea Cubeba 50%	Mandarin 50%
Nutmeg 25%	Lavender 50%
Clary Sage 25%	

Tangerine 50%	Orange 50%
Frankincense 30%	Spruce 30%
Basil (Sweet) 20%	Nutmeg 20%

Mist Sprays

Fill a fine-mist spray bottle with purified water, then add the essential oils. Tighten the cap and shake well. Mist numerous times and breathe in the vapors deeply.

Frankincense . . . . 75 drops	Sandalwood . . . . 50 drops
Orange . . . . 50 drops	Frankincense . . . . 50 drops
Nutmeg . . . . 25 drops	Spruce . . . . 50 drops
Pure Water . . . . 4 ounces	Pure Water . . . . 4 ounces

Cedarwood (Atlas) . . . 60 drops	Lavender . . . . 60 drops
Litsea Cubeba . . . . . . 60 drops	Vetiver . . . . 50 drops
Clary Sage . . . . 30 drops	Anise . . . . 40 drops
Pure Water . . . . 4 ounces	Pure Water . . . . 4 ounces

Elemi . . . . 60 drops	Copaiba . . . . 70 drops
Litsea Cubeba . . . . . . 50 drops	Orange . . . . 50 drops
Petitgrain . . . . 40 drops	Frankincense . . . . 30 drops
Pure Water . . . . 4 ounces	Pure Water . . . . 4 ounces

This exercise can be a valuable means of understanding how honest we are with ourselves to help us lessen inner conflicts and create a state of inner peacefulness and well-being.

- Choose a method for your aromatherapy session: application, diffuser, or mist sprays. Select and use a formula (see below).

- Do Relaxation Exercise (see page 90). Allow yourself to reach a quiet state of mind, then examine the actions you take and the motives behind them. Each session should last 20 to 30 minutes.

Application

Apply one of these formulas to the upper chest, back of the neck, and shoulders until the oil is fully absorbed into the skin. Breathe in the vapors deeply.

Spruce . . . . 4 drops	Bay . . . . 4 drops
Labdanum . . . . 4 drops	Tangerine . . . . 4 drops
Litsea Cubeba . . . . . . 2 drops	Patchouli . . . . 2 drops
Carrier Oil . . . . 2 teaspoons	Carrier Oil . . . . 2 teaspoons

Geranium . . . . 4 drops	Peru Balsam . . . . 5 drops
Bois de Rose . . . . 3 drops	Lemon . . . . 5 drops
Sandalwood . . . . 3 drops	Carrier Oil . . . . 2 teaspoons
Carrier Oil . . . . 2 teaspoons	

Copaiba . . . . 5 drops	Frankincense . . . . 4 drops
Pepper (Black) . . . . . . 3 drops	Cedarwood (Atlas) . . . 4 drops
Tangerine . . . . 2 drops	Spikenard . . . . 2 drops
Carrier Oil . . . . 2 teaspoons	Carrier Oil . . . . 2 teaspoons

Diffusers

Depending on the type of diffuser you have, place the essential oils on the diffuser pad or in the glass bottle to disperse the aroma into the air. Breathe in the vapors deeply.

Spruce	50%		Tangerine	50%
Palmarosa	30%		Spruce	30%
Petitgrain	20%		Citronella	20%

Bois de Rose	50%		Tangerine	40%
Lemon	30%		Bay	30%
Geranium	20%		Myrtle	30%

Mist Sprays

Fill a fine-mist spray bottle with purified water, then add the essential oils. Tighten the cap and shake well. Mist numerous times and breathe in the vapors deeply.

Spruce	50 drops		Peru Balsam	60 drops
Lemongrass	40 drops		Lemon	30 drops
Palmarosa	40 drops		Myrtle	30 drops
Cedarwood (Atlas)	20 drops		Spikenard	30 drops
Pure Water	4 ounces		Pure Water	4 ounces

Bois de Rose	60 drops		Tangerine	60 drops
Citronella	30 drops		Copaiba	40 drops
Tangerine	20 drops		Sandalwood	20 drops
Patchouli	20 drops		Bois de Rose	20 drops
Clove	20 drops		Vetiver	10 drops
Pure Water	4 ounces		Pure Water	4 ounces

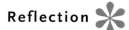
The path you have followed in prior years brought you to where you are now. The path you are on now will determine where you will be in life in future years. Are you presently on the right path?

- Choose a method for your aromatherapy session: application, diffuser, or mist spray. Select and use a formula (see below).

- Do Relaxation Exercise (see page 90). Allow yourself to reach a peaceful and quiet state. Then, reflect on your path. Repeat this exercise as many times as you feel necessary. Each session should last 20 to 30 minutes.

Application

Apply one of these formulas to the back of the neck, upper chest, and temple area until the oil is fully absorbed into the skin. Breathe in the vapors deeply.

Litsea Cubeba ...... 4 drops	Bay .... 4 drops
Pepper (Black) ...... 3 drops	Lemongrass .... 4 drops
Cedarwood (Atlas) ... 3 drops	Patchouli .... 2 drops
Carrier Oil .... 2 teaspoons	Carrier Oil .... 2 teaspoons

Elemi .... 4 drops	Frankincense .... 4 drops
Petitgrain .... 3 drops	Spikenard .... 4 drops
Hyssop Decumbens .. 3 drops	Myrrh .... 2 drops
Carrier Oil .... 2 teaspoons	Carrier Oil .... 2 teaspoons

Vetiver .... 4 drops	Spikenard .... 4 drops
Hyssop Decumbens .. 4 drops	Orange .... 4 drops
Chamomile (Roman) . 2 drops	Patchouli .... 2 drops
Carrier Oil .... 2 teaspoons	Carrier Oil .... 2 teaspoons

Fir Needles .... 4 drops	Lemon .... 4 drops
Litsea Cubeba ...... 4 drops	Basil (Sweet) .... 4 drops
Frankincense .... 2 drops	Patchouli .... 2 drops
Carrier Oil .... 2 teaspoons	Carrier Oil .... 2 teaspoons

Diffusers

Depending on the type of diffuser you have, place the essential oils on the diffuser pad or in the glass bottle to disperse the aroma into the air. Breathe in the vapors deeply.

Frankincense	50%	Litsea Cubeba	50%
Cinnamon Leaf	30%	Frankincense	20%
Fir Needles	20%	Ginger	30%

Lemon	40%	Chamomile (Roman)	50%
Bay	40%	Tangerine	50%
Orange	20%		

Spruce	40%	Lavender	30%
Tangerine	40%	Petitgrain	30%
Fir Needles	20%	Mandarin	30%
		Ginger	10%

Mist Sprays

Fill a fine-mist spray bottle with purified water, then add the essential oils. Tighten the cap and shake well. Mist numerous times and breathe in the vapors deeply.

Litsea Cubeba	50 drops	Fir Needles	40 drops
Mandarin	50 drops	Spruce	40 drops
Patchouli	30 drops	Frankincense	40 drops
Ginger	20 drops	Lemon	30 drops
Pure Water	4 ounces	Pure Water	4 ounces

Bay	40 drops	Lemon	50 drops
Orange	30 drops	Grapefruit	30 drops
Petitgrain	30 drops	Vetiver	30 drops
Lavender	30 drops	Ginger	30 drops
Peru Balsam	20 drops	Frankincense	10 drops
Pure Water	4 ounces	Pure Water	4 ounces

Mandarin	40 drops	Litsea Cubeba	35 drops
Lemon	40 drops	Peru Balsam	35 drops
Frankincense	25 drops	Fir Needles	30 drops
Patchouli	25 drops	Basil (Sweet)	25 drops
Peru Balsam	20 drops	Ginger	25 drops
Pure Water	4 ounces	Pure Water	4 ounces

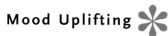

Massage one of these formulas on the upper chest, back of the neck, shoulders, and down the back until the oil is fully absorbed into the skin. Breathe in the vapors deeply. For best results, massage for 30 minutes.

Peppermint	8 drops	Geranium	5 drops
Copaiba	5 drops	Tangerine	5 drops
Lemon	4 drops	Vetiver	5 drops
Thyme	3 drops	Citronella	5 drops
Carrier Oil	4 teaspoons	Carrier Oil	4 teaspoons

Bois de Rose	6 drops	Frankincense	5 drops
Ylang-Ylang	5 drops	Mandarin	5 drops
Benzoin	5 drops	Cypress	5 drops
Basil (Sweet)	4 drops	Bay	5 drops
Carrier Oil	4 teaspoons	Carrier Oil	4 teaspoons

Peru Balsam	6 drops	Petitgrain	5 drops
Bay	5 drops	Bergamot	5 drops
Bergamot	5 drops	Geranium	5 drops
Basil (Sweet)	4 drops	Labdanum	5 drops
Carrier Oil	4 teaspoons	Carrier Oil	4 teaspoons

Mandarin	4 drops	Hyssop Decumbens	5 drops
Spearmint	4 drops	Palmarosa	4 drops
Grapefruit	4 drops	Petitgrain	4 drops
Frankincense	4 drops	Vanilla	4 drops
Spikenard	4 drops	Chamomile (Roman)	3 drops
Carrier Oil	4 teaspoons	Carrier Oil	4 teaspoons

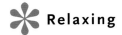

Relaxing

Massage one of these formulas on the upper chest, back of the neck, shoulders, down the back, and the bottoms of the feet until the oil is fully absorbed into the skin. Breathe in the vapors deeply. For best results, massage for 30 minutes.

Celery . . . . 5 drops	Spikenard . . . . 4 drops
Orange . . . . 5 drops	Celery . . . . 4 drops
Frankincense . . . . 5 drops	Neroli . . . . 4 drops
Copaiba . . . . 5 drops	Peru Balsam . . . . 4 drops
Carrier Oil . . . . 4 teaspoons	Carrier Oil . . . . 4 teaspoons

Lemongrass . . . . 5 drops	Vetiver . . . . 5 drops
Mandarin . . . . 5 drops	Elemi . . . . 5 drops
Sandalwood . . . . 4 drops	Marjoram . . . . 4 drops
Petitgrain . . . . 4 drops	Lavender . . . . 4 drops
Elemi . . . . 2 drops	Cedarwood (Atlas) . . . 2 drops
Carrier Oil . . . . 4 teaspoons	Carrier Oil . . . . 4 teaspoons

Orange . . . . 5 drops	Bois de Rose . . . . 5 drops
Labdanum . . . . 4 drops	Litsea Cubeba . . . . . . 4 drops
Copaiba . . . . 4 drops	Chamomile (Roman) . 4 drops
Basil (Sweet) . . . . 4 drops	Mandarin . . . . 4 drops
Chamomile (Roman) . 3 drops	Ylang-Ylang . . . . 4 drops
Carrier Oil . . . . 4 teaspoons	Clary Sage . . . . 3 drops
	Carrier Oil . . . . 4 teaspoons

Surrender Your Stress

Stress is the body's response when life's demands become overwhelming. It is especially produced on occasions when we suppress our natural instincts or withhold our feelings. If the stressed state is allowed to linger, it causes considerable damage to the body. The adrenal glands can become exhausted, resulting in impaired physical and mental functioning, reduced energy levels, fatigue, and depression. Stress may be responsible for an increase in blood pressure, immune-system suppression, heart disease, and other organ and nervous system disorders.

One of the great paradoxes is that with the advancement of modern technology—intended to make life easier and improved—stress-related illnesses are increasingly rising. It has been estimated that as many as 75 percent of all medical complaints are stress-related.

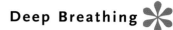

Breathing is the foundation of life. However, in most large cities, the air pollution from industry and vehicle emissions is so great that it discourages people from breathing deeply. In addition, stress has the same effect, causing a person to breathe shallowly. Deep breathing is essential to relieve stress and maintain good health and well-being. By using essential oils and practicing deep breathing exercises daily, you should notice favorable results.

Application

Apply one of these formulas to the upper chest and abdomen until the oil is fully absorbed into the skin. Breathe in the vapors deeply.

Eucalyptus . . . . 4 drops Peppermint . . . . 4 drops Sandalwood . . . . 2 drops Carrier Oil . . . . 1 teaspoon	Fir Needles . . . . 4 drops Cajeput . . . . 4 drops Cedarwood (Atlas) . . . 2 drops Carrier Oil . . . . 1 teaspoon
Tea Tree . . . . 4 drops Spearmint . . . . 4 drops Copaiba . . . . 2 drops Carrier Oil . . . . 1 teaspoon	Copaiba . . . . 4 drops Grapefruit . . . . 3 drops Anise . . . . 3 drops Carrier Oil . . . . 1 teaspoon
Myrtle . . . . 4 drops Eucalyptus . . . . 4 drops Cedarwood (Atlas) . . . 2 drops Carrier Oil . . . . 1 teaspoon	Hyssop Decumbens . . 5 drops Tea Tree . . . . 4 drops Cedarwood (Atlas) . . . 2 drops Carrier Oil . . . . 1 teaspoon
Sandalwood . . . . 3 drops Frankincense . . . . 3 drops Spruce . . . . 3 drops Peppermint . . . . 1 drop Carrier Oil . . . . 1 teaspoon	Lavender . . . . 4 drops Sandalwood . . . . 3 drops Marjoram . . . . 2 drops Spearmint . . . . 1 drop Carrier Oil . . . . 1 teaspoon

Diffusers

Depending on the type of diffuser you have, place the essential oils on the diffuser pad or in the glass bottle to disperse the aroma into the air. Breathe in the vapors deeply.

Lavender 40%	Hyssop Decumbens .. 50%
Eucalyptus 30%	Frankincense 50%
Hyssop Decumbens .. 30%	

Fir Needles 50%	Cypress 25%
Tea Tree 20%	Spearmint 25%
Eucalyptus 20%	Cajeput 25%
Juniper Berry 10%	Lemon 25%

Peppermint 30%	Myrtle 30%
Tea Tree 25%	Lime 30%
Lavender 25%	Cubeb 20%
Spruce 20%	Fir Needles 20%

Mist Sprays

Fill a fine-mist spray bottle with purified water, then add the essential oils. Tighten the cap and shake well. Mist numerous times and breathe in the vapors deeply.

Cajeput .... 40 drops	Copaiba .... 50 drops
Juniper Berry .... 25 drops	Eucalyptus .... 30 drops
Rosemary .... 25 drops	Peppermint .... 30 drops
Tea Tree .... 25 drops	Petitgrain .... 30 drops
Spearmint .... 25 drops	Clove .... 10 drops
Copaiba .... 10 drops	Pure Water .... 4 ounces
Pure Water .... 4 ounces	

Lavender .... 50 drops	Lavender .... 50 drops
Cedarwood (Atlas) ... 50 drops	Helichrysum .... 50 drops
Spearmint .... 50 drops	Hyssop Decumbens .. 50 drops
Pure Water .... 4 ounces	Pure Water .... 4 ounces

Petitgrain .... 30 drops	Frankincense .... 50 drops
Myrtle .... 30 drops	Hyssop Decumbens .. 50 drops
Spruce .... 30 drops	Lemon .... 50 drops
Frankincense .... 30 drops	Pure Water .... 4 ounces
Cubeb .... 30 drops	
Pure Water .... 4 ounces	

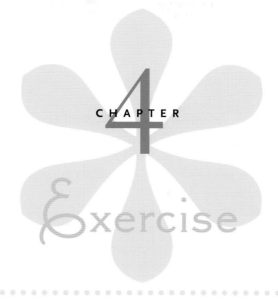

CHAPTER 4

Exercise

To shape your body the way you want it to be, you need to adopt a dual approach. First, you need to develop and tone your muscles. Second, and just as important, you need to maintain a healthy level of body fat so that those sleek, toned muscles are visible to the outside world.

Perhaps the single most widespread reason that people exercise is to achieve and maintain a healthy body weight. But losing weight through exercise isn't a matter of simply burning off calories while you are working out. Resistance training in particular helps you lose body fat in more subtle ways.

First, let's look at the importance of aerobic exercise in body shaping. Aerobic activities, or sustained exercise that makes you sweat and keeps your heart pumping, help eliminate that extra body fat that can cover up even well-developed muscles.

The amount of fat you burn during aerobic exercise depends on your fitness level. A trained athlete burns fat sooner after exercise starts than someone who is moderately fit; a "couch potato" takes even longer to start burning fat, and even then, burns it at a slower rate than a fit individual. Even during nonaerobic physical activities or at rest, a sedentary person burns fat at a much slower rate than someone who is active.

Having extra body fat slows down the metabolism, which makes it less efficient. Aerobic exercise temporarily raises the metabolism, so you have more energy and are also burning more calories.

Find an aerobic activity you like (otherwise you won't stick with it), then get up and do it for 30 minutes to an hour most days of the week. You'll look better, feel better, be healthier, and have more energy!

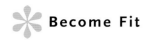

Become Fit

Fight Adult–Onset Diabetes

Adult-onset diabetes, or type 2 diabetes, is a debilitating, often fatal disease that strikes about eighteen hundred Americans every day—that's more than 650,000 new cases a year! The majority of victims are over forty years old. Approximately nine out of ten cases of diabetes are type 2. Ironically, most if not all of these cases are preventable.

Adult-onset diabetes affects the body's ability to use sugar. This disease disrupts normal metabolism both at rest and during physical activity.

As people grow older, they tend to become less active, lose muscle, and gain body fat. This is especially true in modern American culture. Those who fail to maintain their muscle mass as they age through an active lifestyle, resistance training, or both, increase their risk of developing diabetes. To understand why, let's take a look at how the body manufactures and stores energy for its daily needs.

We make use of the sugars and starches that we consume by changing them into glucose. Glucose is carried in the bloodstream to the body's various tissues, but mostly to the muscles. For glucose to enter the muscle, insulin (a hormone made by the pancreas) must be present.

In a healthy person, any glucose that is not immediately needed for energy is stored in the muscles. If there is more glucose available than the muscles can accommodate, then the excess glucose finds its way to the liver, where it is converted to fat.

If you do not have very much muscle tissue, you lack glucose storage sites. The level of glucose in the bloodstream ("blood sugar") can become abnormally high. This forces the pancreas to work harder to produce more insulin, trying to get the glucose out of the bloodstream and into the muscle cells. Eventually the pancreas can wear out from overuse. The result is an impaired ability to manufacture insulin, or type 2 diabetes. The body's ability to use and store glucose is damaged. Diabetes, if left uncontrolled, can lead to heart disease, kidney failure, nerve dysfunction, stroke, high blood pressure, high cholesterol levels, and ulcers of the feet.

So what does exercise, including aerobic activities and weight training, have to do with diabetes? Aerobic activities and weight lifting build muscle faster than any other form of exercise. Remember, if you've developed your muscles, then you have plenty of storage space for glucose. Your pancreas has less work to do, and you are less likely to develop diabetes. If you are already diabetic, weight training is an essential part of controlling the disease so that you can still live a normal life.

Fight Osteoporosis

Osteoporosis is the progressive weakening of the bones due to mineral loss. It causes bones to become less and less dense, creating a stooped posture and increasing the risk of broken bones. This latter risk especially must be taken seriously. For example, if you fail to protect your bone density, a simple fall in your golden years can break your hip, and few individuals over sixty-five or seventy ever completely recover from a broken hip. Very often, in fact, a broken hip starts a downward spiral in health that leads to death within two or three years. Women are especially vulnerable to osteoporosis, but men can be affected too.

Doing some form of weight-bearing exercise regularly is crucial to the prevention of osteoporosis. Calcium is deposited in the bones in proportion to the amount of stress (load) placed on them. Bones adapt to such exercise by becoming denser and stronger so they can provide sufficient support for the muscles. Lifting weights is the fastest, most effective way to preserve and increase bone mass (other than using prescription drugs) because it is also the fastest, most effective way to build muscle.

For weight lifting to affect bone density, you must lift enough weight to overload the muscle—you have to train to the point of "muscle failure." We'll show you how in this book. But for now, please note that training to muscle failure does not mean you need to spend a lot of time in the gym. It is a matter of technique, not time. If you begin even a modest program of resistance training and stick with it for the rest of your life, you're helping to guarantee that you'll maintain your health and vitality to a ripe old age.

For your bones to get the maximum benefit possible from weight training, it is a good idea to become aware of some other things you can do to decrease your risk of osteoporosis.

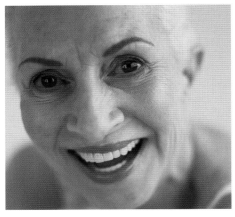

It is also useful to be aware of the uncontrollable risk factors in the development of osteoporosis. If you fit into any of the following categories, there's all the more reason to do everything you can to minimize your controllable risks, especially through exercise.

- Fair-skinned people
- Small-boned people, who have less bone mass to begin with naturally
- Thin-boned people, who are not as strong because they are not required to support a higher body weight. (This is not a good reason to put on weight, just make up for it through weight training!)
- People with a family history of osteoporosis
- People over the age of 40, especially women who have passed through menopause. Estrogen helps prevent bone mineral loss, and after menopause, estrogen production nearly ceases.

A long-term commitment to exercise and weight training is the single best decision you can make to prevent osteoporosis.

Exercise and Heart Disease

There are a number of "risk factors" for coronary artery disease (heart disease). Some of them you have control over; a few you don't. The controllable risk factors are:

1. High cholesterol, which can be managed by eating a low-cholesterol diet, exercising regularly, and taking medication if necessary. Weight training and aerobic exercise help you lose body fat and thus reduce cholesterol. In addition, regular aerobic exercise increases your high-density lipoproteins (HDLs; the "good cholesterol"). HDLs sweep the low-density (LDLs; "bad cholesterol") out of your bloodstream, thus lowering your risk of heart disease.

2. High blood pressure, which can also be managed by diet, aerobic exercise, stress reduction, and medication if necessary. Because aerobic exercise lowers

your overall blood pressure, it helps reduce your risk of stroke as well as heart disease.

3. Cigarette smoking, which can be managed only by quitting.

4. Lack of exercise, for which the cure is, of course, to exercise regularly.

5. Obesity, which is managed by diet, counseling, and exercise. Both aerobic exercise and weight training help you lose body fat. Loss of body fat, in turn, reduces your risk not only of heart disease, but also of stroke, adult-onset diabetes, and some cancers.

The heart disease risk factors that you can't control are fewer:

1. Family history or an inherited predisposition for heart disease.

2. Age of 45 or more—Menopausal women are at greater risk after their bodies stop producing estrogen. Estrogen replacement therapy can reduce this risk, but long-term use of estrogen can increase other health risks. The best solution is to change bad lifestyle habits.

3. Gender—Males are at higher risk.

Don't be at all discouraged just because you fall into some of the above groups. Even if you're an older adult from a family with a history of heart disease, your chances of avoiding heart disease are good as long as you eat a very low fat, mostly vegetarian diet, do regular aerobic exercise, don't smoke, maintain a healthy weight, and manage your stress.

On the other hand, even if you're young, female, and not aware of any family history, you're not immune. Protect yourself by avoiding the controllable risk factors as well.

You may have noticed that exercise shows up as a solution to four out of the five controllable risk factors. You can see how important exercise is in preventing heart disease! A sedentary lifestyle is a major risk factor for developing cardiovascular disease. Doing regular exercise, especially aerobic exercise, is one of the most important steps you can take to reduce your risk of heart disease. So, in addition to your weight-training regimen, find an aerobic activity you like and do it for at least 20 (preferably 30) minutes most days of the week. Some different types of aerobic exercise are brisk walking (walk as if you have some place to be and are running late), jogging, running, cycling, step aerobics, and aerobic exercise classes.

The heart is a muscle. For it to remain strong and healthy, it needs to be worked, just like the other muscles in our body. Aerobic exercise strengthens the heart. It takes time for your heart to actually become stronger, but its functions (oxygen delivery out to the rest of your body) improve almost immediately. When your heart becomes stronger, more oxygen can be circulated to your body with less work (fewer heartbeats). Eventually your heart rate (heartbeats per minute) lowers because your heart has become more efficient at supplying your body with the oxygen it needs to live. A slower heart rate (fewer beats per minute) means your heart may last longer because it doesn't have to work so hard.

Weight training, as important as it is, doesn't have the heart-strengthening benefit of aerobic exercise. So your exercise program must be comprehensive and address physical fitness through a variety of means. There are in fact three major cornerstones of physical fitness: aerobic exercise, resistance training, and flexibility work (stretching). If you do all three, not only are you on track to live a long, disease-free life, but you're also helping ensure that you'll feel as good as possible while you're at it.

Fight Arthritis

Resistance exercise eases the pain of osteoarthritis and rheumatoid arthritis.

Lifting weights strengthens the muscles and joints. When exercises are performed correctly, range of motion in the joints increases. Full range of motion means the joints are more flexible. Weight training also decreases the risk of injuries, which aggravate the afflicted joints, because stronger muscles make better shock absorbers and better joint stabilizers.

People with arthritis are often obese, partly because arthritis makes them so inactive. Obesity aggravates the effects of arthritis. An exercise program that includes strength training and walking can improve arthritis symptoms by helping the sufferer lose weight.

If you have arthritis, check with your doctor before starting any exercise program.

Manage Stress

When we are under stress, our bodies release certain hormones and chemicals that increase our heart rate, metabolism, blood pressure, respiratory rate, and muscle tension. This heightened state is often referred to as the "fight or flight" response. In most stressful situations we cannot fight or flee, so our bodies don't have an appropriate way to handle these conditions.

Unfortunately, the chemicals created by our bodies under stress have a negative impact on our immune systems. Too much stress is not good for our health.

If you are under continuous stress, whatever the source, your body's reaction can result in any number of physical or emotional symptoms, or

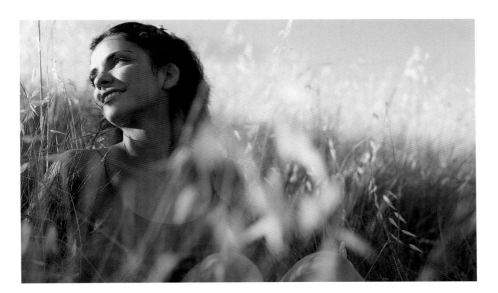

both. Headaches, stomachaches, ulcers, digestive problems, and insomnia are a few examples of physical problems related to excessive stress. If you don't have a way to reduce your stress and it becomes chronic, there is evidence it can lead to or worsen coronary artery disease, high blood pressure, and the risk of stroke.

Some emotional problems brought on by stress include edginess, aggression, a decline in libido, depression, anxiety attacks, loss of a sense of well-being, feelings of ill will, and boredom.

How can you avoid these dangers? First, if something is a continual source of stress in your life, try to resolve or eliminate it. If that isn't possible, learn to accept it. Second, increase your stress threshold—your ability to take stressful situations in stride. The best way to become more stress-resistant is to take good care of your health. Most important, get regular exercise. Also, eat a healthy diet, don't drink or smoke, and cut back on caffeine. Devote some time each week to some form of genuine relaxation. Develop close relationships with friends and family. The more people you know and care about, the greater your resources for emotional support. Make long-term commitments to someone and something. Long-term goals often make short-term problems easier to handle.

Strengthen the Immune System

The human immune system appears to function better when we exercise regularly. According to recent studies, physically fit people get fewer colds and upper respiratory tract infections. This is probably because even moderate exercise increases the circulation of the natural "killer" cells in your bloodstream, such as T-cells and immunoglobulin. These cells protect our bodies from foreign invaders. The increase lasts only a few hours, but apparently that's long enough to ward off some infections. Don't overdo it, though; too much exercise is probably worse than not enough.

Build Bone and Muscle Strength

After the age of 25, we lose from a quarter to a half pound of muscle each year in the absence of exercise. This loss of muscle, and the corresponding loss of bone mass, has a terrible impact on the quality of life of older people. Their posture stoops, their bones become brittle, they become weak, they lose their balance, and they are easily injured.

Aerobic exercise and strength training are the most effective ways to prevent this degenerative process from occurring. By lifting weights, it's possible to actually reverse the shrinkage and build more muscle and bone mass.

Strong muscles help maintain good posture, they enhance the ability to balance, and they help prevent injuries. As you exercise, you not only strengthen your muscles and build bone mass, you also strengthen the connective tissue (tendons and ligaments) within the working joints. Strong connective tissue and denser muscles make better shock absorbers. They stabilize the joints. They hold the body erect and keep it in proper alignment. In all these ways, they lessen the potential for injury.

More muscle strength is helpful for all physical activities. The stronger you are, the more successful you are at sport performance, and the easier everyday activities become.

Muscle atrophy (shrinkage) often contributes to pain in the body. For instance, weak muscles in the lower back and abdominals are a key factor in low back pain. Another example is neck pain. If you sit at a desk all day, neck strength can decrease up to 30 percent between 9 A.M. and 5 P.M. This can lead to neck pain. If the muscles and connective tissue in and around the neck are strong, this strength decrease may have less impact, which translates to less, if any, pain. Also, strong muscles may lessen the pain caused by chronic health problems such as arthritis.

It's harder to be independent and self-reliant if you don't have the strength to support those attitudes. Both the act of working out and the results you get from the process provide positive reinforcement and can help improve your self-image and self-concept.

Think ahead—when you're in your eighties, you'll want to look up and out at the world, not down at the ground. Start weight training now, so that all your years can be experienced fully.

Too many people make the excuse that they are too tired to exercise or they need to save their energy. What these people don't realize is that exercise actually energizes the body and reduces fatigue—those who exercise regularly have more energy for the rest of their activities than those who do not! There are several reasons for this paradoxical effect. For starters, exercise increases your body's ability to utilize oxygen, which improves stamina, creates more vigor, and enhances your concentration. Also, regular exercise helps reduce muscle tension, a major cause of fatigue. And, on the cellular level, exercise encourages your body to manufacture more mitochondria, which is the place in the cell where energy is produced.

Exercise helps improve your psychological response to stress, and unmanaged stress is probably the number one cause of fatigue in the United States today. Also, the extra energy generated by exercise can help you accomplish more and deal with the everyday pressures of life, which means you'll avoid some of the things that have tended to cause you stress.

Exercise helps you to relax, and regular exercise helps you to sleep better. A good night's sleep is always great for increasing energy levels.

Exercise improves self-image and gives you a feeling of accomplishment. These psychological factors have a huge impact on your energy levels. When

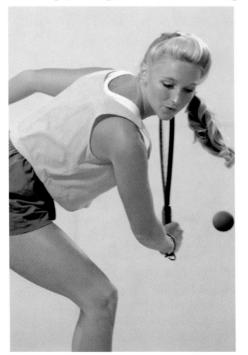

you feel good about yourself, you're more likely to want to go out into the world and explore life's possibilities.

Exercise invigorates your body in both the short term and the long term. The biggest short-term gain comes right after a bout of aerobic exercise. Your metabolism is higher than before you exercised, and you're burning calories at an accelerated rate. The longer and harder you exercise without overdoing it, the greater the temporary metabolic boost.

Lifting weights also boosts energy by improving glycogen storage—the means by which your body makes sugar available for energy. The carbohydrates in your food are broken down into glucose molecules and stored in the muscles as glycogen. Think of your muscles as the gas tank in your car. With a bigger gas tank, you can store more fuel; thus, your car will run for a longer period of time.

Similarly, the more muscle you have, the more space you have to store glycogen and the longer your body will run before experiencing fatigue. You'll have more energy to get you through the day, without experiencing an afternoon slump. In fact, glucose metabolism can improve by as much as 23 percent after just four months of regular strength training. On the other hand, if you don't have much muscle available for glycogen storage, not only will you have less energy available, but you'll also have a greater tendency to put on fat. Your body will circulate the excess glu-

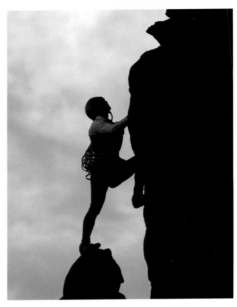

cose back to your liver, where it is converted into fat and then stored in your body's fat cells.

Stimulate Your Mind

Regular exercise increases the amount of oxygen delivered to the brain and improves mental agility. Your brain makes up only 2 percent of your body weight but uses a full 25 percent of the glucose and oxygen you take in! Exercise increases your body's ability to take in and utilize oxygen. When you exercise, you saturate your body with oxygen, and hence more oxygen becomes available for brain power. If you don't exercise, then as you get older your heart gets sluggish. Your arteries start to clog up. Blood flow to the tiny capillaries that nourish the brain cells can slow to a mere trickle. If you want to remain mentally alert and agile as you age, do some kind of exercise most days of the week.

Exercise also activates the sections of your brain that control movement and balance. A long-term exercise regime, including resistance training, can keep your motor skills strong into old age, allow you to stay coordinated, and help you maintain your balance.

Exercise Tips

Don't Waste Time

When you work out in the gym or at home, you don't want to waste your time. Each workout should make a difference—not a big difference, but a difference nonetheless. The benefits of exercise are cumulative. Every workout does a little something to improve the muscle and bone. If you want your muscles to grow bigger, denser, and stronger, you have to train them harder than what they're used to.

To spark the physiological process that changes the muscle, you have to overload the muscle. If the muscle doesn't reach fatigue each time you train, then the workout is not hard enough. Of course, "hard" is a relative word. For a beginner, light weights and short training sessions can still equal a hard workout.

The overload principle is even more important when it comes to increasing bone mass. Bone mineral density will not increase unless there's a great deal of stress placed on the bones. Bones adapt to stress by becoming denser and stronger.

So make each workout matter. Even if you spend just 20 minutes training, make those 20 minutes as potent as possible. A good, hard workout—one where you train your muscles to failure or nearly to failure—will invigorate and empower you, and give you more energy and self-confidence.

Timeline

Optimally, everyone should take one day a week off from all forms of vigorous exercise. At the least, take a day off every week from aerobic exercise and a different day off from resistance training. This break is necessary for your muscles, connective tissue, and joints to recover. This short amount of total rest will not have any negative effect on your fitness level; on the contrary, time off from a heavy training schedule actually improves fitness.

When physically conditioned, you can safely exercise aerobically 20 minutes to an hour 6 days of the week, and you can lift weights safely up to five or six times per week. Also, each major muscle group in your body except the abdominals needs a 48-hour rest before you train that muscle group again. This allows time for the physiological adaptations to take place within the muscle. If you train the same muscle group every day, you'll certainly create negative results.

From time to time, it's also important to take more than a day off from lifting weights, preferably a few days. We're not suggesting that you become a couch potato during these periods. Instead, try "active rest" or cross-training—engage in alternative forms of exercise. For instance, swim laps in place of lifting weights, or go for a brisk walk or a jog instead of training your legs in the gym.

The idea is to make a change in your training program that gives your body a chance to recover before beginning another rigorous training cycle. Participate in activities that challenge the body and mind in creative and different ways. Whatever you choose to do, the idea is to cut back on the daily demands of intense exercise to prevent overtraining. The result from "active rest" will be an increase in both your fitness and your enjoyment of your exercise program. You'll also be less susceptible to the injuries that often result from overtraining.

Listen to your body. There are going to be days when you are scheduled to train and you don't feel up to it. Listen, but make sure you are not just looking for an excuse to be lazy.

Allow yourself to progress slowly in your workouts. Push yourself, but not to the point where you risk injuries. And be sensible! The long-term benefits are well worth it. Following are some guidelines to help you answer the question: How much exercise is too much?

If exercise is causing you pain and you're ignoring your body's need for rest, then you're overdoing it. You may be psychologically addicted to exercise, or "exercise dependent," to the point of unhealthiness. An early indication of exercise dependency is how a person deals with an injury. Someone who is exercise dependent tries to work through the injury instead of taking the necessary time off to let it heal.

Exercise shouldn't be the focus of your life. If your workouts interfere with family, work, or life's everyday obligations, you are spending too much time at the gym. If you do something every day of your life (besides eating and sleeping), eventually you're likely to

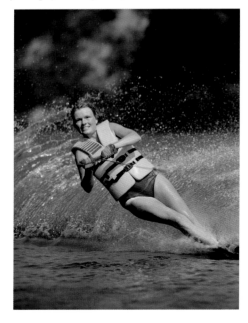

get bored with the activity and lose interest in it. This is a common occurrence with exercise. When people first start to exercise, they love the way it makes them feel—to the point where some people overdo it and forsake life's other activities. Eventually, because they can't keep up the pace they've set for themselves, they quit. Training is like anything in life—if we have too much of a good thing, it no longer interests us. With exercise, there is also the potential for developing overuse injuries.

If you become compulsive about exercise, your commitment to it may not last very long. Let exercise and its many benefits enhance your life, not rule it.

Often, overexercisers feel edgy or even depressed if they miss a training session. Many are obsessed with staying thin, often maintaining a body weight that is too low for optimum health. Overexercisers work out to have a "perfect body" instead of better health, and they often lie about how much they exercise.

Some symptoms of overtraining include:

- Elevated resting pulse rate
- Loss of appetite
- Recurring colds, other illnesses, or rashes
- Insomnia
- Lethargy in other activities besides working out
- Frequent nightmares
- A feeling of being tired or drained
- Recurring injuries
- Continued soreness in the same muscle

If you have an elevated resting pulse rate and two or more of the other symptoms, you're probably overtraining. If your resting pulse rate is normal, then your problems are probably not due to overtraining; look instead for psychological factors in your life that could be causing the symptoms.

People who are addicted to exercise usually won't acknowledge it, not even to themselves. Such denial is typical of all forms of compulsive behavior. But there is a point where even the compulsive exerciser becomes injured or exhausted and has to take some time off. If this time off leads to behavioral changes such as moodiness, irritability, or depression, it's time to do some self-examination. Exercise should be seen as a way to become and stay healthy, not an obsession for its own sake.

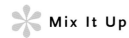

Mix It Up

Once your body becomes accustomed to an exercise program, it's time to give your muscles new challenges by changing your program and making it harder. You'll know when this time has come by how your workouts feel. You'll also probably notice that your progress has slowed or maybe even stopped. You may even have reached some of your goals by this point in your training—now it's time to set some new ones!

You'll be moving from exercises and movement techniques that are less stressful and physically complex to exercises and movement techniques that are more stressful and physically complex. Be sure to progress in a way that is challenging but without threat of injury. The following are a number of ways you can progressively make your workout more demanding. These methods guarantee that your workouts will continue to deliver results.

The Long Run

Making exercise an ongoing part of your life—for the rest of your life—will take some planning and effort. Here are some ideas and suggestions that may make it easier for you to stay committed and to exercise for the long run.

First, find a time of day for exercise that you can be consistent with. Pick a time that fits your schedule and lifestyle. Once you have that time in place, be as consistent as possible. But if your schedule must change occasionally, be flexible.

Now and then, take 2 or 3 days off from serious exercise.

Keep an Exercise Diary

When you "train for life" (training to be healthy and fit at all stages of your life), it's imperative to focus on the positive changes, big and small, that occur as a result of exercise. Recording these changes can make them more real and meaningful. Therefore, we recommend you keep a record of your progress as follows.

Heart Rate

Note the decrease in your resting heart rate as a result of aerobic exercise.

For three mornings in a row, do the following: Set your alarm at the same time each day. Before even sitting up, find your pulse at your neck or wrist and count how many times it beats in 10 seconds, then multiply by 6. (For more accurate results, count for 20 seconds and multiply by 3.) This number is your resting heart rate in beats per minute. If the number is different each morning, add up the total of all 3 days' rates and divide by 3 to get an

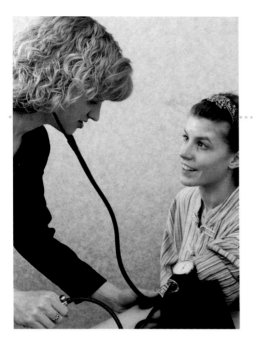

average. Be sure to have the clock within reach and visible without having to get up to turn on the light.

Blood Pressure

Note the decrease in your blood pressure as a result of exercise, and any changes in your eating habits.

You must go to a health practitioner to find out if your blood pressure has decreased. This is well worth the effort. Elevated blood pressure is a risk factor in both heart disease and stroke. Any decrease in your blood pressure means you're lowering your risk of developing both of these diseases.

Joint Flexibility

Measure the increase in joint flexibility as a result of the stretching exercises you have been doing (see Chapter Five).

To discover any increases in the range of motion in your muscles and joints, become aware of how much easier it is to bend, stretch, and reach. Make notations of these increases.

Increasing Strength

Record strength increases as a result of weight lifting. Note increased joint stability as well.

To record strength increases, do timed push-ups, curl-ups, and wall sitting. These three tests will give you an idea of the increases in muscle strength in the arms, chest, and shoulders (push-ups); trunk flexors and abdominals (curl-ups); and thigh and buttocks muscles (wall sitting).

Wall sitting means simply sitting with your back flat against a wall, knees at right angles and feet planted firmly on the floor. Your arms hang at your sides. Time yourself and see if you can sit in this position for one minute, then two, and so on.

Then, time how many push-ups you can do in one minute and how many curl-ups you can do in one minute.

Resting Metabolism

Measure the increase in your resting metabolism as a result of weight lifting.

To measure increases in your basal metabolism, you must first buy a digital thermometer. Upon waking, but before getting up, place the digital thermometer under your arm for 10 minutes. The number showing on the digital readout is your basal temperature.

Take this measurement for four mornings in a row. Add the four numbers and divide the total by 4. The result is your basal temperature. If this number is below 96.7 degrees, you probably have a sluggish metabolism. Note the increase in your basal temperature as you become more fit.

Improved Body Mass Index

Record your improved body mass index as a result of exercise.

The body mass index (BMI) is a method of measuring fatness level based on a person's height and weight. Used by both doctors and exercise professionals, it enables individuals to determine whether they are at risk for diseases that are weight-related, such as heart disease, hypertension, and type 2 (adult onset) diabetes.

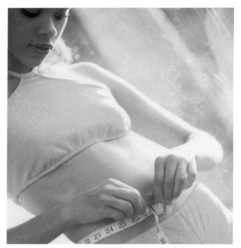

Here is how to calculate your BMI. Multiply your weight in pounds by 700, then divide the result by the square of your height in inches. For example, for a person 5 feet 7 inches (67 inches) tall weighing 128 pounds, the calculation would be as follows:

128 lbs. x 700 = 89,600

67" x 67"= 4,489

89,600 ÷ 4,489 = BMI of 19.95

If your BMI is above 30, or above 27 and you have a family history of obesity, then your risk of developing these weight-related diseases is moderate to very high. If your BMI is 25–27 and you have no family history of obesity, your risk is low to moderate. If your BMI is 25 or less, your risk is low to very low.

In general, a healthy person has a BMI below 25.

Be aware, however, that BMI does not take into account a person's body composition—his or her ratio of fat to lean tissue. Also, it does not consider a person's gender; men are heavier than women and will tend to have a higher BMI without being less healthy. Nevertheless, BMI is well suited for determining risk in sedentary people who have yet to develop much muscle tissue. Body-fat testing is the preferred method for determining risk in athletic and fit individuals.

Fat-to-Lean Ratio

Keep track of your improved body composition (fat-to-lean ratio) and your girth measurements. Note how much your physical appearance has improved. To record changes in body composition, you must have a percent body fat test done by a fitness professional. The most accurate method for testing percent body fat is hydrostatic, or underwater, weighing. You sit in a tank, up to your neck in water. You're strapped into a chair so you won't float to the top. You then inhale a breath, followed by exhaling as completely as possible all the air from your lungs. While you're holding your exhale, an attendant lowers you, head and all, into the water for 5 seconds. The attendant registers your underwater weight during this time. Very few people get it right the first time, so the test usually takes 45 minutes to an hour to complete. It's an expensive test (about one hundred dollars), and can be done only in labs and clinics that have the proper apparatus.

Skin-fold caliper testing is also accurate, second only to hydrostatic testing. Armed with calipers, a fitness professional pinches the fat on your body at seven different sites. The seven numbers are then plugged into a formula, and the resulting figures tell you how much body fat you have, compared to lean body tissue. This test only takes a few minutes to do, if performed by a person who is familiar with the procedure. For skin-fold caliper testing to be accurate, it should not be administered right after a workout. Also, you should be relatively dehydrated (nothing to eat or drink for 2 hours before the test) and your skin should be perfectly dry. The tester has to know where and how to pinch you, how to use the calipers, and how to apply the formula. Health clubs and gyms usually have staff available to administer skin-fold tests. The test shouldn't cost more than twenty dollars.

The third method of testing body fat percentage is bioelectrical impedance. To be tested, you lie on your back with an electrode attached to your foot and hand. A machine sends a signal from one electrode to the other. The faster the signal travels, the more muscle you have. This is because water conducts electricity, and muscle is about 70 percent water. Fat, on the other hand, is about 7 percent water, so the signal does not travel as fast through fat. The test takes just minutes, and under ideal conditions, is nearly as accurate as caliper testing. The major drawback to this test is that if you're at all dehydrated, the test can overestimate your body fat. To avoid the possibility of dehydration, you're not allowed alcohol or caffeine

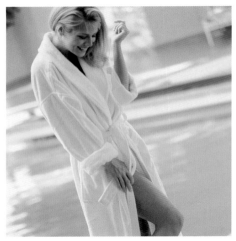

within 24 hours of the test. Bioelectrical impedance is expensive (about fifty dollars). Many health clubs and sports medicine clinics offer the service.

Changes in girth measurements can be recorded in two ways. One, notice if your clothes are fitting you better. Two, actually take your own measurements. I recommend you measure and record the size of your upper arms (both arms), chest, waist, hips, thighs (both), and calves (both).

Energy Level

Note how much more energy you have now, compared to before you started working out.

Keeping track of increased energy is easy. Just feel how much more energy you have for exercise and everyday life.

Set Goals

Besides being a powerful motivator, keeping records also helps you to set goals for yourself. Having goals in life helps keep life interesting and challenging. The same is true in regard to long-term health and fitness. Set goals that can be met by taking small and doable steps. Have realistic expectations. Don't think you're going to change your body overnight.

Once you've met your current goals, it will be time to set new ones. But let's not overlook the forest for the trees. The process by which we meet our goals is every bit as important and challenging as the goals themselves. The process makes up our day-to-day experiences; it's the "stuff" of life.

Affirm that you're improving in life, and you will improve. The power of positive thought is much greater than we can imagine. Turn each negative around into a positive and your life will turn around as well.

A healthy body encourages both a healthy mind and a healthy spirit. When you start taking responsibility for your own health and well-being, life becomes more meaningful and more enjoyable.

Visualization

Visualization can help you clarify your intentions in your own mind, and program your subconscious to help achieve your goals. It enables you to take some control over the "pictures" of reality created by your mind and to direct those pictures in a positive way. This can lead to more control in all areas of your life.

Here is a simple visualization process: Sit quietly with your eyes closed, either cross-legged on the floor or in a chair with your back supported and your feet flat on the floor. Give yourself a minute or two to relax. One effective way to relax is to focus on each part of your body in turn, starting from your face and gradually working down to your feet. Another way is to breathe deeply and steadily, focusing your attention on your breath as it flows in and out. When you feel relaxed, allow an image to come into your mind's eye of yourself, your body, or your behavior as you would like yourself to be. Make the picture as clear as you can, filling in all the details you can think of. Think of it not as a future ideal but as a present reality. If you like, while holding the image in your mind, you can silently repeat to yourself affirmations, phrased in the present tense, expressing your ideals, such as "I am slender and strong," "I have control over how I look," or "I eat foods that nourish and strengthen my body." Invent your own affirmations, ones that feel right for you. Stay with your images for as long as you like, then take some deep breaths and gradually

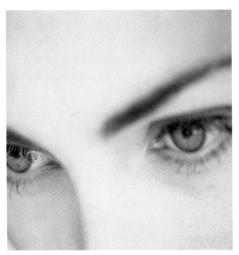

open your eyes. Carry your images with you in your daily life. As you're doing the exercises in this book, you might want to conjure up the body image you've visualized, or as you're shopping for groceries recall your diet visualization.

Trust and believe in yourself. Maintain a positive attitude. What you think directly affects your body; the mind has a great deal of power. Use that power to your benefit!

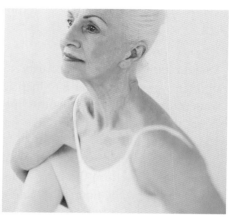

On its most surface level, yoga is a challenging, fun discipline that keeps the body fit. It regulates the internal organs and balances the circulatory, respiratory, and hormonal systems. Yoga alleviates stress, aids in the healing of physical injuries and illnesses, and helps us reclaim our general sense of well-being.

But yoga gives us a sense of well-being that is quite different from the "endorphin high" experienced in Western-style exercise. As we practice yoga, we sense a mastery of our world. As we practice the strength-building poses, we become stronger both physically and mentally. And as we become more flexible in our bodies, we become more flexible in our attitudes.

Practicing yoga also heightens our sense of emotional well-being. Many medical doctors and psychotherapists contend that emotional trauma is not held just in our hearts and minds, but also in our bodies. This must be true, as many yoga students experience emotional release while doing the poses. Some people suddenly remember hurts from long ago and are able to immediately process them. While they are practicing the poses or in the relaxation phase that follows, many students report spontaneous feelings of love or forgiveness; others have profound insights. All students report increased inner peace and relaxation, which is reflected in their faces. As we release and heal these pent-up emotions, we allow more space for our true, loving natures to shine forth. In other words, yoga amplifies our sense of inner love, joy, and harmony.

If our minds are active, then maybe it is a good idea to have active bodies as well. But let's harness that activity for our highest good, just as we harness the power of a waterfall to generate electricity. Through yoga poses we can reach that same meditative place others are reaching by sitting—and we will have much more fun!

The rewards you reap from practicing yoga will surprise you, far surpassing your most optimistic dreams for physical well-being, joy, and inner peace. Health will replace injury, gratitude will replace worry, self-confidence will replace fear. Your joie de vivre will multiply manifold. All aspects of your life will be transformed.

Yoga Tips

Consider all of the following tips as they would apply to all of the poses. The tips provide advice on form and will maximize the benefits of your practice sessions. Move into the poses slowly and deliberately.

Remember to breathe!

Lengthen your back and lift your sternum (your breastbone).

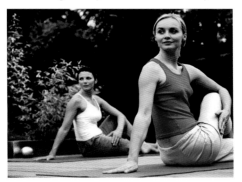

Only bend as far forward as you can with your back straight. The more you can lift your sternum, the more your upper back will straighten, and the more you can lengthen your back, the straighter your lower back will be. Keeping the back straight strengthens the muscles and allows your posture to improve quickly. If you round your back when it should be straight, you train your spine to curve, which is definitely not the result you are looking for.

Move from the hip crease. The hip crease is the hip joint, the place where the front of the hip and the leg meet.

Straighten your knees and your elbows. If you can't straighten your knees, try to lengthen your hamstrings (the muscles on the back of the thighs) and lift your quadriceps (the muscles on the front of the thighs). If your elbows don't straighten, lengthen your arms as much as possible. Work on these things—and remember, you are just practicing!

Keep your head in line with your spine. In other words, don't tilt your head backwards as you do the poses, or you will give yourself a neckache.

Keep your throat, neck, shoulders, and jaw soft. Soft means relaxed. Try to be conscious of this; you will feel more relaxed throughout your practice.

These poses are designed for people with normal limitations. You should start slowly and not overdo it.

One side may be more challenging than the other side, so you should do that side twice. Well . . . it's a suggestion.

Loose, comfortable clothing or workout clothes are best for yoga practice.

Bare feet are essential unless you are in some of the resting poses.

Some days it will be easy to do yoga; other days it may be tough getting started.

Yoga Warm-Ups

Warm up with the first 6 poses before each daily yoga practice. After completing the designated sessions take Corpse Pose to complete your practice.

Knees to Chest

Simply lie on your back, bring your knees to your chest, and hug them.

Cat Pose

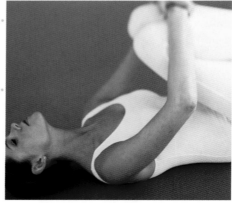

Kneel on all fours, shoulders over your wrists and knees under your hips. Exhaling, tuck your pelvis down and round your spine toward the ceiling in an upward arch. Inhaling, reverse the movement, dropping your abdomen and lower back while broadening your chest forward and up. Repeat 4 to 8 times.

Desk

Lie on your back, feet hip-distance apart and as close to your hips as possible. Lift your hips as high as possible and keep them lifted. If you can, clasp your hands underneath your back, and roll your shoulders under.

Child's Pose

From a kneeling position, widen your thighs, place your buttocks on your heels, and bring your torso toward the floor. Rest your forehead on the floor. If your body doesn't reach your heels, place a folded blanket or two on your feet. Rest with your arms in front of you or beside you. Breathe into your lower back, and with each exhalation, allow your body to relax a little more.

Lower Back Stretch

Sitting on the floor, widen your legs so they are wider than hip-distance apart. From the hip crease, bend forward and allow your entire body to relax. Drop your head and completely relax your neck. If you are not completely comfortable, try putting a rolled blanket or towel at the hip crease and lean over again.

Standing Forward Bend

Standing with your feet parallel, about 6 to 12 inches apart, inhale your arms out from your sides over your head. Exhaling, bend forward with your knees slightly bent, arms straight out front then toward the ground. Inhaling, bend your knees more and raise your chest and head; exhale and straighten your legs slightly—but not completely folding over from the hips. Inhaling, come up with your knees slightly bent, leading with your chest. Raise your arms out to the sides then overhead, back out to the sides resting on either side of your torso. Repeat 4 times.

Corpse Pose

Lie on your back with your legs hip distance apart. Relax your arms away from your sides. If you have trouble with your lower back, place a rolled-up blanket under your knees. Cover your eyes with a small towel or with your yoga tie and insert earplugs if you wish. With each exhalation, relax a little bit more.

Daily Yoga Practice Sessions

Practice Session One

(Hold each pose through 5 complete breaths inhaling and exhaling)

Staff Pose
Lie down with your buttocks against the wall or as close to the wall as possible. Extend your legs up the wall. Work on straightening your knees and flexing your feet toward you.

Wide-Angle Pose
From Staff Pose, simply widen your legs. Slowly—you don't want to overstretch your inner thigh muscles. Flex your feet toward you. Gravity is your friend. Allow it to bring your legs down as they are ready. To take pressure off your inner thighs, roll up blankets and place them under the top of your thighs.

Bound Angle Pose
Bring the soles of your feet together. Firmly press your feet together. If you did not use the blanket roll-ups in Wide-Angle Pose, you may want to add them here.

Knees to Chest
Bring your knees to your chest.

Dead Bug Pose
Bring your thighs to the sides of your torso. Position your feet as if you are going to walk on the ceiling. Place an old necktie, towel or strap around each foot and pull your legs toward you. If this is too easy, from the inside of the legs, place your hands on the arches of your feet and pull your legs toward you.

Practice Session Two

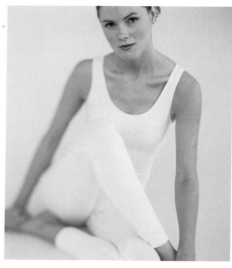

(Hold each pose through 5 complete breaths inhaling and exhaling)

Seated Wide-Angle Pose

In this pose and the following four poses, sit on some folded blankets or against a wall to help straighten your back and relieve stiffness in your hips. Stretch your legs out to the side. Lengthen your back and lift your sternum. Place your hands or fingertips behind you to help lengthen your back. Keeping your back straight, bend slightly forward from the hip crease. If you like, you can walk your fingers forward.

Wide-Angle Variation

From the same position, lengthen your back, lift your sternum, and slightly twist your torso toward your right leg. From the hip crease, bend over your right leg. Once you've gone as far as you can with your back straight, release and switch sides.

Archer Pose

Sitting, extend your legs in front of you. Bend your right knee and strap the ball of your right foot. Straighten your knee and lift your leg toward the ceiling, flexing your toes toward you. Continue to lengthen your lower back and lift your sternum. DO NOT compromise your straight back and straight knee for height.

Full Forward Bend

Sitting on folded blankets with your legs extended in front of you and your toes flexed toward you, strap the balls of both feet. With your back and knees straight and your sternum lifted, bend forward from the hip crease. Go slowly! This is not a contest to see how far down you can get—a long straight back is most important.

Wide-Angle Forward Bend

Sit on the floor and widen your legs so they are wider than hip distance apart. From the hip crease, bend forward and allow your entire body to relax. Drop your head and completely relax your neck. If you are not completely comfortable, try putting a rolled blanket or towel at the hip crease and bend forward again.

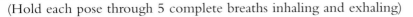

(Hold each pose through 5 complete breaths inhaling and exhaling)

Reclining Hamstring Stretch

Lie on your back with your legs extended. Grab your right foot with your hand, or strap the ball of your right foot, lift your leg toward the ceiling and, if possible, straighten your knee. Flex your toes toward you keeping the foot of the extended leg flexed as well. Naturally, you have to do both sides!

Reclining Inner Thigh Stretch

Assume setup as for the previous pose. Lift your right leg up and then bring your leg out toward your right shoulder. You can stay in this pose longer if you place a folded blanket or towel under your upper thigh. Switch sides.

Double Inner Thigh Stretch

Use the same setup as Reclining Inner Thigh Stretch, but this time bring both legs to the side at the same time. Double the props if necessary.

Supported Chest Opener

Roll up a blanket and lie down over it, placing the roll-up directly behind your sternum. You may need to experiment with blanket height to determine what is most comfortable. If you would like, you can also place a pillow or folded blanket under your head. Close your eyes and relax.

Practice Session Four

(Hold each pose through 5 complete breaths inhaling and exhaling)

Leg Balance—Front Angle

Stand with your feet about 6 inches apart, raise your right leg out in front of you with your leg slightly bent, foot flexed. If you would like, use a towel or strap placed across the ball of your right foot to help elevate and hold the leg. Keep your back and both knees straight, if possible. Release and switch sides. This pose is easier for some people and for others the next pose is easier. Whichever one is harder for you, do it twice!

Leg Balance—Side Angle

Stand with your feet about 6 inches apart and raise your right leg out to the side with your leg extended straight, foot flexed. If you would like, use a towel or strap placed across the ball of your right foot to help elevate and hold the leg. Keep your back and both knees straight, if possible. Release and switch sides.

Tree Pose

Stand with your feet hip-width apart. Shift your weight onto your left foot. Lift your right foot and press your foot into your thigh and your thigh into your foot. When you feel aligned and strong bring your hands together in front of your chest in prayer position. Hold for 5 breaths. Release and switch sides.

Standing Wide-Angle Pose

Stand with your feet be 2 to 3 feet apart. Keeping your back and legs straight and your sternum lifted, lift your arms overhead. Start to bend forward from the hips, arms extended and back flat. Place your fingertips or hands on the floor (or as close to the floor as you can get.) Continue to lengthen your back and lift your sternum.

Practice Session Five

(Hold each pose through 5 complete breaths inhaling and exhaling)

Upward Arm Stretch

Stand tall with your feet hip-distance apart and your hands as high over your head as possible, palms facing each other. Stretch all the way from your lower back making sure that your shoulders are down and not scrunched up toward your neck. Breathe and continue to stretch upward.

Backward Arm Stretch

Assume the same position as Upward Arm Stretch but pivot your arms so that your palms face behind you. Allow your elbows to straighten if possible. Lift your chest, keep rolling your shoulders down, and continue to lift your chest.

Forward Arm Stretch

Stand tall with your feet hip-distance apart and bring your hands to your chest, palms facing forward, elbows out. Interlace your fingers and on the inhale extend your arms straight out in front and continue to stretch and breathe.

Wide-Angle Forward Bend

Sit on the floor and widen your legs so they are wider than hip-distance apart. From the hip crease, bend forward and allow your entire body to relax. Drop your head and completely relax your neck. If you are not completely comfortable, try putting a rolled blanket or towel at the hip crease and bend forward again.

Practice Session Six

(Hold each pose through 5 complete breaths inhaling and exhaling)

Triangle Pose

Stand with your feet parallel 3 to 4 feet apart. Extend your arms parallel to the floor, palms down. Pivot the right foot 90° to the right and angle your left foot slightly toward the right. From the hip crease, laterally extend toward the right. On an inhale, raise your left arm, extending your torso to the right, and bring your right hand to your calf, ankle, or floor or place a block next to your calf to use as a support. Keep the right side of your torso extended. If you can, look up at your thumb. Breathe! Release and switch sides.

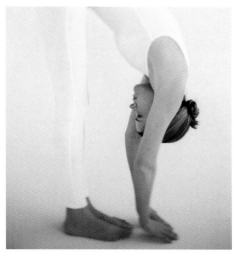

Warrior II

Use the same beginning stance as for Triangle Pose. Keeping your torso erect, bend your knee until your calf and thigh are at right angles to each other and extend your arms with your palms facing down. If you can, relax your shoulders a little more. Release and switch sides.

Side Angle Pose

Start with the same setup as Warrior II. Bend the forward knee into a right angle. Moving from the hip crease, extend your upper body laterally over your thigh. Place your right hand beside the pinky-toe-side of your forward front foot. Extend your left arm straight up toward the ceiling. Breathe. Release and switch sides.

Practice Session Seven

(Hold each pose through 5 complete breaths inhaling and exhaling)

Downward Facing Dog

Kneel on all fours, shoulders over your wrists and knees under your hips. Turn your toes under. Press your palms to lift your hips high and come up on your toes keeping your knees bent. Keep your torso angled downward. Press your sitting bones toward the ceiling and lengthen through your shoulders. Straighten your legs, keep your buttocks lifted, and lower your heels toward the ground. Work on straightening your arms and legs, and lengthening your back as much as possible.

Plank Pose

Lie flat on your stomach with your toes curled under and your hands under your shoulders. Press your palms on the floor and draw all of your arm muscles and your shoulders up toward the ceiling. Lift your buttocks so they are in line with your spine, and straighten your arms and legs. Make sure that your shoulders are over your wrists and hands. Keep your abdomen moving toward your spine and press through your heels while keeping your spine, buttocks and legs on an even plane. If you are feeling strong, you can do some push-ups from this pose.

Child's Pose
From a kneeling position, widen your thighs, place your buttocks on your heels, and bring your torso toward the floor. Rest your forehead on the floor. If your body doesn't reach your heels, place a folded blanket or two on your feet. Rest with your arms in front of you or beside you. Breathe into your lower back, and with each exhalation, allow your body to relax a little more.

The 5-Second Pre-Headstand
Kneel down. Place the backs of your clasped hands against the wall and the sides of your forearms on the floor. Your elbows are directly under your shoulders. Come up on your toes and walk toward the wall. Lift your shoulders to their absolute maximum. Your head hangs down. Walk in some more and keep lifting your shoulders! This pose is quite difficult, so hold it only for a few seconds. Rest in Child's Pose and try the pre-headstand two or three more times.

Practice Session Eight
(Hold each pose through 5 complete breaths inhaling and exhaling)

Warrior I
Stand with your feet parallel 3 to 4 feet apart. Extend your arms out to the sides, parallel to the floor, palms down. Pivot the right foot and thigh 90° out then pivot your left foot so your left hip faces forward. Square your torso to the wall in front of you. Bend your front knee until your calf and thigh are at a right angle to each other. Inhaling, take your arms overhead with your palms facing each other. If you can, relax your shoulders a little more while keeping your spine lengthened. Release and switch sides.

Warrior III
Return to Warrior I. Shift your weight to your right leg. Now—extend your left leg straight behind you, keeping your leg even with your hips and your front hipbones even, and flex your toes toward you. Keep your arms against your torso or out in front of you, parallel to the ground. Hold for as long as you can. Don't forget to breathe. Bring your leg down, re-establish Warrior I, and then extend your left leg.

Forward Arm Hang
Stand with your feet hip-distance apart and place your thumbs in your hip crease and bend forward from that crease. Release your thumbs and allow your arms to hang down, or hold your elbows. Relax your neck. You can bend your knees to get a deeper lower back stretch.

(Hold each pose through 5 complete breaths inhaling and exhaling)

Cobra

Lie on your stomach and place your hands on the sides of your chest. To protect your lower back, firmly press your pubic bone into the floor. Keep your legs straight and firm. Raise your chest, curving your upper back inward and extending your chest outward. Lift your sternum. Keep your lower rib cage on the floor. Your arms should be at the side of your torso. Keep your head in line with your spine. Do not tilt your head backward or you will give yourself a neckache.

Locust Variation 1

Lie on your stomach with your arms and legs extended. To protect your lower back, press your pubic bone into the floor and straighten and firm your legs. Lift and extend your right arm and right leg. Release, then lift and

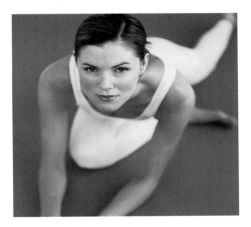

extend your left arm and left leg. Rest and repeat several times.

Locust Variation 2

Lie on your stomach with your arms and legs extended. To protect your lower back, press your pubic bone into the floor and straighten and firm your legs. Lift and extend your right arm and left leg. Release, then lift and extend your left arm and right leg. Rest and repeat several times.

Full Locust

From the same position, lift both arms and both legs. Be sure to press your pubic bone into the floor, and straighten and firm your legs.

Desk

Lie on your back with your feet hip-distance apart and as close to your hips as possible. Lift your hips slightly, clasp your hands underneath your back, and roll your shoulders under. Now lift your hips as high as possible and keep them lifted. Hold as long as you can. Rest and try again.

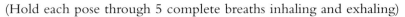

(Hold each pose through 5 complete breaths inhaling and exhaling)

Feet on the Floor Twist

Lie on your back, legs bent, feet together and on the floor, and arms extended to your side. Keeping your legs together, bring them to the right side. Come back to the center and twist to the left.

Foot on Knee Twist

Lie on your back with your legs straight, toes flexed toward you and arms extended to each side. Place your right foot on your left knee. Turn toward the right, moving your knee toward the floor—not necessarily all the way to the floor. Keep your left shoulder on the floor. Come back to the center and change sides.

Seated Twist 1

Sit on the floor with your legs out in front of you. Square your torso to the front. On an inhalation, straighten your spine and on an exhalation twist toward the left, twisting from the very bottom of your spine—placing your left hand behind you pushing with your right hand to the top of your right thigh or knee. Repeat the inhalation/straighten, exhalation/twist series several times. Release and switch sides.

Seated Twist 11

Sit on the floor with your legs separated in a v-shape. Square your torso to the front. On an inhalation, straighten your spine and on an exhalation twist toward the left, twisting from the very bottom of your spine—placing your left hand behind you pushing with your right hand to the top of your right thigh or knee. Repeat the inhalation/straighten, exhalation/twist series several times. Release and switch sides.

Practice Session Eleven

(Hold each pose through 5 complete breaths inhaling and exhaling)

Boat with Strap

Sit on the floor with your legs out in front of you. Place a strap around the balls of your feet and 2 feet from the floor. Lean back slightly so your torso forms a v-shape with your legs. Lengthen your back, lift your sternum, squeeze your thighs together, and press your feet into the strap. If this is too easy, do the pose without the strap.

Leg Lifts

Lie on your back with your left and right legs straight. Raise your right leg and then slowly lower it toward the floor. Continue several times and then switch sides.

Yoga Sit-Ups

Lie on your back. With your knees bent and feet hip-distance apart, place your hands behind your head and try to touch your knees with your elbows—more than once! Only bring your back halfway to the floor after touching your elbows to your knees.

Yoga Sit-Ups 2

From the previous position, bring your right foot to your left knee. Sit up and try to touch your right knee with your left elbow—several times. Switch the foot position, bringing the right elbow to the left knee. Only bring your back halfway to the floor after touching your elbow to your knee.

Practice Session Twelve

(Hold each pose through 5 complete breaths inhaling and exhaling)

Standing Forward Bend

Standing with your feet parallel, about 6 to 12 inches apart, inhale your arms out from your sides over your head. Exhaling, bend forward with your knees slightly bent, arms straight out front then toward the ground. Inhaling, bend your knees more and raise your chest and head; exhale and straighten your legs slightly—but not completely folding over from the hips. Inhaling, come up with your knees slightly bent, leading with your chest. Raise your arms out to the sides then overhead, back out to the sides resting on either side of your torso. Repeat 4 times.

Quadriceps Stretch

Assume Downward Facing Dog. Bending your left leg slightly pressing your weight into your arms, bring your right knee forward between your hands. If you can't get it all the way to meet your hands then use one of your hands to place it. Your right leg should be at a 90° angle with your hands on either side. Now bring your left knee to the floor, placing both hands on the top of your knee to steady yourself, and lift your torso so that it is erect. You will now be in a kneeling position. Start to sink your hips toward the floor. Your left side will feel awfully lonely if you don't do both sides.

Lunge

Assume Downward Facing Dog. Bending your left leg slightly pressing your weight into your arms, bring your right knee forward between your hands. If you can't get it all the way to meet your hands then use one of your hands to place it. Your right leg should be at a 90° angle with your hands on either side. Now straighten your back leg, pressing through the heel and sinking your hips a little further down. Keep breathing. Release and switch sides.

Standing Hamstring Stretch

Stand with your feet parallel about 2 feet apart. Extend your arms parallel to the floor, palms down. Pivot the right foot and thigh 90° out then pivot your left foot so your left hip faces forward. Square your torso to the wall in front of you and elongate your back. Lengthen your lower back and lift your sternum. Fold over your front leg keeping it as straight as possible. As you progress, you will be able to place your hands on the floor or a block while maintaining a straight back. Release and switch sides.

Practice Session Thirteen

(Hold each pose through 5 complete breaths inhaling and exhaling)

Seated Hamstring Stretch

Sit on the floor and widen your legs so they are wider than hip-distance apart. Lengthen your back, lift your sternum, and raise your arms overhead. Bend slightly forward from the hip crease, keeping your back elongated—do not round your back! Go as far toward the floor in front of you as possible. It is okay if your knees are bent slightly—this is an intense stretch for your hamstrings and you do not want to force yourself. Over time you will be able to straighten your legs. Make sure to do both sides.

Rock the Baby

Sit on the floor with your knees slightly bent and feet on the floor, keeping your back as straight as possible. Bring your left leg up, close to your chest. Place your left foot in your right hand and your left knee in your left hand. Move your leg from side to side, as though you are rocking a baby. Over time, these babies like to be held close to the chest and parallel to the floor. Make sure you rock this baby's twin brother or sister!

Practice Session Fourteen

(Hold each pose through 5 complete breaths inhaling and exhaling)

Standing Forward Bend

Standing with your feet parallel, about 6 to 12 inches apart, inhale your arms out from your sides over your head. Exhaling, bend forward with your knees slightly bent, arms straight out front then toward the ground. Inhaling, bend your knees more and raise your chest and head; exhale and straighten your legs slightly—but not completely folding over from the hips. Inhaling, come up with your knees slightly bent, leading with your chest. Raise your arms out to the sides then overhead, back out to the sides resting on either side of your torso. Repeat 4 times.

Lunge

Assume Downward Facing Dog. Bending your left leg slightly, pressing your weight into your arms, bring your right knee forward between your hands. If you can't get it all the way to meet your hands then use one of your hands to place it. Your right leg should be at a 90° angle with your hands on either side. Now straighten your back leg, pressing through the heel and sinking your hips a little further down. Keep breathing. Release and switch sides.

Warrior I

Stand with your feet parallel 3 to 4 feet apart. Extend your arms parallel to the floor, palms down. Pivot the right foot and thigh 90° out then pivot your left foot so your left hip faces forward. Square your torso to the wall in front of you. Bend your front knee until your calf and thigh are at right angles to each. Inhaling, take your arms overhead with your palms facing each other. If you can, relax your shoulders a little more while keeping your spine lengthened. Release and switch sides.

Warrior II

Stand with your feet parallel 3 to 4 feet apart. Extend your arms parallel to the floor, palms down. Pivot the right foot 90° to the right and angle your left foot slightly toward the right. Bend your knee until your calf and thigh are at right angles to each other and extend your arms with your palms facing down. If you can, relax your shoulders a little more. Release and switch sides.

Standing Forward Bend 2

Stand with your left side facing the chair. Place your left foot on the chair seat, bending the knee. Make sure your left foot is aligned with the right foot, which is about 12 inches from the chair seat. From the hip crease, bend forward. Hold onto your elbows and allow your head to hang down. Release and switch sides.

Forward Arm Hang

Stand with your feet hip-distance apart and place your thumbs in your hip crease and bend forward from that crease. Release your thumbs and allow your arms to hang down, or hold your elbows. Relax your neck. You can bend your knees to get a deeper lower back stretch.

Child's Pose

From a kneeling position, widen your thighs, place your buttocks on your heels, and bring your torso toward the floor. Rest your forehead on the floor. If your body doesn't reach your heels, place a folded blanket or two on your feet. Rest with your arms in front of you or beside you. Breathe into your lower back, and with each exhalation, allow your body to relax a little more.

(Hold each pose through 5 complete breaths inhaling and exhaling)

Hero Pose

Kneel, with your knees together and lower your buttocks to your feet. If you need to use props kneel with your knees hip-distance apart, and place a rolled-up towel or blanket between your calves. If you are immediately uncomfortable, come up and add another towel. You may have to experiment with the thickness of the rolls. Eventually, your props will become lower and your knees will come together.

Arm Variations 1

Stretch your arms straight overhead, palms facing each other. Lengthen your arms as though you are stretching all the way from your hips. Lift your sternum, but relax your throat, neck, and shoulders, and keep reaching for the ceiling.

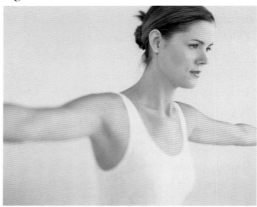

Arm Variations 2

Interlock your fingers, then face your palms outward. Stretch your arms overhead, so your palms face upward. Work on straightening your elbows and on stretching all the way from the waist. Relax your throat, neck, and shoulders as you try to lift higher.

Arm Variations 3

Bring your arms behind your back, holding a tie between your hands. Lift your arms as high as you can. Keep lifting your sternum. As you gain flexibility, bring your hands closer together on the tie. Or forget the tie and interlock your fingers.

CHAPTER

5

Stretching

The primary reason for stretching is to keep your muscles limber, increase joint mobility, and maintain full range of motion in your joints. Stretching also helps reduce muscle soreness and prevents injuries.

Think of your muscles as a willow tree, able to bend in the wind. The more able you are to move and bend freely, the less likely you are to "break" or injure yourself. Weight lifting contracts your muscles; flexibility work keeps them limber and supple. Stretching enhances physical and athletic skills and aids in the reduction of stress.

The ability to relax your muscles is also very important in developing flexibility. Relaxation is the opposite of tension. Your ability to relax is important because it enhances your ability to decrease tension and its neg-

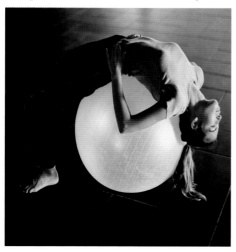

ative consequences. Relaxation is an important part of any stress-reduction program. Also, stretching exercises encourage a union of body, mind, and spirit.

Mobility and pain-free movement of the muscles are critical factors in how you live your life. When you suffer from pain or discomfort, it can hinder your daily activities. Stretching can facilitate mobility, improve muscle mechanics, and allow you greater opportunities every day. To master the basics of stretching, you need to understand its fundamental concepts.

 Goals

A stretch is a specific position sustained to increase and maintain the length of a muscle or a muscle group. It lengthens tendons, warms up ligaments, and prepares joints for work. As a result, there is:

1. Additional flexibility throughout the body;

2. Decreased tightness or stiffness;

3. Improved awareness of muscles and their capabilities during any daily activity or sport;

4. Increased coordination and agility in daily or recreational activities;

5. Decreased blood pressure and a "fit" cardiovascular system;

6. Enhanced circulation, which provides muscles with oxygen and other nutrients for the support structures of the human frame;

7. Quicker removal of waste products (lactic acid, carbon dioxide, nitrogen, cellular metabolites) from the muscles;

8. Reduced pressure on joint cartilage and spinal discs, which reduces the arthritic wear-and-tear process (osteoarthritis or degenerative disc disease);

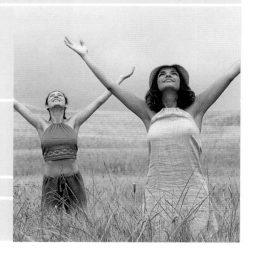

9. Reduced inflammation and joint pain often seen in numerous types of arthritic conditions (rheumatoid arthritis, gout, Reiter's syndrome);

10. Less stress on the nervous system;

11. Facilitation of overall health and sense of well-being.

 Flexibility

Flexibility means having the freedom to move. It is a major part of everything you do. By following a specific routine geared to your physical makeup, you can dramatically improve your flexibility by stretching. This added mobility is critical because even the easiest tasks require movement: rising out of bed in the morning, stepping into the tub or shower, reaching into a cupboard or closet, leaning over to tie your shoes, lifting a baby out of a crib, getting something from a car trunk, working at a job, climbing up the stairs, and exercising safely and effectively.

As a result, stretching can be considered even more important than exercising. However, stretching coupled with exercise is the key to lifelong health and well-being.

Exercise

Exercise is a specific work or activity geared towards:

1. Strengthening muscles;
2. Improving cardiovascular function;
3. Strengthening the immune system;
4. Stimulating body chemicals (epinephrine, endorphins);
5. Reducing stress;
6. Rehabilitating from injury;
7. Improving ability and stamina for additional work or play.

The human frame requires preparation in order to perform work safely, and exercise is a form of work. Stretching helps you prepare for any activity by altering your muscle resilience or tone. You should stretch both before and after work or exercise. Stretching before (as part of a warm-up) prepares tissues for work, and stretching after (cooling down) helps tissues recover from the strain or stress of the work or exercise.

Work It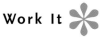

All the stretches in this book are static stretches, which are controlled and slow. In a static stretch, as you stretch a muscle in a slow and gentle fashion, you increase its tension. In a few milliseconds, the spinal cord reflexively tells the muscle to shorten in order to protect the muscle from being over-stretched. It takes 6 to 10 seconds for the brain and spinal cord to perceive that the stretch is safe and, suddenly, the mild pulling sensation you feel of the muscle shortening to resist the stretch is gone. In the next 20 to 24 seconds, the stretch has its beneficial effects. That is why a stretch must be held for at least 30 seconds.

A good rule to follow is that if you feel the uncomfortable stretching sensation for more than 10 seconds, you are stretching too far and too fast. You should ease off slightly until the sensation is gone and then hold the stretch for 30 seconds.

It is important that you do not bounce when you stretch. This kind of stretching, known as ballistic stretching, creates more than double the amount of tension of a static stretch. Even though it is done in many aerobic classes and workout videos, it may actually cause nerve damage and tear muscle fibers. It also does not improve flexibility.

Timing

Ideally, stretching should be done when the body is warm. That way, there is sufficient blood flow carrying important minerals, such as calcium and magnesium, throughout the tissues before you begin to stretch. Optimum muscular relaxation is also the key to effective stretching. Mid-morning, after lunch, and early evening are excellent times to stretch, since the body has already been moving around and has the required nutrients supplied (assuming from a proper diet). Realistically, though, most individuals cannot stop in the middle of the day to engage in "lengthy" stretching routines, nor will they take time in the evening to stretch, because they are tired or have other commitments. It is with this thought in mind that we developed the shower stretch routine.

In the Shower

Since most people shower daily, it is a good place to incorporate stretching. Most people do not mind spending an extra 5 to 10 minutes in a warm shower to do something good for their bodies. If you bathe instead of shower, you can stretch in the living room or bedroom after you bathe. A morning stretch prepares the muscles and the human frame for the stressors encountered daily. It also significantly reduces the chance of injury or the recurrence of pain from previous injuries.

Warming Up

Wherever you do your stretching, you must perform some minimal movement first. In the shower, this can be washing your body. Elsewhere, it can be marching in place, riding a stationary bike, or anything that gets the blood flowing without causing strain. A warm-up consists of 2 to 5 minutes of movement plus a stretching routine. The goal is to get the blood flowing without challenging the body to new heights. Both average people and professional athletes can injure themselves if they engage in too vigorous movements before stretching. "Cold" muscles, tendons, and ligaments are not prepared to deal with the sudden onset of strain, which can cause ankle sprains, pinched spinal nerves, or ruptured Achilles tendons. The warm-up stretching routine should consist of 15 to 20 percent of the total workout time. For example, if you exercise for 60 minutes, you need 9 to 12 minutes of warm-up.

Cooling Down

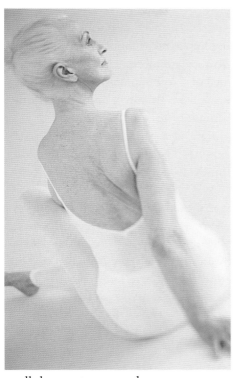

After every activity, especially taxing ones, you should do a cool-down stretch routine, similar to the warm-up stretch, to relax the muscles that were just exercised. The cool-down helps eliminate the metabolic buildup of waste, such as lactic acid, nitrogen, and carbon dioxide, from the muscles to enhance muscle repair and recovery. Otherwise, the metabolic waste will cause muscle stiffness, which affects the movement of the joints.

By cooling down, you will help reduce the muscle soreness that may occur after a particularly stressful activity as well as prevent blood pooling, dizziness, heart palpitations, and nausea. If you incorporate deep abdominal breathing during the cool-down, you will increase the cellular waste removal even more.

A cool-down should consist of 5 to 15 percent of the total workout time. For example, if you exercise for 60 minutes, you need 3 to 9 minutes of cooling down. Ideally, if you stretch during your exercise (e.g., during weight-lifting sets, you stretch the muscle that you are training for 30 seconds after each set), it will make your cool-down much more efficient.

The Need for Stretching

We should not forget the emotional stress that occasionally affects us. If you have had a particularly stressful day, you should do a basic head-to-toe stretching routine to help you relax and get a proper night's sleep. Without proper sleep, you cannot think as clearly, and the stress you experience is multiplied. As a result, you can become more irritable, angry, and frustrated. If sleep deprivation continues, you can experience burnout, chronic fatigue, insomnia, pain, and, at worst, a complete nervous breakdown. Stretching can be an important component in alleviating the stress and helping the body to recover.

 ## Stretching in Spurts

Surprisingly, little stretching time is required to make noticeable gains. An average morning stretching routine in the shower takes about 5 to 10 minutes and produces great results. At work, you may stretch specific tight muscles two to four times a day for 2 minutes (total of 4 to 8 minutes). If you exercise three times a week for an hour each time, you would warm up with 10 minutes of stretching and cool down for 5 minutes (total of 15 minutes).

Let's say that 1 or 2 days a week you are in a particularly stressful state and, consequently, stretch for 10 to 15 minutes. On average, then, you might stretch about 25 minutes a day. That constitutes approximately 1 to 2 percent of your day.

Since stretching is a passive activity, it should be considered relaxing as opposed to something that requires effort. Remember, exercise is work, stretching is not. You can stretch while sitting or lying in front of the television. The average person watches television for more than 2 hours a day, or 8 percent of the day. If you stretched only while watching television, you would quickly rise to an expert level of flexibility. Even if you were to stretch only during the commercials, you would attain a good level of flexibility in a very short time.

But you should have fun with stretching. Let it be a form of meditation. Use it to relax, unwind, contemplate, get away from the world for a few minutes, or plan your next day. It can be both physically and psychologically rewarding.

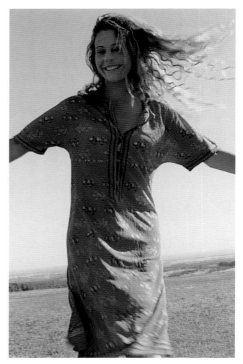

Techniques

Jaw

Open Mouth Stretch

Stand in a comfortable position. Open your jaw to its limit without straining. Hold for 30 seconds. Breathe deeply. If you are prone to temperomandibular joint syndrome (TMJ), do not push this stretch too hard.

Jaw Protrusion Stretch

Stand in a comfortable position. Hold your head up and stick your lower jaw comfortably forward. Hold for 30 seconds. Breathe deeply.

Neck

Neck Turn

Stand comfortably. Keeping your chin and jaw parallel to the ground, look over your right shoulder so that your face is 90 degrees from your torso midline. Hold for 30 seconds. Breathe deeply. Repeat on the other side. This stretch can make checking lanes when driving much easier.

Neck Tilt

Stand comfortably. Lean your right ear toward your right shoulder. Keep your nose pointing straight ahead. Do not force the stretch or point your nose to your shoulder. Hold for 30 seconds. Breathe deeply. Repeat on the other side.

Neck Tilt with Slight Extension

Stand comfortably. Tilt your right ear to your right shoulder and turn your face to the left, or upward, about half an inch. Slightly extend your neck backward about half an inch. Hold comfortably for 30 seconds. Breathe deeply. This will stretch the front left side of your neck. Repeat on the other side. This stretch helps your posture. If you feel a pinch in your neck or experience dizziness, consult your chiropractor immediately. Never lean your head straight back into extreme extension!

Shoulder

The muscle stretched in the following routine is commonly overlooked or forgotten. Yet, when stretched properly, it can provide substantial relief of neck pain.

Front Press Out

Sit up straight in a chair or stand with your feet shoulder-width apart. Clasp your fingers and push your palms away from your body. Once your elbows are straight, you will feel a stretch to the top and back of your shoulders. Hold comfortably for 30 seconds. Breathe deeply.

Deltoid Stretch

Stand comfortably with your feet shoulder-width apart. Keeping your left arm straight, reach it across your body. Use your right hand to pull your elbow into your chest while your face and shoulders are pointing straight ahead. Hold comfortably for 30 seconds. Breathe deeply. Repeat on the other side. For a deeper stretch, bend your left arm at the elbow and twist your torso to the right. This stretches the back of your left shoulder rotator cuff muscles (the deltoids, commonly referred to as "delts"). Repeat on the other side. Always do this stretch first in any shoulder flexibility program.

Internal Rotation Stretch

Stand with your feet shoulder-width apart, knees slightly bent, and shoulders back. Hold both arms straight with your palms facing in. Turn your palms inward to stretch the muscles that rotate your shoulders backward. Hold comfortably for 30 seconds. Breathe deeply.

Rotator Cuff Stretch

Stand comfortably with your feet shoulder-width apart. Bend your left arm at the elbow and place the top of your wrist (back of your hand) at your side above your waist. Use your right hand to hold your left elbow and bring it forward. When you become more flexible, your left elbow should almost point in front of you. For a greater stretch, twist your torso to the right. Hold comfortably for 30 seconds. Breathe deeply. Repeat on the other side.

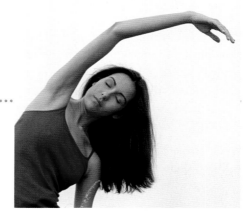

Arm over Head Stretch

Stand comfortably with your feet shoulder-width apart. Keeping your back and neck straight, gently pull your right elbow over your head. In order to reduce neck strain, do not force your head forward. For a greater stretch, lean your torso to the left. Hold comfortably for 30 seconds. Breathe deeply. Repeat on the other side.

Lower Chest Stretch

Stand at arm's length from a doorway or wall. Stretch your arm out against the support until it is at a 45-degree angle above your shoulder or the horizontal plane. Keep your palm flat against the support and your arm straight to stretch the bicep at the elbow, which indirectly helps the movement of the front of your shoulder. When you begin, you may find that your torso and face are toward the wall. As your flexibility increases, your torso will point away from the wall.

Reach Stretch

Stand facing a wall with your arm straight out at shoulder height and fingers outstretched so that your fingertips touch the wall. Let your finger slowly walk up the wall; you may have to move closer to the wall as your fingers climb higher. Go as high as comfortably possible. Stop. Hold for 30 seconds. Breathe deeply. Mark this level off with a pencil so that you can monitor your progress. Repeat on the other side. This stretch is also called the "wall walk."

Tall Stretch

Stand comfortably with your feet shoulder-width apart or until you feel balanced. Point your toes slightly out. Raise your hands over your head with your palms inward and your arms shoulder-width apart. Stretch comfortably upward, standing up on your toes if possible. Hold for 30 seconds. Breathe deeply. You can do this stretch lying down on the bed or floor with your toes pointed. If you are prone to calf cramps, don't point your toes.

Middle Chest Stretch

Stand at arm's length from a doorway or wall. Stretch your arm out against the support until it is parallel to the floor. Keep your palm flat against the support, elbow straight, and fingers pointing backward. The closer your body is to the support and the more you twist your torso away from it, the greater the stretch will be on your chest. Hold comfortably for 30 seconds. Breathe deeply. Repeat on the other side.

External Rotation Stretch

Stand comfortably with your feet shoulder-width apart, knees slightly bent, and shoulders back. Hold your arms straight out in front of you with your palms facing inward. Then turn your elbows outward to stretch the muscles that rotate your shoulder forward and inward. Hold comfortably for 30 seconds. Breathe deeply.

Upper Chest Stretch

Stand at arm's length from a doorway or wall. Stretch your arm out against the support until it is at a 45-degree angle below the horizontal plane. Keep your palm flat against the support, fingers pointed downward, and elbows straight. The closer your body is to the support and the more you twist your torso away from it, the greater the stretch will be on your chest. Hold comfortably for 30 seconds. Breathe deeply. Repeat on the other side.

Squatting Chest Stretch

With your feet shoulder-width apart and your toes pointing straight ahead or slightly outward, place both hands on a desk, tabletop, or chair. Keep your elbows straight and palms down or inward—not outward. Slowly squat down to a comfortable level. Make sure that your stance is solid so that you do not slip and strain your shoulders. Hold for 30 seconds. Breathe deeply. The deeper your squat, the greater the stretch on your chest.

Chest

Shoulder Blade Squeeze

Stand comfortably with your feet shoulder-width apart. Place your hands behind your back and join your fingers together. If your hands are below your waist, you will stretch your middle and upper chest. If your hands are above the horizontal plane, you will stretch your lower chest. Squeeze your shoulder blades together and hold comfortably for 30 seconds. Breathe deeply.

Arm

Wrist Extension Stretch

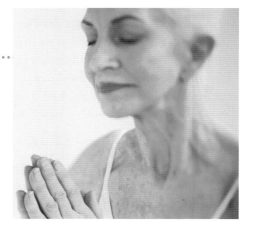

Stand comfortably with your feet shoulder-width apart. Put your hands together in a prayer position and press your wrists downward until your forearms form a 90-degree angle with your hands. You may not be able to do this at first, but as your flexibility increases, you will be able to push your wrists farther down. Hold comfortably for 30 seconds. Breathe deeply.

Wrist Flexion Stretch

Stand comfortably with your feet shoulder-width apart. Place the backs of your hands together at the level of your stomach and press. Press your forearms downward, if possible. Slowly raise your hands up to a comfortable level. Hold for 30 seconds. Breathe deeply. This stretch move is also known as a "reverse prayer" stretch.

Bottom of Wrist Stretch

Stand with your feet shoulder-width apart. Keeping your forearms parallel to the floor, tilt your wrists 10 to 15 degrees up toward your elbows. With your hands out, point your thumbs up. Hold comfortably for 30 seconds. Breathe deeply. This is a good stretch for the inside of the forearm.

Top of Wrist Stretch

Stand comfortably with your feet shoulder-width apart. Keeping your forearms parallel to the floor, tilt your wrists 20 to 30 degrees inward toward your body. Try to point your fingers to the floor. Hold comfortably for 30 seconds. Breathe deeply. This stretch is for your outside forearms.

Open Hand Stretch

While standing or sitting comfortably, spread your fingers as wide as possible. Imagine that you are trying to grasp a basketball that is too big for your hand. Hold for 30 seconds. Breathe deeply. Repeat with the other hand. This stretch is for your palms and fingers.

Closed Hand Stretch

While standing or sitting comfortably, make a tight fist by clenching your hand. Hold for 30 seconds. Breathe deeply. If your hand begins to cramp, you are squeezing too tightly. Repeat with the other hand. This stretches the back of the hand.

Wrist Extension Stretch

Stand comfortably with your feet shoulder-width apart. Hold the fingertips of your left hand with your right hand. Your fingertips can be pointing up or down. Press the palm of your left hand forward and straighten your elbow. Hold comfortably for 30 seconds. Breathe deeply. Repeat on the other side.

Wrist Flexion Stretch

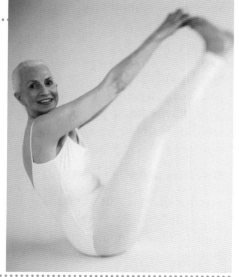

Stand comfortably with your feet shoulder-width apart. Bend your left palm down and secure your fingertips with your right hand. Your fingertips can be pointing up or down. Press the left wrist forward and straighten the elbow. Hold for 30 seconds. Breathe deeply. Repeat on the other side. This is an excellent stretch for tennis elbow.

❋ Back

Knee-to-Chest Stretch

Lie down on the floor or a firm surface (not on a soft bed, as it can strain the ligaments of the lower back). Bring your left knee as close to your chest as possible. Pull from above or below your left knee to help bring it closer to your chest. If you feel a pinch on the top of your hip, you are going too far. Hold comfortably for 30 seconds. Breathe deeply. Repeat with your right leg. This stretch can also be done standing up. It helps to open the base of the back and hip joint.

Figure–4 Stretch

Lie flat on your back. Cross one foot over the other knee so that your ankle is resting on your lower thigh muscle. Wrap your hands under the back leg and slowly pull your leg toward you. Breathe deeply. Hold comfortably for 30 to 60 seconds. Feel the stretch in the buttock muscle of the leg that is crossed in front of you.

This gluteal muscle stretch (formerly called a "piriformis stretch") is a more advanced hip stretch and should be done after the Knee-to-Chest Stretch. The Figure–4 Stretch also places stress on the sciatic nerve, so stretch slowly and cautiously.

Knee-to-Opposite Chest Stretch

Stand up comfortably against a wall, or lie down on a firm surface. Slowly bend your left knee to your torso and then move it towards your right side. Use your right hand to help move your left leg. Hold comfortably for 30 seconds. Breathe deeply. Repeat with your right leg. This stretch can be done standing up or lying down. This stretch works the piriformis muscle (lower buttock muscle) and external rotators of the hip by internally rotating the hip.

Cat Stretch

Get on your hands and knees on a mat or carpet. Keep your feet together. Press the center of your back upward toward the ceiling. Hold comfortably for 30 seconds. Breathe deeply. Always follow this stretch with a Back Arch.

Back Arch

Remaining in the hand-and-knee position from the previous stretch, press your abdomen toward the floor. Do not press your lower abdomen to the floor, or you might place stress on the lower back joints and cause pain or irritation to this region. Hold comfortably for 30 seconds. Breathe deeply. This is an excellent stretch for those who sit all day or have slouching problems.

Pelvic Tilt

Lie on your back on the floor with your knees bent. Contract your buttocks and press your lower back to the floor. This automatically raises your pelvis 1 to 5 inches off the floor. Do not force this stretch. Let your pelvis rise as naturally as possible. Hold comfortably for 30 seconds. Breathe deeply.

Lying Back Extension

Lie on your stomach. Gently raise your head and upper body off the ground. Support your body with your elbows. Do not arch your back farther than is comfortable, or you may aggravate any lower back problems that already exist. Hold comfortably for 30 seconds. Breathe deeply. If this causes pain in your lower back, buttocks, or legs, stop immediately and contact a doctor as soon as possible.

Side of Leg Stretch

Stand approximately 18 inches away from a wall. Use the arm closer to the wall as support against it. Cross your outside leg over your inside leg. Keep the foot of your outside leg flat on the floor. Allow your inside hip to move toward the wall, and guide it with a little pressure from your outside hand on your outside hip. Keep your spine straight. Hold comfortably for 30 seconds. Breathe deeply. Repeat on the other side. As you become more flexible, you may lean your torso away from the wall, or roll your outside foot so that its bottom faces away from the wall, and hold for 60 seconds to maximize the stretch.

Sitting Twist (on floor)

Sit on the floor with your right leg crossed over your left. Use your right elbow to apply very gentle leverage against your right knee. Rest your left hand on the floor for support. Hold comfortably for 30 seconds. Breathe deeply. Do not use this stretch to crack or adjust your back. This stretch works the buttocks and spinal rotator muscles on the side of the straight leg. Repeat with the other leg.

Ankle Reach

With your legs spread apart, lean over the hamstring you wish to stretch. To stretch the inside of your hamstring, lean straight forward. Keep your head up, back straight, and knees slightly bent at all times. Do not round your back. Hold comfortably for 30 seconds. Breathe deeply.

One Leg Stretch

Stand close to a chair or wall so that your spine is straight. Hold the foot of your left leg with your left hand and feel the stretch in the front of your thigh. Support yourself with your right hand, if necessary. Hold comfortably for 30 seconds. Breathe deeply. Repeat on your right leg. Avoid using the opposite hand to hold your ankle, because this places a great deal of stress on your knee, shoulder, and neck. Do not lock the knee of the support leg; keep it slightly bent.

T-Stretch

Hold your left ankle with your left hand. Lean your body forward so your torso and thigh are approximately parallel to the floor. Keep a slight bend in your support leg, and keep your neck in line with the plane of your body. Hold comfortably for 30 seconds. Breathe deeply. Repeat on your right leg.

Lunge Against Wall

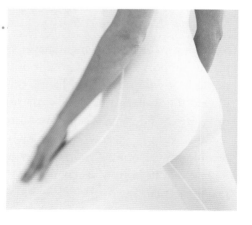

Keep your spine straight, head raised, and palms against a wall for support. Bend your front knee 90 degrees, and keep your foot flat on the ground. If possible, rest your rear knee gently on the floor to prevent bouncing during the stretch. Keep your rear ankle bent to help support you. Press your pelvis toward the wall. Feel the stretch at the front of the hip of your back leg. Hold comfortably for 30 seconds. Breathe deeply. Repeat on the other side.

Thigh

Side Lunge

Stand with your feet wider than shoulder-width apart. Point your toes slightly outward. Keep your feet flat on the floor and balance yourself by placing your hands on your thighs. Bend one knee and slowly move your body to that side. Do not lean forward. Hold comfortably for 30 seconds. Breathe deeply. This will stretch the groin muscle. Lean to the other side.

Supine Groin Stretch

Lie on your back. Bend your knees at 90 degrees and join the soles of your feet together. Move your knees away from each other toward the floor. Hold comfortably for 30 seconds. Breathe deeply. If you feel undue stress in the groin or hip area, place a pillow under each knee to minimize the stress.

Lying Hamstring Stretch

Try this stretch only if you have easily progressed through the previous hamstring stretches, or if you can raise your legs straight up at 90 degrees. Lie on the floor and raise one leg up 90 degrees. Bend the opposite knee at 90 degrees to reduce stress on your lower back. Clasp both hands either (1) above the knee to stretch the entire hamstring or (2) below the knee to stretch the upper hamstring at the pelvis.

Hamstring Stretch to Bench

Place the heel of one foot on a bench, chair seat, or box. Stand far away enough from the platform so that your raised leg is straight. Slowly bend forward at the waist and lean your body weight over your raised leg. Place one hand on the thigh or knee of the raised leg. This stretch allows you to isolate one hamstring at a time. Never round your back as you lean forward. Hold comfortably for 30 seconds. Breathe deeply. Repeat with your other leg.

Straight Leg Stretch

Place your hands on the back of a chair or against a wall for support. Keep your front knee bent with your shin straight. Keep both feet flat on the floor and your spine straight. Keeping your back leg straight, slide it back until you feel the stretch in the back of your lower leg behind the knee. Hold comfortably for 30 to 60 seconds. Breathe deeply. Repeat with your other leg. This stretch works the muscle that runs down the back of the leg to form the Achilles tendon at the heel.

Note: Muscles that are more fibrous, such as tendons, require more time (30 to 60 seconds) to stretch effectively.

 ## Front of the Lower Leg/Calf Region

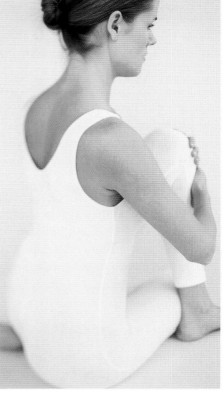

Standing Shin Stretch

Rest the top of one foot on the seat of a chair or on a box so that your knee is bent at 90 degrees. For a deeper stretch, press down on the heel of your back leg with the hand of the same side. Hold for 30 seconds. Breathe deeply. Repeat with your other leg.

Half-Kneeling Shin Stretch

Kneel so that your legs are bent at 90 degrees. Extend your ankles and keep your feet together. You should be at arm's length from a wall so that you can use it as support, if needed. Do not sit back; otherwise, it will strain your knees. Hold for 30 seconds. Breathe deeply.

Inner Ankle Stretch

While standing or sitting, point the toes of one foot, straighten your ankle, and then point your toes outward to stretch your inner ankle. Hold for 30 to 40 seconds. Breathe deeply. Repeat with your other ankle.

Outer Ankle Stretch

While standing or sitting, point the toes of one foot, straighten your ankle, and then point your toes inward to stretch your outer ankle. Hold for 30 to 40 seconds. Breathe deeply. Repeat with the other ankle.

Bent-Knee Calf Stretch

This stretch is similar to the Straight Leg Stretch (see page 181) except that your back leg is slightly bent. Perform the Straight Leg Stretch until you feel a mild stretch in the calf of your back leg. Then bend the knee of your back leg about 5 degrees to stretch the deeper calf muscles. Hold for 30 seconds. Breathe deeply. Repeat with your other leg. This stretch is also called a "soleus stretch."

Calf Stretch on a Step

Use the railing and wall for support as you place the front half of your feet on a step. Prop your heels below the step. Keep your knees slightly bent for a deep calf muscle stretch or straight for an outer calf muscle stretch. Hold comfortably for 30 seconds. Breathe deeply.

Inner Calf Stretch

This stretch is similar to the Calf Stretch on a Step, except, with your toes out, you stretch the inner calf muscles. Hold comfortably for 30 seconds. Breathe deeply.

Outer Calf Stretch

This stretch is similar to the Calf Stretch on a Step, except, with your toes in, you stretch the outer calf muscles. Hold comfortably for 30 seconds. Breathe deeply.

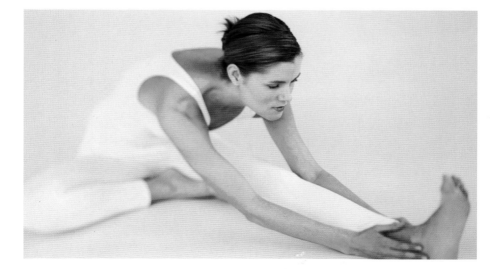

When to Stretch

You should stretch before and after every training session. Of course, you can stretch anytime, but it is essential to do some stretches before and after every workout. Stretching should be slow and controlled, with no bouncing or pulsing. Push yourself in your stretches. Do stretch to the limit of movement, but not to the point of pain. Breathe deeply and relax into the stretch. Once you've reached your full stretch, hold it for 20 to 30 seconds. As you go in and out of each stretch, be sure to use slow, fluid movements.

At the end of each workout, do 5 more minutes of stretching from the post-workout stretches below. That will be enough to maintain your flexibility, and you'll feel the difference that stretching makes. The benefits of stretching, as with all forms of exercise, are long-term. One stretching session will not prepare you for a particular workout.

 ## Post-Workout Stretches

Back and Hamstring Stretch

Lie on your back. Extend your right leg. Wrap both hands around your left leg, above the knee, and pull your left leg toward your chest. Hold and breathe for 20 seconds. Repeat with the other leg. This stretch can also be done with both legs at once.

Buttocks Stretch

Sitting on the floor with your legs crossed, lean your elbows either on top of your legs or on the floor, and press forward. Hold and breathe for 20 seconds.

6

Weight Training

If you work out with weights every day, you're setting yourself up for joint injury and muscle depletion. That's true even if you don't train the same muscle group two days in a row, because those muscles will still be taxed as assisting or stabilizing muscles and won't ever get the full rest that they need.

Resistance Training

Working out with weights, or "resistance training," builds a better physique and a healthier body. Resistance training can tighten and tone your muscles, increase your size by adding inches where you want them, and help you control your weight so you can lose inches where you don't want them. In short, lifting weights is the most effective and the quickest way to create a positive change in the shape of your body.

Women often don't want to train with weights because they are afraid they'll bulk up. In fact, because women don't have high levels of muscle-building hormones, they will find it very hard to add on enough muscle mass to look bulky.

The method of training required to develop bulky muscles is called "bodybuilding." The *30-Day Revitalization Plan* focuses on "body shaping," or "body sculpting." The exercises are basically the same, but the training methods are different. Body shaping requires less time and lighter weights than a bodybuilding training regimen. Body shaping is much less time- and energy-intensive—you can develop a great shape by training three to four times a week for 45 minutes to an hour. Another big difference between these two methods of training is that bodybuilders usually train with a particular event or goal in mind, whereas body shaping with free weights is about being healthy and having a strong, attractive body over the long term.

Getting Started

The single most important way to prevent injury is simply to use good form while exercising.

Free Weights

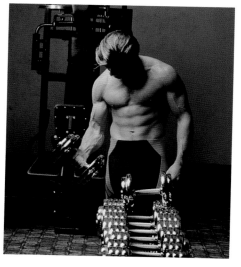

Free weights fall into three categories: barbells, dumbbells, and weight-stack equipment, where gravity is the source of resistance. Once you learn the proper use of the three types of equipment, correct lifting techniques, and some basic exercise theory, using free weights will help you build a strong and shapely body.

Exercising with free weights more effectively duplicates how human beings move naturally. With free weights, more muscles are involved, as you balance and stabilize the weights. This effort targets not just the primary working muscle in a given exercise, but also the smaller accessory muscles. Even the lifting of weights off their rack requires a wide range of balancing and stabilizing actions. Working out with dumbbells and barbells takes greater effort and gives you a more complete workout. Machines stabilize the weights for you, so balance and coordination are not enhanced and accessory muscles are not involved.

When you lift a barbell or dumbbell, the resistance is greater at the beginning of the movement; then, to some extent, momentum helps with the rest of the movement. Think of lifting a grocery sack off the counter as matching the movement in a bicep curl; the initial effort is the greatest. Machines, on the other hand, generally work with equal resistance throughout the lift, which does not match real-life movement mechanics. A free-weight workout, by duplicating the natural lifting movement, results in a greater degree of functional fitness, better preparing you to lift or maneuver heavy objects outside the gym.

When you work out with dumbbells, there is a specific way to lift the weights off the floor and into the starting position, and a specific way to put them back down again.

Most dumbbell exercises are done on a bench. Before you begin, have the dumbbells on the floor beside the bench. Pick up one dumbbell at a time and place it on the top of your leg, then do the same with the other. Next, lift one knee up so you're simultaneously pushing with the thigh and lifting with your hand. In this way, bring the dumbbell up to shoulder level. Then do the same with the other dumbbell. Next, if the exercise calls for it, lower your back onto the bench.

When you're finished with your set, bring the dumbbells back to your shoulders; then, one at a time, put them back on top of each leg. Next, pull yourself up into a sitting position (the weight of the dumbbells helps you do this). From the sitting position, place each dumbbell, one at a time, back onto the floor.

This will all seem unnecessary, unless you are working with heavier weights. Still, it's best to use this proper method, even if the dumbbells you are using now aren't that heavy. You won't have to relearn technique when you graduate to heavier weights.

Body Mechanics

The most important factors for a safe exercise routine are holding your body properly and performing the exercise movements correctly. Exercises done with these things in mind also deliver the best results. Never compromise safety for the sake of a quicker workout, an easier workout, or any other reason.

While performing any weight-lifting exercise, keep in mind these basic safety rules. Read and reread them frequently. Remember, safety first, and safe form equals effective form.

Sticking Points

Anyone who lifts weights is bound to run into a "sticking point" occasionally in certain exercises—a part of the lift that you can't move through without "cheating." About 99 percent of weight lifters take the easy way out and cheat on their form. But there is a better way.

The usual way individuals respond to a sticking point is by sacrificing good form. They either use momentum and swing the weight through the range of motion, or they contort their body in such a way that the weight can be jerked through the sticking point. Both methods can lead to injury, and neither of them makes you stronger. Swinging, jerking, and contorting simply do not lead to functional strength—they lead to more swinging, jerking, and contorting . . . and to injury.

The real solution to training through a sticking point is simple: Reduce the resistance, and practice moving through the limited range of motion at the point where the sticking occurs. For real strength gains to be made, the weaker part of the muscle (think of it as the weakest link in a chain) must be the target of controlled, partial repetitions.

No one likes to reduce the amount of weight he or she is lifting. But in this case, it works. As soon as the weaker part of the muscle gets stronger, you can return to training with a full range of motion without having to cheat.

Joint Conditioning

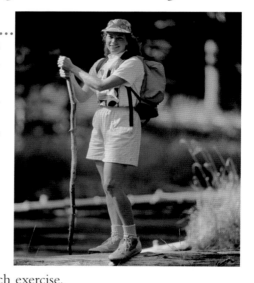

Weight training strengthens not only the muscles and bones but also the connective tissue in the joints. The connective tissues most affected by weight lifting are tendons, which hold muscle to bone. The stronger the tendons, the stronger the joints. Strong joints increase joint stability, which plays an important role in injury prevention, both in and out of the gym.

As a general practice, lift the weights through the joint's full range of motion as instructed in each exercise.

Even after your muscles and joints are conditioned, avoid the temptation to lift too heavy a weight. You must always consider not only your muscular strength (how much resistance the muscles can handle) but also your joint strength (how much resistance the connective tissue can handle). Good form is compromised when you try to lift more than your body can handle. Poor form usually leads to injury or at the least, to a less potent workout. Poor form is the biggest enemy to building shapelier, stronger muscles safely.

Besides increasing your likelihood of injury, training with poor form develops "artificial strength," where you think you're developing strength in one particular muscle group, while in reality you're depending on other muscle groups to assist with an exercise. That cuts into your true strength gains.

Rest—An Elemental Need

Working out with weights creates microscopic muscle contusions (ruptures) and causes muscle spasms. Lactic acid also builds up. These processes are part of muscle development; they are signs that you have stimulated the muscle and had a good workout.

When you rest, events occur at the cellular level that cause the muscle and joint structures to change. Without the needed rest, these cellular changes don't have a chance to take place. The result may be injury, or at the very least, a reduction in strength gains.

It's not necessary to understand all of these physical processes, but it may be helpful to understand a few. It's during the resting phase that contractile proteins within the muscle increase in size and number. That increase is what makes the muscle stronger. Tendons (the connective tissues associated with muscle) become thicker and stronger, making the joint more stable and durable. The number of capillaries within the muscle increases in order to handle the increased amount of oxygen flowing to the muscle. Bones become denser and stronger in order to handle the new stress placed on them by the muscle.

A 48-hour resting phase is as necessary to muscle development as the training itself. All the weight-training programs in this book are designed to give the primary working muscles a 48-hour rest before training them again. If you expect to make real progress, you must not train the same muscle or muscle group within a 48-hour period.

Recognizing and Managing Injuries

There are four kinds of soreness or pain that can result from lifting weights. The first two below are signs that you're doing it right; the other two mean that you've injured yourself.

The "Burn"

Lactic acid builds up in your muscles as you work them. The lactic acid is what prevents you from doing more reps. It also causes a slight burning sensation in the muscle; thus the expression "No pain, no gain!" As soon as you finish your set and oxygen returns to the muscle, the lactic acid is dispersed and the sensation disappears.

Soreness

It is normal for your muscles to feel sore for 48 to 72 hours after a hard workout. Good ways to relieve soreness are slow stretching, warm compresses, a hot bath, rest, or massage. If the soreness persists for more than 3 days, you may have strained a muscle.

Strains

A strain (or "pulled muscle") usually appears suddenly. It results when the muscle or tendon is overstretched, resulting in tiny tears. If you follow our safety rules and avoid overtraining, strains should not occur.

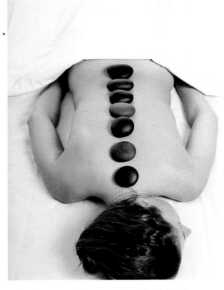

Should you strain a muscle, first and foremost, stop your workout. You'll need at least a few days' rest—more if the strain is severe. When you do start lifting weights again, start out considerably lighter than usual, until you're sure you have completely recovered. The formula for treating strains is RICE—rest, ice, compression, and elevation. Of these, rest and ice are the most important. Aspirin also helps ease pain and reduce swelling. If the strain persists or seems serious, see your doctor.

Muscle strains heal well with proper attention and rest. But if you don't treat a strain or give yourself time to recover, the injury can become chronic.

Sprains

A sprain is a severe injury and is very rare in weight training. It occurs when the ligament is pulled or twisted beyond its maximum range of motion, most often happening in the ankles. A sprain always happens suddenly and is accompanied by severe bruising and swelling. If you suspect you have a sprain, see your doctor. In the meantime, use the RICE treatment mentioned in the discussion of strains.

Don't be scared off by the above cautions. If performed correctly, weight training is one of the safest forms of exercise.

Warming Up

Why warm up? There are important physiological reasons why warming up prevents injury and increases the benefits of your workout—we'll cover those in just a minute. But equally important, warming up prepares us psychologically for a workout. We go into the gym, or wherever it is we train, with a mood and mindset created by whatever has happened to us so far that day. We might be frustrated because we were stuck in traffic, we may be feeling angry or sad, we could be anxious because of job stresses, or we might be worried about an important exam we're about to take. A warm-up helps put us in the present. We become body conscious, and a body-mind connection is made that will result in a more effective as well as a more enjoyable workout.

Physiologically speaking, a warm-up elevates the core temperature and individual muscles of your body, which makes exercise safer. Cold, stiff muscles and joints are at higher risk of injury than those that have been properly warmed up.

A warm-up also increases respiration and heart rate and stroke volume. How fast you breathe, how fast the heart beats, and the amount of blood passing through the heart muscle each time it beats are all measures of how much blood is circulating from your heart to the rest of your body. The red blood cells in the bloodstream are what carry the oxygen to your muscles. Warming up allows more oxygen to be delivered more efficiently to the working muscles.

Without this rich supply of oxygen, your muscles won't work very effectively. One reason is that lactic acid, a by-product of muscle activity, builds up and prevents any further work. Oxygen disperses lactic acid and allows exercise to continue. Energy enzymes cannot function at full capacity in the presence of lactic acid. A good warm-up, and the oxygen it delivers to your muscles, increases the effectiveness of these enzymes by dispersing lactic acid. By warming up, you are more energized.

Another good reason to warm up is that a warm, oxygenated muscle has greater flexibility. Flexibility helps prevent injuries.

Finally, warming up before a workout improves the viscosity of the synovial fluids that surround movable joints. Think of the Tin Man in The Wizard of Oz. He could move just fine once his joints were oiled. It's similar with people. A warm-up lubricates our joints, which allows us to move freely. Full, easy range of motion in all our movable joints is a key factor in preventing joint injury.

How much of a warm-up should you do? Five to 10 minutes on a stationary bike, treadmill, or step climbing machine is enough. Do your warm-up exercise at an intensity that makes you break into a sweat. The more power necessary for a sport or activity, the more important the warm-up.

A warm-up is sometimes based on the dynamic movement of a specific sport or activity. Specific warm-ups use movements that are similar to the movements of a particular sport. In the case of weight lifting, a warm-up can consist in part of a weight-lifting exercise that works the same muscles you will be training that day. Go ahead and start your prescribed exercise, but use a very light weight and do 10 to 15 reps. After this initial warm-up set, you'll be ready to start your routine using heavier resistance.

If you lift weights with cold, tight muscles, you're inviting injury. There won't be enough oxygen in the muscles to enable them to perform, and your energy enzymes will be slogging around in an acid bath. Both will cause early muscle fatigue, which leads to poor body mechanics and to possible joint and muscle injury.

The bottom line: Without a warm-up, your workouts will be less potent, more dangerous, and not nearly as much fun.

 ## Cooling Down

After aerobic exercise, cooling down might mean just going more slowly— switching from a run to a walk to slow down your heart rate. After a weight-lifting workout, the best way to cool down is to stretch all the muscles you trained in that session.

Breathe slowly and deeply while cooling down. To ensure the deepest relaxation, be aware of your body's releasing the muscle's tension. The cool-down is a good time to do a visualization exercise or to repeat to yourself one of your affirmations.

A cool-down period has both physical and psychological benefits. Psychologically, it reduces stress. A cool-down allows time for the body and the mind to relax.

Physiologically, a cool-down does a number of important things. Cool-down stretching increases flexibility and helps retain full range of motion in the joints, which decreases the risk of joint injury. It also improves muscular balance and postural awareness.

In general, a cool-down helps reduce muscle soreness by increasing the blood supply and nutrients going to the muscles and joints.

All workouts need a cool-down, but the higher the intensity level of a workout, the more important the cool-down becomes.

 ## At Home

Working out at home is convenient and can save you lots of time, but it presents its own special challenges. When you work out at a gym, it's easier to focus on the task at hand, because you don't have the distractions that often occur at home. There is no phone to answer, no favorite TV program competing for your attention, no children wanting you to play. Because your home is a more relaxed environment, it will probably be more difficult for you to concentrate on your workout. Here are some suggestions to make it easier:

Choose a time when there are as few distractions as possible. Hopefully this coincides with a time when your energy level is high. If you really feel like a vigorous workout, it's of course easier to follow through and do it.

Be flexible, but try to train at the same time each day. Our bodies long for and respond well to routine. If possible, have a designated area for your workout, a place where you can leave your equipment. Make sure your workout area is bright and airy with good air circulation. A mirror is helpful. It provides instant feedback on body form and function. Music is great, and unlike at a gym, at home you get to play what you like. Music motivates people. Virtually all gyms play upbeat music to inspire their patrons to "move." The same philosophy works at home.

Methods

Shape-Training Exercises

Thighs and Buttocks

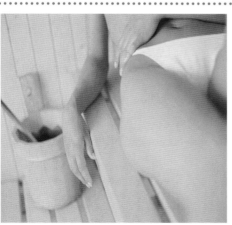

The thighs and buttocks are the two most difficult areas of the body to train. The muscles involved are the largest in your body; it requires a lot of energy to train them hard enough to make a difference.

There is also the knee tracking factor. The knees have to track correctly in order to avoid injuring them. Knees are a hinge joint and should move back and forth in only one plane of motion. It takes a certain amount of muscle strength and body awareness to keep the knees properly aligned. Knees tend to turn out or cave in.

Finally, there is the lower back to consider. Almost all leg and buttocks exercises involve the erectors or lower back muscles, either as primary working muscles or as stabilizers. Often the weaker erector muscles prevent us from working our leg and buttocks muscles to full capacity. Those who begin with relatively undeveloped lower back muscles will find they must ease up on some of the lower body exercises until their backs are strong enough to handle the load.

Thus, training the lower body is not only more physically demanding than training other muscle groups, but it also requires a higher degree of mental focus in order to prevent injury.

If you carefully follow the directions for each exercise, your lower-back muscles and knee joints will be protected and not at risk for injury.

Knee Extension

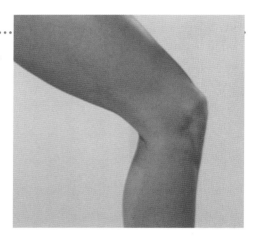

Works quadriceps (commonly referred to as "quads")—front of upper leg.

• Starting Position

Follow directions on the equipment and adjust it to fit your body. The roller pads should be even with your ankle bones. Your feet should be relaxed, your toes pointing straight ahead.

• Movement

A. Exhale, and straighten out your knees, bringing your legs almost parallel to the floor.

B. Inhale, and slowly lower your legs four-fifths of the way down.

Notes

Don't kick up your legs or drop them down. Strive for controlled, even movements.

Don't lock your knees at the top of the movement (avoid hyperextending the knees).

Lower your legs only four-fifths of the way down to avoid hyperflexion (overstretching) of the knees.

Curl

Works hamstring—back of upper leg.

• Starting Position

Follow directions on the equipment and adjust it to fit your body. The roller pads should be resting on the area between your Achilles tendons and your lower calf muscles.

- **Advanced Variation**

When your knees are fully flexed, lift your thighs off the bench by squeezing your buttocks muscles. Do not perform this variation if you have lower back problems.

- **Movement**

A. Exhale as you bend your knees, bringing your feet toward your buttocks.

B. Inhale as you slowly lower your legs four-fifths of the way down.

Notes

Don't lower your legs any farther than four-fifths of the way down, to avoid hyperextension of the knees.

Strive for a controlled, even movement.

Squat

Works thighs, buttocks, and lower back.

Squats are a high-risk exercise and must be performed with caution.

- **Starting Position**

Step under the bar and place the bar across your upper trapezius muscles (commonly referred to as "traps") located between your shoulders. Step back away from the rack. Stand with your feet hip-width apart, toes pointing straight ahead. If you're very tall, you may have to position your feet wider than hip width, and your feet may have to be turned out slightly. Your knees should be relaxed, not locked, your back straight (allowing for the natural curve), and your chin level. Look up with your eyes only.

- **Movement**

A. Inhale, lowering your body as if you were sitting down in a chair. Go down until your thighs are parallel to the floor (if you're able). Your shoulders should never go farther forward than mid-thigh.

B. Exhale as you straighten your body, pressing your heels into the floor and squeezing your buttocks as you do so.

Notes

Don't allow your knees to come together.

Keep your feet flat on the floor throughout the exercise.

Strive for controlled, even movements.

During the lowering phase of the lift, don't allow your shoulders and the barbell to go any farther forward than above the middle of your thighs.

At the start of the movement, your hips should tilt back slightly, as if you were sitting down in a chair.

- **Variation: Front Squat**

Feet and knees are together. The bar rests across the front of your deltoids (shoulder muscles; commonly referred to as "delts") and chest in a cross-arm position. This variation targets the quads (front of your upper legs) more than does a standard Squat. The Front Squat is not for beginners; it requires a good sense of balance and front shoulder development.

Dip

Works thighs and buttocks.

- **Starting Position**

Step under the bar, and place the bar across your upper traps with your feet hip-width apart. Then step forward and place one foot on an elevated surface. You will be on the ball of the back foot, which is extended behind you. Position yourself so that your front knee will be directly over your front ankle at the lowest point of the movement. Point both feet straight ahead.

- **Movement**

A. Inhale as you lower your body by bending your front knee and pressing your back knee toward the floor.

B. Exhale, lifting back to the starting position.

Notes

Stay on the ball of the back foot throughout the entire exercise.

Strive for controlled and even movements.

At the bottom of the movement, make sure your front knee and ankle are aligned.

One-Leg Dip

Works thighs and buttocks.

This is an advanced exercise because it requires considerable balance and coordination.

- **Starting Position**

Step under the bar and place it across your upper traps. Place the top of one foot and ankle across a bench behind you. The other leg will be in front of your body. Position this leg so that the knee is directly over the ankle at the lowest point of the exercise. This foot is pointing straight ahead.

• Movement

A. Inhale, and lower your body by bending both your knees.

B. Exhale, and lift back up to the starting position.

Notes

Strive for controlled, even movements.

Keep your front knee and ankle aligned at the lowest point of the exercise.

Your front foot remains pointed straight ahead throughout the exercise.

Lunge

Works thighs and buttocks.

• Starting Position

Step under the bar and place it across your upper traps. Step back from the rack and stand with your feet hip-width apart. Both feet should be pointing straight ahead.

• Movement

A. Inhale as you lunge forward, simultaneously pressing your back knee toward the floor.

B. Exhale, coming back to the starting position.

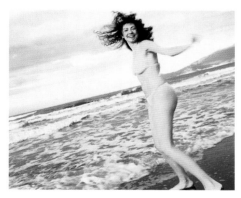

Notes

Lunges require a degree of agility. If you find the movement difficult, stick with dips until you develop more body awareness.

Strive for controlled and even movements.

When you step back after each lunge, step into a hip-width stance.

Position yourself so that the lunging knee is directly over the ankle at the lowest point of the movement.

Step–Up

Works thighs and buttocks.

• Starting Position

Face a flat bench with a set of dumbbells in your hands, or with a barbell across your traps.

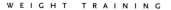

- **Movement**

A. Exhale as you step up onto the bench with your right foot, then immediately step up with the left foot.

B. Inhale, and step down (backward) with your right foot, followed by your left.

Notes

Always begin your step down on the same foot with which you began the step up.

If you're holding dumbbells, don't allow your arms to swing.

Place your entire foot on the bench you're stepping onto.

Do this exercise slowly to avoid losing your balance and falling.

 Adduction
....

Works the inner thighs.

- **Starting Position**

Follow directions on the equipment and adjust it to fit your body. Hip and inner thigh flexibility are factors that must be considered in this adjustment.

- **Movement**

A. Exhale, and squeeze your legs all the way together.

B. Inhale, and slowly open your legs four-fifths of the way back to the starting position.

Notes

Don't allow your legs to jerk open. Strive for controlled, even movements.

Don't allow your buttocks to lift off the bench when squeezing your legs together.

When you train your chest muscles, you also work the deltoid muscles. Please be extra careful when performing chest exercises, because the deltoids are vulnerable and easily injured. If you exceed the proper range of motion, you could hurt your shoulder.

Chest

Chest exercises with free weights are performed while lying on your back. When lowering the weight, never lower your elbows more than approximately 2 inches below your shoulders. If you do lower the weight beyond this point, you're crossing an "anatomical barrier." You'll place extreme stress

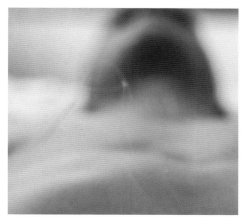

on the deltoid muscle and the shoulder joint, without further benefit to the chest muscles.

Never hyperextend (or "lock") your elbows at the end of a lift. This rule applies to other joints also, and to all weight-lifting exercises. Locking the joints transfers the resistance (weight) from the working muscle to the joints, which in turn puts undue pressure on the bones and connective tissue. Hyperextending your joints will not increase the benefit of the exercise to the muscle and may lead to injury.

When performing exercises for the chest, try to keep the shoulder blades (scapulae) pulled together. This may not be easy at first if you're a beginner. Retracting the scapulae in this way opens and expands the pectoral plate (chest muscles; commonly referred to as "pecs") and shortens the distance the weight has to travel. This increases the amount of power you can exert during the lift.

Avoid arching your lower back. This is a general rule and should be applied to all lifts. Arching is cheating, and when you cheat two things happen (or don't happen). First, you increase the likelihood of injury. When you arch your back, you're using your whole upper body instead of focusing the effort on your chest muscles. The result can be a back strain. Second, arching uses leverage to lift the weight, and cuts into your true strength gains. Keep your back flat (allowing for your natural curve) by placing your feet on the bench or flat on the floor close to the bench. Without the added artificial advantage of arching, you may have to reduce the amount of weight you're lifting, but you'll get more training benefits and see quicker improvement in your chest and shoulders.

If you have a shoulder injury, you may want to avoid some or all of the chest exercises, particularly the wide-grip variations. Start with lighter weights and be sensitive to which exercises cause pain in your shoulder.

Bench Press—Standard Grip

This is the best overall exercise for developing muscle and building strength in the pectoral (chest) muscles.

- **Starting Position**

Lie on the bench, with your feet either on the bench or flat on the floor, the bar over the bridge of your nose, and your hands 2 1/2 to 3 feet apart. Retract the scapulae (pull your shoulder blades together), and lift the bar up and out from the rack. If you're a beginner, don't focus on pulling your shoulder blades together; just allow your shoulder blades to move freely.

- **Movement**

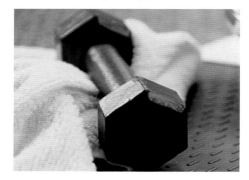

A. Inhale as you slowly lower the bar toward your chest, just over your sternum.

B. Exhale as you push the bar up and back in a very slight arc toward the rack.

When doing incline and decline presses (see Variation), you will lower the bar to a point over the nipple line, and push straight up.

Variation

The bench press is a very versatile exercise; there are four ways you can alter the effect. Your grip can be narrowed to target the inner chest or widened to work the outer chest and deltoids. To focus on the upper part of the pectoral plate, use an incline bench. Use a decline bench in order to target the lower pecs.

Low-Pulley Cable Fly

This exercise is great for shaping and strengthening the lower and outer portions of your chest.

- **Starting Position**

Stand with your feet hip-width apart, your back straight, and your pelvis in a neutral position. With your hands facing forward, take a pulley handle in each hand, allowing the resistance of the weight to extend your arms out at your sides. This will place your hands about 20 inches beyond your legs. Your elbows should be slightly bent.

Dumbbell Press—Flat Bench

- **Starting Position**

Lie on the bench, with your feet on the bench or flat on the floor. Hold a dumbbell in each hand, palms facing forward. Arms are straight up over the chest, elbows slightly flexed. Retract the scapulae.

Movement

A. Inhale as you slowly lower the dumbbells to approximately shoulder level.

B. Exhale as you press the weights straight up to the starting position.

Notes

Don't arch your back.

Keep the dumbbells directly over your chest, not over your face or stomach.

Don't bend your wrists.

At the bottom of the movement, don't lower your elbows any farther than approximately 2 inches below your shoulders.

Squeeze your chest muscles at the top of the movement.

Don't lock your elbows at the top of the movement.

Fly — Incline Bench

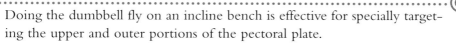

Doing the dumbbell fly on an incline bench is effective for specially targeting the upper and outer portions of the pectoral plate.

Starting Position

Lie on the bench with your feet flat on the floor. Hold a dumbbell in each hand, palms facing each other and toward your feet. Your arms should be straight up over your chest, your elbows slightly flexed. Retract the scapulae.

Movement

A. As you inhale slowly, open your arms until your hands are approximately 2 inches below your shoulders.

B. Follow a semicircular path, as if you were hugging a giant tree, back to the starting position. As always, exhale during the lift.

Notes

Keep the dumbbells in line with your chest (do not move them in the direction of your head or your feet).

Don't bend your wrists.

Don't arch your back.

Keep your elbows slightly flexed throughout the exercise.

Squeeze your chest muscles at the top of the movement.

Pullover

The pullover is effective for targeting the inner chest.

- **Starting Position**

Lie on the bench with your feet on the bench or flat on the floor. Hold a single dumbbell at arm's length (elbows slightly flexed) above your chest, with both hands, palms up, wrapped around one end of the dumbbell.

- **Movement**

A. Allowing your elbows to bend only slightly, lower the dumbbell slowly toward the floor (over your head) until your arms are parallel with your ears. Inhale during this part of the movement.

B. Keeping your arms almost straight, slowly raise the dumbbell back up to the starting position (exhale).

Standard Push-Up

Push-ups are an all-time great exercise for the chest, shoulders, and arms. Although push-up bars are great because they help you steady yourself, this exercise requires no equipment and allows you to get a good chest workout.

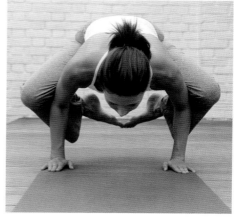

- **Starting Position**

Lie face down on the floor with your hands beside your shoulders.

With your legs together, flex your feet so that the balls of your feet are on the floor.

- **Movement**

A. Exhale, while keeping your torso straight, and push your body up until your arms are fully extended (don't lock your elbows).

B. Inhale and slowly lower yourself until your nose touches the floor.

Notes

Be sure to keep your torso straight (this helps to contract your abdominal muscles; commonly referred to as "abs").

Don't lock your elbows.

Keep your elbows near your sides.

Inexpensive push-up bars are recommended, for all varieties of push-ups, to take the pressure off your wrists. When using push-up bars, you should not go down until your nose touches the floor. Instead, stop at the point where your shoulders are about 1 inch lower than your elbows.

To make the push-up more difficult, place your feet on a stool, chair, or bench.

Variations

Most women find that push-ups from the knees are sufficient to effectively exercise the chest muscles. This variation is performed exactly the same as a standard push-up, only instead of lifting from your feet, you're lifting from your knees.

To emphasize the inner chest and triceps, do push-ups with your hands close together.

To target the outer chest and deltoids, do push-ups with your hands placed about 8 inches out from your shoulders.

Deck

Works chest and front shoulders—the anterior deltoids.

● Starting Position

Adjust the seat so your arms are extended straight out from your shoulders.

● Movement

A. Exhale as you push your arms together until the equipment pads nearly touch.

B. Inhale as you slowly open your arms, without jerking the weight, until your arms are flush with your chest, and no farther.

Note

When returning the weights to the starting position, don't allow your arms to go any farther back than your shoulders.

Back

To train your back effectively, you must be aware of the great variety of muscles that make up this area of your body.

There are the smaller muscles in the upper back—the rhomboids, infraspinatus, and teres major. The upper and midback also contain the larger, more powerful trapezius and latissimus dorsi (commonly referred to as "lats") muscles. Finally, there are the lower back or erector muscles. These are usually the weakest of all the back muscles and the most vulnerable to injury.

We divide the back muscles into four quadrants. The upper back muscles make up one group, the muscles of the lower back another. The lats, which shape the outer back, are the third quadrant, and the middle and lower traps make up the middle back.

The large, powerful lats and upper traps are the easiest muscles to train, simply because they are so big. The smaller muscles of the upper back—the rhomboids, teres major, and infraspinatus—and the lower and middle traps (middle back) are harder to isolate.

Shaping your back proportionally means bringing out these smaller muscle groups as well as the lats and upper traps. In order to effectively train

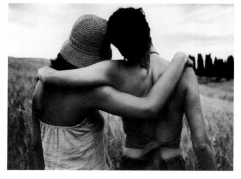

the smaller muscles, you must follow specific refined movement patterns; otherwise, the lats and traps do all the work and reap all the training benefits. The exercises that follow give careful consideration to these movement patterns. If you've had experience training your back, these exercises may be slightly different from what you're used to.

The erectors (lower back) are a notoriously weak muscle group; in many people they are out of shape or even injured. Close attention is paid below to correct (safe) body mechanics in all the exercises, but especially in those that focus on the lower back muscles.

All the back muscles are integral to developing and maintaining good posture. Each muscle has to be trained in conjunction with the others. In this way, you maintain muscle balance and avoid overtraining a particular muscle.

Standard Lat

The most advanced form of lat pull-down is to the rear of the head. All lat pull-down exercises, whether pulling to the front or back of the body, generally work to widen the back.

● Starting Position

Take the bar in a medium grip, palms facing forward. Sit on the bench so the bar will come down behind your head without your having to lean forward at the waist. Place your feet flat on the floor, with knees at a right angle. Elevate your shoulder blades. (This is an exercise refinement that automatically engages the smaller upper-back muscles as you start the working phase of the lift.)

● Movement

A. Exhale and depress your shoulder blades as you slowly pull the bar down behind your head, toward your upper traps. (If you're pulling the bar down in front of your head as a variation, bring it down to your upper chest.) Your elbows should pull straight down to the floor and remain pointing toward the floor throughout both phases of the lift. This exercise refinement takes out most of the external shoulder rotation from the movement and makes the exercise much safer to do.

B. Inhale as you slowly return the bar to the starting position, elevating your shoulder blades at the end of the return.

Notes

Don't arch your back.

Keep your knees at a right angle to stabilize your back.

Keep your elbows pointed straight down to the floor throughout the exercise.

Variations

The grip variations and bar options used in back exercises are nearly endless. It's important to include a variety of bars and grips in your back routines. That way you'll be sure to target all your back muscles, and you'll be able to isolate parts of the bigger back muscles as well. A wide grip targets the outer portion of the lats, a close grip the inner portion and some lower traps. A medium grip is best for working the lat muscles overall. You can hold the bar with an overhand or an underhand grip.

For variety, you can pull the bar down in front of your chest instead of behind your head. Pulling to the front in an underhand grip (palms toward you) is the safest, most effective method for beginners.

Utilize all the bars available to you. Each works the back muscles a little differently. Variety, a key factor in long-term exercise adherence, will keep your workouts interesting and challenging.

Seated Low-Pulley Cable Row

Works lats, middle back, and shoulder girdle.

● **Starting Position**

Take the rowing bar in your hands, and push back into starting position by straightening your legs most of the way (your knees remain slightly flexed throughout the exercise). Be sure your back is straight, your chin level, and your shoulders dropped.

A. Keeping your arms close to your body, exhale and slowly pull the bar toward your sternum. Don't lean back. As you're pulling the bar back, pull your shoulder blades together and expand (open up) your chest.

B. Inhale, and slowly, without jerking the weight, return to the starting position. When you're finished with your set, carefully slide your whole body forward until the tension is off the cable and the plates are restacked. At no time in this exercise should you lean your body forward.

Variations

The grip variations and bar options used in low-pulley rowing exercises are nearly endless. Variety, a key factor in long-term exercise adherence, keeps your workouts interesting and challenging. So utilize all the bars available; each targets the back muscles a little differently. However, in any one workout, once you've begun an exercise with a particular bar and grip, stick with that same bar and grip for all of your sets of that exercise.

Bent-Over One-Arm Row

Primarily works lats. Secondarily, this exercise also works the tricep, shoulder girdle, and rear deltoid muscles. It tends to "thicken" rather than widen the lat muscles, which, developed in this way, help correct bad posture by fortifying the upper torso.

• Starting Position

Place one hand, elbow slightly flexed, and the corresponding knee on a flat bench. Take a dumbbell in the other hand, palm turned toward the body. Be sure your shoulders are squared, your abs tight, and your back flat.

• Movement

A. Exhale and slowly pull the dumbbell straight up until it's beside your chest. Keep your arm close to your body throughout the exercise.

B. Inhale, and slowly, without dropping your shoulder, lower the weight to the starting position.

Notes

Don't arch your back.

Keep your torso still and your abs tight.

Look straight down at the floor throughout the exercise.

Keep your supporting elbow slightly flexed.

Variations

This exercise can be done with both arms at once. To do this, you'll have to decrease the amount of weight you're using. You can also do bent-over rows with a barbell. The body mechanics change with these variations. You'll be standing with your knees bent, your body bent forward at the waist, and your abs tight. If you're using a barbell, pull the bar up to your chest.

T-bar rows are another option. This exercise, done on a piece of gym apparatus designed for that one exercise, matches the body mechanics of barbell rowing.

Upright Rows

Standard upright rows work the upper and middle back and some shoulder muscles.

● **Starting Position**

Stand with your knees slightly flexed, shoulder-width apart, your back straight, and your pelvis tucked in. Hold the barbell in front of your thighs with your hands close together and your palms facing you.

● **Movement**

A. Exhale as you pull the bar up along the front of your body, leading with your elbows, until your upper arms are at a level about parallel with your shoulders.

B. Inhale and slowly return to the starting position.

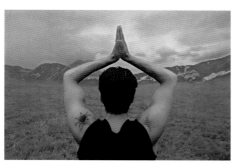

Notes

Keep your chin level.

Don't arch your back.

Keep your shoulders dropped.

Your elbows should be drawn up no higher than your shoulders. (Slightly higher, an inch or so, may be safe for some people.)

Pull-Up (Chin-Up)

Works lats, upper back, shoulder girdle, and rear deltoids.

● **Starting Position**

Place a bench under the bar. Stand on the bench and take hold of the bar in a wide enough grip so that when you're pulling yourself up, your forearms are perpendicular to the floor. Be sure your palms are facing away from your body.

● **Movement**

A. Lift yourself off the bench, exhale, and pull your body up (with the bar in front of your body) until your chin is even with the bar.

B. Inhale, and slowly lower your body until your elbows form approximately a 130- to 140-degree angle.

Notes

Don't lower your body all the way down.

Keep the bar in front of your body for all pull-ups.

Variations

If you're not strong enough to complete a pull-up with your legs hanging, keep your toes on the bench throughout the exercise.

Do a pull-up as above, but reverse your hand grip—palms facing toward your body.

Vary the width of your grips. A wide grip will focus on the outer back; a close grip will work the inner back muscles more.

Dead Lift—Straight Leg

Works lower back, buttocks, and back of thighs.

- **Starting Position**

Grasp the bar in an overhand position with your hands shoulder-width apart, and stand up so you are holding the bar in front of you. Position your feet hip-width apart, with your knees slightly flexed. Your abs should be tight and your pelvis neutral. Keep your back straight and your chin level.

- **Movement**

A. Keeping your back flat and your legs almost straight, inhale as you bend over at the waist, and lower the bar as close to the floor as you can without bending your knees or rounding your back. You must be able to lower the bar to at least below your knees in order for this exercise to be safe.

B. Exhale, keeping your back completely flat, as you lift your body up to an erect position. The bar should practically drag along the front of your legs.

Variation

This exercise can be performed with dumbbells. The movement mechanics are the same.

Dead Lift—Bent Knee

Works lower back, buttocks, and back of thighs.

Although this exercise is very valuable for strengthening the lower back, it can cause injury to that region if performed with too much weight. Start with a very light weight (or even none at all), and work your way up gradually. If you've had lower back problems in the past, consult your ortho-pedist before doing this exercise. Regardless of your history, don't push yourself on this exercise. Do it near the start of your workout, before you tire yourself out with other exercises, and give it your full concentration. It also helps to do this exercise (or straight-leg dead lifts) regularly. If you feel any discomfort, stop immediately.

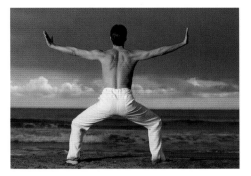

• Starting Position

Stand with your feet hip-width apart. Drop your buttocks so your thighs are roughly parallel to the floor. Grab the bar in an overhand position with your hands shoulder-width apart, and lift the bar up slightly so as to position it over your feet.

• Movement

A. Exhale as you slowly pull the bar up along the front of your legs while straightening your body.

B. Inhale, and slowly reverse the movement. Keep your head up and keep your knees open (don't let them buckle inward).

Notes

Keep your arms straight throughout the exercise.

Keep the bar or dumbbells close to your body throughout the exercise.

Don't lean back when you come up to the standing position.

Variation

This exercise can be performed with dumbbells. The movement mechanics are the same.

Back Extension on Roman Chair

Works lower back muscles.

• Starting Position

Position yourself face down on the Roman chair. Your hands can be across your chest or resting on your lower back. Your neck should be straight.

• Movement

A. Inhale as you lower your body about one-quarter of the way to the floor.

B. Exhale as you lift your body up parallel to the floor, no higher.

Notes

Strive for controlled and even movements.

Lower your torso only one-quarter of the way toward the floor.

Don't lift up any higher than parallel to the floor.

Keep your neck straight.

✳ Shoulders

The shoulders are one of the most vulnerable and easily injured areas of your body—that is, if you don't train them correctly.

It seems that more people injure their shoulders in the gym than any other muscle/joint combination. There are two ways these injuries happen. Over the long run, people may train their shoulders using an unsafe range of motion. Alternatively, people injure their shoulders in one set (or one rep) of an exercise by overloading the deltoid muscles while using an unsafe range of motion in the shoulder joint.

The solution is to use controlled movements when training the shoulders. This is true for all exercises, but it's especially important when training the shoulders or when the deltoids are actively involved in an exercise. We have to be extra cautious because of the complexity of the shoulder joint. The shoulder is basically designed for mobility; therefore, the deltoid muscles should be developed with their function and ability to move in mind.

Pay close attention to the directions given for each individual shoulder exercise below. Preventing shoulder injury is always a key factor in these instructions. If some movements seem odd or unnatural, that's probably because you learned to exercise in a less safe way.

Protecting the shoulders from injury is paramount to long-term exercise adherence. If you develop shoulder impingement (from overuse or from using an unsafe range of motion) or in any way injure your shoulder joint, you may be unable to train your upper body for weeks, possibly even months, at a time.

Shoulder Press

Works top of shoulder.

● Starting Position

Sit on a bench. If you don't have a strong back, use a bench with a back support. Hold the dumbbells so they are about level with your mouth, palms facing forward. Beginners, turn your palms toward your head.

● Movement

A. Exhale as you press the dumbbells straight up, being careful not to fully extend your elbows. This will keep the stress off the elbows and on the deltoid muscles, where it's supposed to be.

B. Inhale as you slowly lower the weights to the starting position.

Notes

Keep your feet flat on the floor to stabilize your back.

Strive for controlled and even movements.

Don't fully extend your arms as you press up.

Press the dumbbells straight up. Don't bring them together overhead. If you do so, you're placing unnecessary strain on the shoulder joint without further benefit to the muscle.

Variations

Beginners, you can do dumbbell presses with your palms facing in, toward your head.

You can alternate arms instead of doing both at once.

You can perform a shoulder press with one arm while leaning on your side on an incline bench.

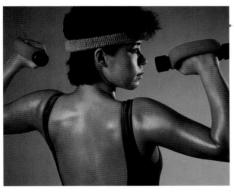

Bar Press

Works top of shoulder. The starting position and movements for this exercise are the same as for the Shoulder Press with dumbbells, only in this exercise, it's the bar that is level with your mouth. Your hands should grasp the bar far enough apart so that your forearms form right angles with the bar (i.e., your forearms should be perpendicular to the floor). You can press either to the front or to the back of your neck. Beginners, press to the front.

Lateral Raise

Works outer shoulder.

● Starting Position

Stand with your legs hip-width apart. Let your spine remain neutral (but allow for its natural curve). Keep your chin level. Do not bend forward at the waist. Keep your abdominals tight. Hold a dumbbell in each hand, with arms hanging down beside you.

● Movement

A. Exhale as you lift the dumbbells straight out to your sides to about shoulder height.

B. Inhale as you slowly lower the dumbbells to the starting position.

Notes

Keep your wrists straight.

Strive for controlled and even movements.

Don't lean forward at the waist.

Keep your hips stable; don't rock back and forth.

Don't bring your arms above your shoulders. If you do, you're placing unnecessary stress on the shoulder joint without further benefit to the muscle.

Front Shoulder Raise

Works front of shoulders.

- **Starting Position**

Stand with the dumbbells held in front of your thighs with your arms straight, your elbows slightly bent, your palms facing thighs, your knees relaxed, and your pelvis and spine neutral.

- **Movement**

A. Exhale as you raise your arms to shoulder level, no higher.

B. Inhale as you slowly lower the weights back to the starting position.

Notes

Keep your wrists straight.

Strive for controlled and even movements.

Don't arch your back.

Don't swing your body back and forth. Keep your trunk motionless.

Don't lift your arms higher than shoulder level.

Variation: Alternate–Arm Raise

You'll probably have to do this anyway when you graduate to more intense training workloads. Alternate reps, not sets—that is, work the left side, then the right, the left, the right, and so on—until you've completed the prescribed number of reps with each arm.

Variation: Half-Prone Front Shoulder Raise

In this variation, your palms face each other; otherwise, follow directions for standard Front Shoulder Raises.

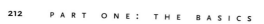

Variation: Front Shoulder Raises with Internal Shoulder Rotation

Perform these exercises as you would a standard Front Shoulder Raise but, as you're lifting your arms up, gradually twist them (movement originates at the shoulders) so your thumbs are nearly turned toward the floor at the top of the movement. Don't twist farther or faster than is comfortable.

Variation: Front Shoulder Raises with Palms Turned Out

In this variation, your palms are turned out (facing up as you lift, and away from your thighs); otherwise, follow directions for standard Front Shoulder Raises.

Variation: Front Shoulder Raises with Olympic Plate

In this variation of the standard Front Shoulder Raise, instead of holding dumbbells, you are holding a single Olympic plate between your hands (hold it with one hand on each side of the outer rim).

Delt Raise

Works back of shoulders.

● **Starting Position**

Lie prone (face down) on an incline bench that is positioned at about a 30-degree angle. Hold a dumbbell in each hand with your arms hanging straight down and your elbows slightly bent. Your neck should remain neutral.

● **Movement**

A. Exhale as you raise the dumbbells out to your sides, to shoulder height only.

B. Inhale as you slowly lower the dumbbells to the starting position.

Notes

Strive for controlled and even movements.

Raise your arms no higher than shoulder height.

Keep your wrists straight.

Keep your neck straight.

Keep your elbows only slightly bent (relaxed), not fully bent.

Variation: Standing Rear Delt Raise

This is an advanced way to perform the exercise, because your abdominal and erector muscles are stabilizing the trunk of your body. While performing the exercise, you lean forward at the waist at approximately a 30-degree angle. The movement is the same as on an incline bench.

Variation: Seated Rear Delt Raise

Sit on the end of a stable bench, feet placed on an elevated surface. Lean forward and rest your chest on the tops of your thighs; then follow the directions for the standard Delt Raise.

Press

Works top and front of shoulders.

- **Starting Position**

Sit on a bench with a back support. Place your feet flat on the floor. Hold the dumbbells in front of you, close to your body; they'll be level with your mouth. Your palms should be facing toward you.

- **Movement**

A. Exhale as you press both dumbbells up to arm's length, gradually turning them as you go so that at the top of the movement, your palms are facing away from you. Don't lock your elbows.

B. Slowly lower the weights to the starting position, gradually turning your palms back in as you do.

Notes

Strive for controlled and even movements.

Don't fully extend your arms.

Don't bring the weights together overhead.

Keep your feet flat on the floor.

 Biceps

Most people find the biceps the easiest muscles in the body to train, probably because biceps exercises match common everyday movements. Each time you pick up a bag of groceries, you're essentially doing a biceps curl. Consequently, out of all the upper-body muscles, biceps are the muscles that are usually the least atrophied in sedentary people.

Biceps are also fun to train. During a workout, your biceps are always in full view; thus you're able to instantly see what you're doing right or wrong and make corrections accordingly. Biceps exercises don't require as much knowledge of body mechanics as do other exercises (e.g., squats). That, of course, makes them much easier to perform.

Biceps development brought on by everyday activities can eventually increase the likelihood of elbow problems. That's because the other muscles in the upper arm, the triceps, are not built up as much by everyday

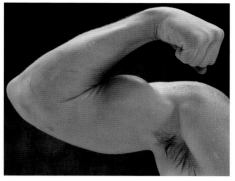

movements. In order for the triceps to contract (work), you have to straighten out your elbow against resistance, which is not a move we often make in everyday life. If you're training your biceps with weights, this imbalance can be amplified, and it's especially important to include a triceps workout in your program too.

The concept of "following the carrying angle" applies to biceps exercises in particular. It means that at the beginning and end of each repetition, the shoulder, elbow, and wrist are in a plumb line to the floor. Following the carrying angle will maximize the effort (and the benefit) of each repetition.

All the biceps exercises in this book involve only one movement, with the exception of one hammer curl variation. You'll start and finish each exercise either with the palms facing up (forward), or with the palms in a half-prone position, facing in toward the body. Exercises done in the half-prone position emphasize the strength of the biceps and are a valuable part of your program. However, less muscle is involved in half-prone exercises, so combining the two positions in one exercise may compromise results. Do one exercise at a time, and don't rotate your hands while performing the exercise, except when performing hammer curls.

Hammer Curl

Works front of upper arm.

● Starting Position
Stand with your knees relaxed, pelvis tucked in, shoulders dropped, chin level, and feet approximately shoulder-width apart. Hold a dumbbell in each hand with your palms turned in toward your body.

● Movement
A. Exhale and flex (bend) your elbows as you bring the dumbbells about three-quarters of the way up toward your shoulders.

B. Inhale as you return to the starting position.

Preacher Curl

Works front of upper arm.

• Starting Position

Sit on the preacher bench with both arms hanging over the top of the arm pad. Hold your hands shoulder-width apart. Your elbows should be slightly bent.

If you have weak wrists, use a specialized curl bar. Otherwise, the straight bar is preferable, because using a straight bar increases the contraction of the biceps.

• Movement

A. Exhale and bend your elbows as you bring the bar up, until your forearms are perpendicular to the floor.

B. Inhale as you return to the starting position. Be careful to keep your elbows slightly bent.

Notes

Keep your wrists straight.

Keep your elbows bent at the bottom of the movement.

Strive to use slow, controlled movements.

Keep your arms parallel to each other on the preacher pad.

Stop when your forearms are perpendicular to the floor (at peak contraction) for maximum benefit.

Variation: One–Arm Preacher Curl (with dumbbell)

Preacher curls can be performed with dumbbells too. The movement is exactly the same. In this variation, hang just one arm over the preacher pad at a time. Alternate sets—a full set with the right arm, then a full set with the left arm, and so on.

Variation: Hammer Curls

Hammer curls can also be done on a preacher bench. Keep your palms turned in (facing to the side) throughout the exercise unless performing the advanced variation.

Concentration Curl

Works front of upper arm.

• Starting Position

Sit on the edge of a bench, both feet planted firmly on the floor, knees open wide. With your right hand, hold a dumbbell between your legs at arm's length, with the back of your upper right arm resting against your inner right thigh, near your knee. You will be leaning slightly forward.

- **Movement**

A. Exhale and curl the dumbbell up by bending your elbow until the dumbbell is three-quarters of the way to your shoulder.

B. Inhale as you slowly lower the weight to the starting position.

Notes

Don't bend your wrists.

Keep the upper portion of your working arm vertical.

Variation

Perform Concentration Curls holding the dumbbell in a hammer curl position. Advanced exercisers may use the rotating position described in the Hammer Curl variation.

Pulley Cable Curl

Works front of upper arms.

- **Starting Position**

Grasp a cable handle in each hand, palms facing up. Center yourself in between the two pulleys. Lift both arms until they're even with your shoulders. Drop your shoulder blades. Bend your elbows slightly. Stand with a straight back and drop your knees.

- **Movement**

A. Exhale and bend your elbows, bringing the handles about three-quarters of the way in and down toward your shoulders.

B. Inhale and slowly return to the starting position.

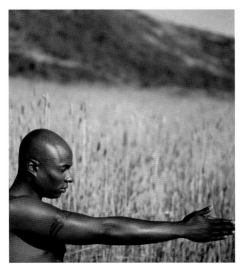

Notes

Keep your wrists straight.

Keep your shoulder blades dropped.

Stop at three-quarters of the way in, at peak contraction, for maximum benefit.

Don't lean forward at your waist.

Strive for controlled and even movements.

Low-Pulley Cable Curl

Works front of upper arms.

• Starting Position

Hold the cable bar in both hands. Extend your arms straight down from your shoulders. Your elbows should be slightly bent, your back straight, and your knees dropped slightly.

• Movement

A. Exhale as you bend your elbows, bringing the bar about three-quarters of the way up toward your shoulders.

B. Inhale and slowly lower the bar back to the starting position.

Notes

Keep your wrists straight.

Don't lean backward.

Strive for controlled and even movements.

Stop three-quarters of the way up, at peak contraction, for maximum benefit.

 ## Triceps

The most important thing to keep in mind when performing triceps exercises is not to lock your elbows. The safest grip when doing triceps work with dumbbells is a half-prone position with your palms faced in toward your body. This position also presents a mechanical advantage that may lead to quicker muscle development.

Black Eye (French Press)

Works back of upper arm.

• Starting Position

Lie back on a flat bench, feet flat on the floor or on the bench. Beginners, hold a dumbbell in your right hand with your arm extended toward the ceiling. Use your left hand to support your upper right arm, near the elbow. Do not lock your right elbow.

• Movement

A. Inhale as you slowly lower the dumbbell to your shoulder, keeping your elbow pointed toward the ceiling.

B. Exhale as you lift the dumbbell back up to the starting position.

C. Perform one complete set, then switch hands and repeat.

Notes

Strive for controlled and even movements.

Don't lock your elbow as you lift up the dumbbell.

Don't allow your working arm to move; keep your elbow pointed toward the ceiling.

Variations

Perform the Black Eye as above, but with both arms at once. This variation is the more advanced version because you give up the support of the other arm.

Perform the exercise using a barbell. Hold the bar with your hands shoulder-width apart. Lower the bar to just above your forehead.

Overhead Extension

Works the back of upper arms.

● **Starting Position**

Sit on a bench with a back support. Hold a single dumbbell with both hands in a vertical position over your head, palms up and thumbs wrapped around the handle. Keep your upper arms close to your head, with your elbows pointing toward the ceiling. Extend your arms, but be sure not to lock your elbows.

● **Movement**

A. Inhale as you bend your arms at the elbows so that the dumbbell is slowly lowered behind your neck.

B. Exhale as you straighten your arms and lift the dumbbell back up to the starting position.

Notes

Keep your back straight.

Strive for controlled and even movements.

Don't bounce the dumbbell off your traps as you lower the weight.

Reverse-Grip Bench Press

Works the back of upper arms.

● **Starting Position**

Lie flat on a bench-press rack. Position your body as you would if you were doing a bench press. Grip the bar as if you were doing a biceps curl, palms facing up. Your grip should be just as wide as your rib cage.

• Movement

A. Inhale as you lower the bar down toward your lower rib cage.

B. Exhale as you press the bar back up to the starting position.

Kickback

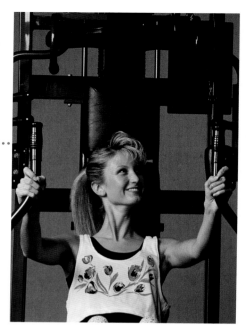

Works the back of upper arms.

• Starting Position

Lean forward, supporting your weight by resting your right hand on a bench; do not lock your right elbow. Make sure your back and neck are straight and your abs contracted. Hold a dumbbell in your left hand, then lift your upper arm so it's parallel to the floor. Your elbow should be bent so the weight is just below your shoulder.

• Movement

A. Exhale as you press the dumbbell back until your entire arm is parallel to the floor.

B. Inhale as you return the weight to the starting position.

Notes

Keep your working elbow lifted and close to your body.

Strive for controlled and even movements.

Keep the elbow of your supporting arm slightly bent.

Straight-Arm Kickback

Works top portion of back of upper arms.

• Starting Position

Stand with a bench at your side and lean forward, resting one hand on the bench and holding a dumbbell in the other hand. Neither elbow is locked. Keep your back straight. The arm holding the dumbbell should be extended down toward the floor.

- **Movement**

A. Exhale as you raise the dumbbell up until your entire arm is parallel to the floor. Don't bend your elbow; the lifting arm should remain straight.

B. Inhale as you return to the starting position.

Note

Strive for controlled and even movements; don't swing the dumbbell.

Straight-Arm Cable Press

Works top portion of back of upper arms.

- **Starting Position**

Stand in front of a bar used for lat pulls, with your arms fully extended at shoulder level. Grip the bar with your palms facing downward.

- **Movement**

A. Exhale as you press the bar down toward your legs.

B. Inhale as you slowly allow the bar to return to the starting position. Don't allow the bar to go any higher than shoulder level.

Cable Rope Pull

Works outer portion of back of upper arms.

- **Starting Position**

Stand in front of the rope. Grip the rope ends with your palms facing down toward the floor. Your elbows should be by the sides of your body.

- **Movement**

A. Exhale as you press the rope down by straightening out your arms, spreading your hands as you do so. Don't lock your elbows.

B. Inhale as you allow the rope to return to the starting position. Keep your elbows by your sides throughout the exercise.

Notes

Strive for controlled and even movements.

Don't allow your elbows to lift; keep them by your sides.

Don't lock your elbows during the rope press.

Variation

This exercise can also be done with the curved (W-shaped) bar.

✳ Calves

Calf training is an integral, but often omitted, part of any workout regimen. It's important to keep the calf muscles strong because these muscles help stabilize the ankles and knees. If you have strong calf muscles you'll be less likely to develop knee and ankle problems and you'll be at less risk for ankle and knee injury. From the point of view of body shaping, your calves are also one of the most visible parts of your body if you ever wear shorts, dresses, or skirts.

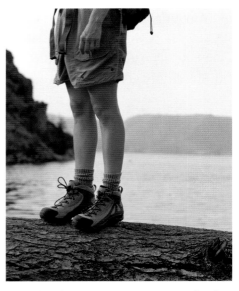

Each time you exercise your calf muscles, be sure to press your heels down as far as possible and lift your heels up as high as you can (the whole time keeping the balls of your feet on the foot pad). By doing this, you're making sure the entire length of the muscle is being worked. Also, keep your back straight when performing standing calf raises, and never bend your knees when doing calf exercises of any kind.

Contrary to popular belief, it's not necessary to turn your feet in or out to target specific areas of the calf muscles. These turned positions place a lot of stress on the knees unless you also externally rotate the hips out as you turn your feet out, and internally rotate the hips in as you turn your feet in. A safer, easier way to target specific parts of the calf is to keep your feet pointing straight ahead and either transfer the greater part of your weight to the inside of each foot, focusing on the area around the big toe (this replaces the turned-in position and emphasizes the inner calf), or transfer the greater part of your weight to the outside of each foot, focusing on the area around the baby toe (this replaces the turned-out position and emphasizes the outer calf). If you want to focus on the center of the big calf muscle (gastrocnemius), distribute your weight evenly across the ball of each foot.

No matter where you concentrate your weights, the balls of your feet always remain flat on the foot pad; some of the weight is merely transferred from side to side (or distributed evenly). Also, the ankles are never tilted in or out; they remain straight throughout the entire exercise, no matter where the focus is placed.

Standing Calf Raise

Works the back of lower legs.

● Starting Position

Follow the directions on the gym equipment. Make sure the shoulder pads are high enough so you can perform your calf exercises with your knees and back straight. Distribute the weight on your feet in one of the three ways described in the introductory part of this section.

● Movement

A. Exhale as you lift your heels up as high as you're able.

B. Inhale as you slowly lower your heels down as far as you can.

Notes

Keep the balls of your feet in place.

Strive for controlled and even movements.

Perform at least one set with each of the three weight distributions.

Keep your back and knees straight throughout the exercise.

Keep your hips stable; don't move them back and forth.

Variation: Standing Dumbbell Calf Raise

Stand with the ball of your right foot on an elevated surface. Wrap your left ankle around your right. Hold a dumbbell in your right hand; balance with your left hand. Perform the calf raises as described above. Then switch legs. Perform at least one set with each of the three weight distributions.

Seated Calf Raise

Works the back of lower legs.

● Starting Position

Follow the directions on the gym equipment. Distribute the weight on your feet in one of the three ways described in the introductory part of this section.

● Movement

A. Exhale as you lift your heels up as high as you're able.

B. Inhale as you slowly lower your heels down as far as you can.

Notes

Keep the balls of your feet in place.

Strive for controlled and even movements.

Perform at least one set with each of the three weight distributions.

Variation: Seated Dumbbell Calf Raises

Sit on a bench with the dumbbells on top of your legs, close to your knees. Place the balls of your feet on the edge of an elevated surface. Perform the Calf Raises as described above. Do at least one set with each of the three weight distributions.

Forearms and Wrists

Even though these exercises may seem unimportant, they're not. The wrists and forearms are often weak links in your body. If the forearm and wrist muscles aren't strong, this may inhibit your ability to work your larger muscle groups to full capacity. For example, weak forearms limit the amount of weight you can lift while doing lat (back) work, because they give out before the larger back muscles do.

Although the wrists and forearms must not be ignored, you needn't feel compelled to work them too often. Three or four sets a week should be enough to keep these muscles strong and in balance with the rest of your body.

Reverse Curl
. . . .

Works forearms.

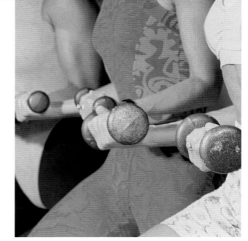

- **Starting Position**

Stand holding a set of dumbbells or a barbell in front of your thighs with your palms facing toward your legs.

- **Movement**

A. Exhale as you bend your elbows and lift up toward your shoulders.

B. Inhale and slowly return to the starting position.

Notes

Strive for controlled and even movements.

Keep your wrists straight throughout the entire exercise.

Keep your back straight.

Works muscles of wrists.

- **Starting Position**

Hold a set of dumbbells or a barbell, and sit on a bench resting your forearms on your thighs so that your wrists are on top of your knees, palms facing up.

- **Movement**

A. Exhale as you curl your wrists up as high as you can.

B. Inhale as you lower the weight so that the backs of your hands again touch the fronts of your knees, in the starting position.

Extension

Works muscles of wrists.

- **Starting Position**

Hold a set of dumbbells, or a barbell, and sit on a bench resting your forearms on your thighs so that your wrists are on top of your knees, palms facing down.

- **Movement**

A. Exhale as you curl your wrists up as high as you can.

B. Inhale as you lower the weight so that the palms of your hands face down and your knuckles touch the front of your knees.

Abdominals

Appearances aside, abdominal exercises are probably the most important exercises for your physical health. When these muscles are strong, they take some of the workload off the lower back; strong abs help to support the lower back, stabilize your body, and protect your back from injury. Moreover, firm, developed abdominals help to hold the internal organs in place, which in turn also takes pressure off the lower back area.

An effective abdominal program is crucial for maintaining erect posture and preventing lower back problems from occurring in the first place. Instead of doing 3 or 4 sets of 8 to 12 reps, as with most other exercises, we recommend you do fewer sets and work to muscle failure on each set. This method seems to be more effective at developing strong abdominal muscles.

For a beginner, muscle failure may occur after just 3 reps. That's okay. As time goes on and as your abs become stronger, that number will increase. If, on the other hand, muscle failure doesn't occur until 100 reps, it's time to increase the training stimulus. Abdominal muscles adapt to repeated training workloads, just as all muscle groups do.

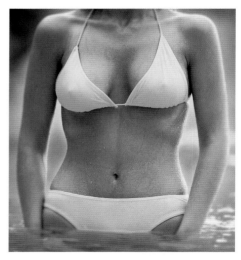

Once your abs are conditioned, you should progressively perform the more advanced exercises. The abdominal exercises in this book are arranged into categories of beginning, intermediate, and advanced exercises. Also, always vary your ab exercises so as to use a variety of movements. That way, you'll be sure to target the entire abdominal plate from a number of angles.

Contrary to popular myth and the advertising campaigns for some abdominal exercise gizmos, abdominal exercises will not help you lose the fat around your midsection. Fat is shed fairly evenly all over your body; you can't "spot reduce." Aerobic exercise (and avoiding fatty foods) will help get rid of the fat. It's also helpful to practice pulling your stomach (abdominals) in and down, as if you are squeezing them shut. Finally, here are two training tips that apply to all abdominal exercises:

- Always keep your knees bent when doing ab work, unless your legs are used in the performance of the exercise. Bent knees tilt the pelvis in such a way that there is less stress and strain on the lower back (erector) muscles and more on the abdominal muscles, where it's supposed to be.

- Imagine that your abdominal area is like the bellows of an accordion. When you're lifting your body (against gravity), always squeeze the bellows (abs) shut.

Sit-ups

• Starting Position
Lie on your back with knees bent and your feet flat on the floor. Place your hands behind your head with your elbows pulled back.

• Movement
A. Exhale as you contract your abdominal muscles and lift your tailbone up off the bench.

B. Inhale as you slowly lower your tailbone back down.

Notes

Don't lift your lower back off the bench, just your tailbone.

Keep your legs perpendicular to the floor.

Strive for controlled and even movements.

Squeeze your abs shut like an accordion as you lift.

Variation of Sit-ups

Beginners, do this exercise with your knees bent. Your thighs will still be pointing toward the ceiling.

● **Movement**

Press your upper body a little higher, then release, in short pulsing movements, exhaling each time you press up. Continue until you cannot do any more pulsing movements.

Notes

Keep your neck straight. Avoid the tendency to roll your head forward when you're pulsing up.

Keep your abs squeezed shut throughout the exercise.

Variation

If you are a beginner, do this exercise with your knees bent and your hands behind your head.

Curl-Up—Center

Works abdominals.

This is a beginning abdominal exercise, with variations for intermediate and advanced exercisers.

● **Starting Position**

Lie on your back with knees bent and your feet flat on the floor. Place your hands behind your head with your elbows pulled back.

● **Movement**

A. Exhale as you slowly lift your shoulders and upper back off the floor as high as you can.

B. Inhale as you slowly lower them down.

Variations

If you're an intermediate exerciser, perform this exercise with your legs bent and your feet off the floor or with your legs straddled over a bench.

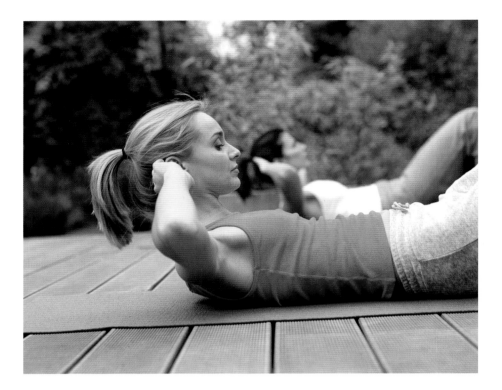

If you are advanced, perform this exercise with your legs pointing straight up toward the ceiling.

Notes

Keep your neck straight.

Keep your elbows pulled back.

Don't arch your back.

Squeeze your abs shut as you lift.

Side Curl-Up

Works abdominals and obliques.

This is an exercise designed for all levels of fitness. To increase the training stimulus, lift your body higher so your elbow comes closer to touching your knee.

• Starting Position

Lie on your back. Place your left hand behind your head and your right hand on the floor. Place the back of your right ankle on top of your left knee.

- **Movement**

A. Exhale as you lift your shoulders and upper back as high as you can, pressing your left elbow toward your right knee.

B. Inhale as you slowly lower your back down.

C. Perform a full set, then reverse positions and repeat steps A and B.

Notes

Strive for controlled and even movements.

Don't arch your back.

Squeeze your abs shut as you lift.

Trunk Curl / Pelvic Tilt Combination

Works abdominals.

This is an intermediate to advanced abdominal exercise.

- **Starting Position**

Lie on your back with your knees bent and your feet flat on the floor. Place your hands behind your head.

- **Movement**

A. Exhale and tilt your pelvis up at the same time that you slowly curl your upper back off the floor.

B. Inhale and slowly lower your entire body back down.

Notes

Strive for controlled and even movements.

Don't lift your lower back off the floor. Stop as soon as your hips are tilted up.

Squeeze your abs shut as you lift.

Knee-Up

Works hip flexors.

This is an advanced abdominal exercise with a super-advanced variation.

- **Starting Position**

Hang by your hands from a bar or rings, with your thighs at a right angle to your chest.

- **Movement**

A. Exhale as you slowly pull your knees up toward your chest, allowing your pelvis to roll upward.

B. Inhale and slowly lower your pelvis and legs back to the starting position.

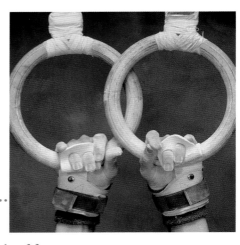

Notes

Don't allow your body to swing.

Strive for controlled and even movements.

Variation

Perform this exercise with your legs straight, or nearly straight, as you become more advanced.

Bar Twist

Works waistline and lower back muscles.

Bar twists are effective for all levels of fitness.

- **Starting Position**

Sit on the edge of a bench with a bar resting across your upper traps in back of your neck. The weight of the bar is dependent on your level of fitness and physical ability.

- **Movement**

Twist your entire upper body from side to side. Breathe normally.

Notes

Twist as far as you can.

Allow your head to turn naturally along with your torso; all movement originates at your waistline. Avoid the tendency to lead with your head.

Don't stop or hesitate as you turn toward the front.

If you're a beginner, use a wooden pole in place of a weighted bar.

CHAPTER

7

Home Spa

To complement the changes in your figure and your mind-set, you will also want to work on your face, skin, hair, hands, and feet. The motivation behind the techniques and recipes presented in the *30-Day Revitalization Plan* is to reinvigorate your natural self. The best way to achieve that goal for your appearance is by cleaning up your face, skin, hair, hands, and feet because looking healthy and natural is the basis of looking good. It does not matter that your features may not be perfect. If your face and skin are radiant; if your hair has a natural glossy shine; and if your hands and feet are well-groomed and smooth, then you are guaranteed to look good.

Face

Because the skin on your face is more delicate than the skin on your body and also much more visible, it is extremely important to treat it with special care. The face often gives away a person's age, with problems ranging from acne in the oil-producing skin of young people to lines and wrinkles of those who have grown older and whose skin retains less moisture. Clear, refreshed, and well-nourished skin along with toned facial muscles is the key to looking your best.

Cleanse

Although ordinary soap removes dirt and kills bacteria that can clog pores, it dries out the skin, doesn't remove all makeup, and is generally too harsh for the face. So it is important to use a gentle cleanser on your face. The first step of your cleansing routine is to exfoliate with a scrub or special sponge. The exfoliating routine for the face, however, is far milder than that for the arms or legs because the skin is much more fragile. Exfoliating removes dry, flaky, excess skin cells that cloud your face and clog pores. If your skin is particularly sensitive and often very red after exfoliating, you can gently exfoliate once a day, preferably at night. After exfoliating, moisten your face with warm but not hot water. Apply a dime-size drop of cleanser to one hand and lather between both hands. Then gently rub both hands over your face in a gentle, upward, circular motion, but avoid rubbing the cleanser too close to your eyes. Rinse with warm water and pat dry with a facial towel, but be careful not to rub. Always use a clean towel to prevent the spread of bacteria.

◎ Walnut Scrub

1/4 cup plain yogurt
1/4 cup finely ground walnuts

Mix yogurt and almonds together. Apply the scrub to your moistened face. Rinse face with warm water and pat dry.

◎ Oatmeal Scrub

2 tablespoons ground oats
2 teaspoons brown sugar
2 tablespoons aloe vera
1 teaspoon lemon juice

Grind oat flakes to a fine powder in a blender or coffee grinder. Mix oats, sugar, aloe vera, and lemon juice to form a smooth paste. Massage onto damp skin. Rinse face with warm water and pat dry.

To use as a body scrub, triple the ingredients.

◎ Gentle Oatmeal Cleanser

1/2 cup oatmeal
Plain yogurt

Mix oatmeal and enough yogurt to form a paste. Apply to face with upward, circular strokes. Rinse face with warm water and pat dry. Refrigerate remaining cleanser for up to 1 week.

◎ Lemon Cleansing Cream

3 tablespoons witch hazel
6 tablespoons soft shortening (not margarine)
1 tablespoon lanolin
1 teaspoon lemon extract
2 drops yellow food coloring for a soothing yellow color

In a food processor or blender, mix witch hazel, shortening, lanolin, lemon extract, and food coloring on low speed until well blended. Increase speed to high, and mix until all ingredients are mashed. Saturate a cotton ball with the cream and apply to face in an upward, circular motion. Rinse face with warm water and pat dry.

◎ Facial Sauna

To further purify your skin and clean out your pores, try a facial sauna.
These formulas increase circulation to skin cells.

Heat a small pot of water. Pour the water into a large, heat-resistant bowl. Add one of the essential-oil combinations shown below, drape a towel over your head, lean forward, and close your eyes. Allow the vapors to come in contact with your face.

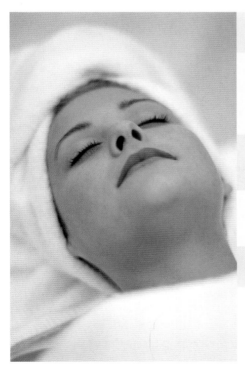

Frankincense	5 drops
Lemon	5 drops
Tangerine	4 drops
Copaiba	6 drops
Bois de Rose	5 drops
Grapefruit	5 drops
Lavender	6 drops
Tea Tree	3 drops
Peppermint	1 drop
Elemi	6 drops
Lime	4 drops
Sandalwood	5 drops
Tangerine	5 drops

Tone

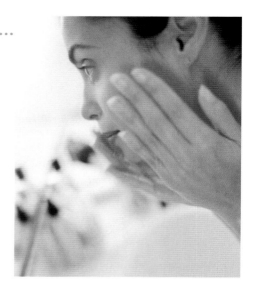

After cleansing your face, apply a toner or astringent to remove excess oil and grease, close your pores, and stimulate blood flow. To apply the toner to your face, saturate a cotton ball—to avoid spreading bacteria—with toner or astringent, and then gently rub on the face with upward, circular strokes.

◎ Rosewater Toner

3 1/2 cups witch hazel
1/2 cup dried rose petals
5 sprigs fresh rosemary

Mix witch hazel, rose petals, and rosemary. Blend well. Strain. Apply strained mixture to face with upward, circular strokes. Rinse face with warm water and pat dry.

◎ Strawberry Refresher

2 tablespoons rubbing alcohol
1/2 cup fresh strawberries
3 tablespoons petroleum jelly
2 drops spirit of camphor

In a food processor or blender, mix all ingredients on high until smooth and creamy. Saturate a cotton ball with the refresher and apply to face. After 20 minutes, remove by rinsing face with warm water. Store remaining mixture in refrigerator for up to one week.

◎ Fresh 'n' Cool Skin Freshener

2/3 cup water
2 tablespoons rubbing alcohol (70%)
3/4 teaspoon borax powder
1 drop green food coloring (optional)
3 drops perfume or cologne
    (optional)

In a food processor or blender, mix water, rubbing alcohol, borax, food coloring, and perfume, if desired, on high until borax is dissolved. Refrigerate mixture until icy cool. After cleansing face, saturate a cotton ball with freshener and apply by patting on face and neck. Rinse face with warm water and pat dry. Store remaining freshener in refrigerator for up to one week.

Moisturize

Even if your skin is oily, you still need to moisturize in order to protect skin cells and replenish lost water and broken barriers. Choose an over-the-counter moisturizer that is most appropriate for your skin type. Are you dry or oily? Neither (normal) or both (combination)? Generally for the face, noncomedogenic moisturizers are best, because they are more delicate and are made without the oils that tend to clog pores. Moisturizers that are fruit or milk-based contain alpha-hydroxy acids, which are great for reducing fine lines and dry skin but can be harsh on sensitive skin. As with your cleanser and toner, you should apply moisturizer to your face in circular, upward strokes.

To protect your skin from sun exposure, which hastens wrinkling, always use a moisturizer with an SPF of at least 15.

◎ Cold Cream

Use this luscious cold cream every night before bed.

4 ounces white beeswax
2 cups almond oil
1¹/₂ teaspoons borax
5 ounces rose water
Red food coloring (optional)

Melt the beeswax. Add the almond oil to the melted beeswax. In a separate pan, heat the borax and rose water, but do not boil. Add the borax and rose water to the beeswax mixture. Stir constantly until cooled to prevent lumps. Add food coloring to make pink. Apply cream to face. Blot with tissues. Reapply and blot again until skin is clean. Store remaining cream in refrigerator for up to one week.

Facial Masks

To bring the luxurious feel of a spa closer to home with the beneficial bonus of even softer facial skin, facial masks are the perfect option. When applying your mask, be sure to work around your hairline, eyes, mouth, and nostrils.

◎ Carrot and Honey Mask

2–3 large carrots
4¹/₂ tablespoons honey

Peel carrots and then steam. Mash. Mix carrots and honey. Apply mask to face. After 10 minutes, rinse face with cool water and pat dry.

◎ Peaches-and-Cream Complexion Mask

1 medium peach
1 tablespoon honey
Oatmeal

Cook peach until soft. Mash. Mix peach with honey and enough oatmeal into a thick paste. Apply to skin. After 10 minutes, rinse face with cool water and pat dry.

◎ Almond Meal Cleansing Mask

1/2 cup blanched almonds
1/2 teaspoon honey
Milk

Chop almonds in a blender until they are a fine meal. Place 1 tablespoon of almond meal in bowl. Store remaining meal. Add the honey and enough milk to form a thick paste. Apply to entire face until smooth. After 10 minutes, remove with warm water and pat face dry.

◎ Cucumber-Egg Mask

1/2 cup unpeeled cucumber pieces
1 egg white
1 tablespoon dry milk

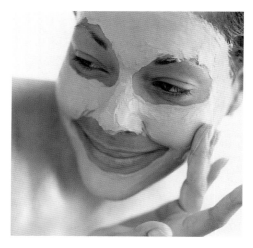

In a blender or food processor, blend cucumber, egg white, and dry milk at high speed until smooth. Saturate a cotton ball with mixture and apply to entire face. After 30 minutes, remove mask with warm water and pat face dry.

◎ Minty-Meal Cleansing Mask

4 tablespoons oatmeal
1 teaspoon dried mint leaves
Hot water

In a food processor or blender, mix oatmeal and mint leaves on high until finely ground. Add enough hot water to make a spreadable paste. Apply mask by gently patting and smoothing mixture onto face. After mask has dried, remove with warm water. Then rinse face with cool water and pat dry.

◎ Lemon and Honey Face Mask

1 fresh egg yolk
1 teaspoon olive oil
3–4 drops lemon juice
1/4 teaspoon honey
1/2 teaspoon plain, uncooked oatmeal
1/2 teaspoon powdered milk
1/2 teaspoon powdered laundry starch

Mix egg yolk, olive oil, lemon juice, honey, oatmeal, milk, and laundry starch until creamy. Smooth over face in upward circular strokes with fingertips. After 15 minutes (10 minutes for dry skin, 20 minutes for oily skin), rinse face with warm water, then splash face with cold water. Pat face dry.

◎ Face Mask for Balancing Oily Skin

1 tablespoon powdered brewer's yeast
Witch hazel or rose water

Mix yeast with enough witch hazel or rose water to make a semi-stiff paste. Apply to clean face with fingertips. After mask dries, remove with warm water, then splash face with cold water. Pat face dry.

◎ Face Mask for Improving Skin Texture

2 teaspoons dried milk powder
1 teaspoon cold water
1 teaspoon almond oil (optional, but recommended for dry, flaky skin)

Mix milk powder, cold water, and almond oil, if desired, until creamy. Apply cream with fingertips in a circular upward motion to clean face. After mask dries, rinse face with warm water.

◎ Face Pack for Normal, Dry, or Sensitive Skin

2 tablespoons brown rice
5 1/2 tablespoons coarse oatmeal
1/2 teaspoon chamomile flowers
White of 1 small egg
1 teaspoon honey
3 drops lemon juice

Bring brown rice, oatmeal, chamomile flowers, and just enough water to cover to a boil. Reduce heat and simmer until cooked. Rub mixture through a sieve and discard residue. To the smooth paste that will result, add egg white, honey, and lemon juice. Apply to face and let dry. After 15 to 20 minutes, rinse face with warm water. Refrigerate remaining paste for up to one week.

Night and Eye Creams

While the skin of the face is much more delicate than the skin of the body, the skin underneath the eyes is even more fragile. The skin under the eyes is extremely thin, often exposing underlying veins as dark circles, and needs its own special attention. To lock in moisture and help in the fight to reduce fine lines and wrinkles, night and eye creams can be very beneficial. Night creams tend to be heavier and oilier than ordinary facial moisturizers, so they might look out of place during the day and will cause makeup to smear. Night and eye creams work wonders on rejuvenating your face while you sleep because day-to-day interferences, such as dirt, dust, and human touch, are less likely to disrupt the creams from working their magic.

◎ Strawberry Night Cream

1/2 cup crushed strawberries
Almond oil or glycerine

Mix strawberries and almond oil or glycerine to create a smooth cream. Before bed, apply to face with circular, upward strokes. Rinse off in the morning with warm water.

◎ Strawberry Facial Cream

1 egg yolk
1 tablespoon wheat germ
2 teaspoons lemon juice
1/3 cup fresh strawberries
1/3 cup vegetable oil

In a food processor or blender, mix egg yolk, wheat germ, lemon juice, and strawberries on high until liquefied. Slowly add vegetable oil. Blend until mixture is creamy. Apply to face with upward, circular strokes. In the morning, rinse face with warm water and pat dry.

Face Toning

Two anatomical structures supply the basic support for facial beauty: One is the facial musculature; the other is the subcutaneous tissue directly under the surface of the skin, which provides the skin with its elasticity. Facial muscles and facial skin are closely connected, which is why the skin is able to follow every movement of the muscles. But it is precisely this close connection that causes the condition and structure of the muscles to have such an impact on how we look. The muscle structures' loss of strength is bound to affect the skin.

And the same holds true for the second facial structure: the tissue that gives the skin its elasticity and its smooth, youthful, and wrinkle-free appear-

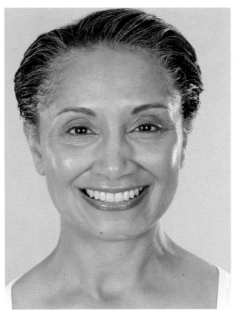

ance. Skin loses its elasticity whenever tissue fiber begins to atrophy (that is, when tissue fiber is reduced in volume).

This is precisely what happens during the aging process—muscle and tissue fiber literally decrease. The facial musculature and the subcutaneous tissue lose tone and volume.

This aging process, however, can be slowed down considerably if a training and exercise program specifically geared to the facial muscles is instituted. This means that, by undertaking a sensible exercise program of the facial musculature, you can slow down the aging process, and already existing "weak spots" can be totally—or in part—regenerated.

Musculature and tissue increases in volume and tone when exercised. Face building is accomplished with a systematic training program, specifically designed to exercise facial musculature. It is important that you complete these exercises correctly and that you adhere to the program as described. In other words, make sure that each step is performed with great care and attention.

Logic tells us that the aging process of the face can be slowed down and that damage due to deterioration can be reversed, either wholly or at least in part, because we have been successful in doing that—and for a long time—with our bodies.

The exercises that follow will effectively return weak muscles—that have turned into something resembling overstretched rubber bands—to a healthy, well-toned condition. As a matter of fact, the exercises will prevent healthy muscles from getting into such a sorry state.

In the course of the exercises, the skin that covers the facial musculature is gently stretched; this happens naturally in reaction to the movement of the muscles.

This gentle stretching is a physiological process that will, in effect, increase and regenerate the production of collagen and elastin, two substances that are important for the elasticity of the skin.

Everyday, automatic movements of facial muscles are not sufficient to keep the elasticity of the muscle fibers in good, firm, youthful condition. If the face is allowed to remain "unmoved," which is the natural state of affairs, muscles and tissues begin to atrophy, and the result is loose, wrinkled skin that has taken on a "wilted" look.

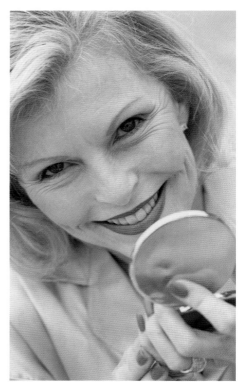

Daily 5- or 10-minute exercises, however, have an almost miraculous effect. After only 2 or 3 months, you will be admired for your youthful, beautiful, clear, firm skin and the well-defined contours of your face. Naturally, face-building exercises can also considerably postpone—and even reverse—the aging process of the skin. With these exercises, it is not uncommon to be able to turn back the clock by as much as 10 to 15 years.

The facial exercises have another benefit: they increase blood circulation to the face, which in turn permits more oxygen and more nutrients to reach the cells of the skin. This increased circulation considerably aids the all-important cleansing process and enhances the skin's ability to absorb moisture.

An increased internal availability of oxygen and good nutrition, with a simultaneous increase in effective cleansing of the tissues, is a sure guarantee for clear, healthy skin without the unsightly enlargement of pores.

Face-building has three main benefits. Loose skin is "lifted": The skin regains a youthful, firm appearance. The elasticity of the skin is improved: The skin is able to cover the musculature firmly and tightly and thereby smooth out those much-feared wrinkles and crow's-feet. The skin is better nourished, with the pores unclogged, and better able to absorb moisture; the fiber of the connective tissues is increased and strengthened. The skin will be firmer, large pores will be decreased, and the skin will regain a rosy, healthy, and firm appearance.

All are advantages that no one wants to miss.

Stand or sit in front of a mirror. Try to do the exercises as accurately as you can. Visualize the muscle. It might be helpful to put your fingers on the muscle so that you can "feel" in which direction the muscle fibers are moving and when a muscle is exercised. Every exercise should be performed with every ounce of energy that you can muster. The maximum tension should be held for at least 6 seconds.

In the beginning, when the musculature is rather weak and loose, the maximum tension that you can create will not be very strong. The force of tension will increase, however, from week to week.

The exercises have to be done regularly, at least five times a week. For the first 2 weeks, do each exercise five times. After 2 weeks, increase the number of repetitions for each exercise by 5. Increase the number of repetitions by 5 more for each of the next 2 weeks until you are completing 20 repetitions for each exercise.

Training will be at its most effective when you have reached 20 repetitions for each exercise, with no more than a 1-second interval between repetitions. Every repetition must be executed with the maximum force. Also, you do not need to pause between exercises. You should not need more than 5 to 10 minutes for five to six exercises.

Visible changes can be expected after 2 or 3 months. Do not, therefore, expect miracles after 2 weeks. We know from various training programs for the body that it takes time to regenerate and rebuild the musculature.

It is important that you continue with your program once a satisfactory result has been obtained, but for maintenance, no more than two to three times a week is necessary.

Placing your fingers over the region to be exercised eliminates the possibility of creating artificial folds or wrinkles. Your fingers should touch the skin only lightly, and under no circumstances should the skin be stretched or pulled.

There are exercises that do not require the aid of fingers, but if a fold or wrinkle seems to increase when you are doing that particular exercise, place one finger on the fold anyway. This little trick will prevent artificial folds from being created.

◎ **Forehead**

For a beautiful forehead, work the eyebrow (musculus frontalis), which lifts the eyebrows and pulls the scalp forward. This action creates the wrinkles on the forehead.

1. Put your fingers across your forehead so that both ring fingers rest comfortably across your eyebrows. Now try, against the pressure of your fingers, to lift your eyebrows and to pull the scalp forward.

2. Hold at the maximum tension for 6 seconds.

3. Release, then repeat four more times.

◎ **Frown lines**

You won't need Botox® if you do this exercise. At the nose and forehead region, where frown lines tend to form, flex the muscle between the nasal and frontal bone (musculus corrugator glabellae), which causes a vertical fold at the top of the nose.

1. Pull your eyebrows tightly together. Avoid the formation of a crease between your eyebrows by pressing with both index fingers lightly above the skin of both eyebrows.

2. Hold at the maximum tension for 6 seconds.

3. Release, then repeat four more times.

◎ **Crow's-feet**

To banish crow's-feet, exercise the area at the frontal bone and frontal–maxillary extension of the upper jaw to the ligaments of the inner lid (musculus orbicularis occuli). This muscle closes the eye and pulls the eyebrow down. Also, it pulls the skin around the eye towards the middle, creating crow's-feet.

1. Position your fingers at the outer edge of the orbital cavity and close your eyes. The fingers are automatically pulled toward the middle of your face. Do not work against the movement of the muscle.

2. Hold at the maximum tension for 6 seconds.

3. Release and repeat four more times.

◎ **Nose to Cheek**

For a beautiful blending from nose to cheek, work the muscle at the inner and outer rim of the orbital cavity (musculus levator labii superioris), whose function is to raise the upper lip.

1. Flare your nostrils while wrinkling your nose. To prevent folds from forming, position your index or middle finger from the inside of your eyes down to the corners of your mouth. The finger pressure will prevent the muscle from moving and thereby create an isometric form of exercise.

2. Hold at the maximum tension for 6 seconds.

3. Release and repeat four more times.

◎ Upper Cheek

For a firm upper cheek and upward-pointing corners of the mouth, flex the muscle at the side of the cheekbone (musculus zygomaticus mayor), which lifts the corners of the mouth to smile.

1. Pull the corners of your mouth up toward your outer cheekbones (as if laughing out loud). In order not to create folds and wrinkles, put your index fingers next to the orbital cavity and slightly touch the labial–nasal fold.

2. Hold at the maximum tension for 6 seconds.

3. Release and repeat four more times.

◎ Chin and Neck

To firm up the area of your chin and neck, exercise the muscle at the lower jaw and the corners of the mouth (musculus platysma), which will tighten the skin at your neck.

1. Tense the musculus platysma. This exercise is greatly supported if you forcefully pull down your lower lip. When this exercise is correctly executed, the neck muscle will be clearly visible.

2. Hold at the maximum tension for 6 seconds.

3. Release and repeat four more times.

Skin/Body

Our remarkable skin is perhaps the most resilient organ of the body. An extraordinary protector and our first line of defense against the assault of the outside world, it can endure harsh weather and a variety of environmental conditions yet can be sensitive and gentle enough to respond to a kind and loving touch.

Covering every inch of our outer body, the skin also performs many other vital functions. Operating as a thermostat, it helps regulate body temperature by conveying signals to the brain via nerve cells. And when healthy, the skin helps the body eliminate about 25 percent of its waste through perspiration.

Often referred to as a mirror of health, the skin is a reflection of the inner condition of the body and the showcase to the world. Closely related to our emotions, it turns pale when we are ill or stressed and is radiant and glowing when we are healthy and happy. Fortunately for us, the skin continually replenishes itself, creating millions of new cells each day.

From before we are born to the end of our life, our skin is always there to protect us.

Baths

Besides being necessary for hygiene, baths are beneficial for good health. The bath formulas that follow help moisturize and scent the skin as well as relax you and restore your energy. Relax and enjoy your bath for no more than 30 minutes; otherwise, your skin will become dehydrated. Always follow a bath with moisturizer to replenish lost nutrients and to seal the skin.

◎ Milk Bath

This delicate blend leaves your skin gently scented and feeling like silk.

Blanched or slivered almonds, enough to make 1/3 cup almond meal
3 cups powdered milk
1/4 cup oatmeal
1/4 cup dried orris root (has a soft violet scent)
1 capsule vitamin E (break open into dry ingredients)
1/3 cup cornstarch

In a blender, food processor, or coffee grinder, grind blanched or slivered almonds to a fine powder. Combine almond meal with powdered milk, oatmeal, orris root, vitamin E, and cornstarch until thoroughly mixed. Scoop 1/2 cup to 1 cup onto a small sheet of muslin or even a face cloth. Pull up the edges of the fabric and tie securely with a piece of string to form a bag. Attach bag to the bathtub faucet, allowing warm water to run over the bag. Store remaining mixture in an airtight container for your next several baths.

Aromatherapy Baths

Fill the bathtub with water as warm as you like. Add one of the formulas listed opposite, dispersing the oils evenly throughout the water. Enter the bath immediately, because the essential oils evaporate quickly.

Lavender . . . . 5 drops	Bois de Rose . . . . 7 drops
Bois de Rose . . . . 5 drops	Patchouli . . . . 4 drops
Vanilla . . . . 5 drops	Litsea Cubeba . . . . . . 4 drops
Carrier Oil . . . . 1 teaspoon	Carrier Oil . . . . 1 teaspoon

Palmarosa . . . . 5 drops	Sandalwood . . . . 7 drops
Mandarin . . . . 5 drops	Mandarin . . . . 5 drops
Cedarwood (Atlas) . . . 5 drops	Frankincense . . . . 3 drops
Carrier Oil . . . . 1 teaspoon	Carrier Oil . . . . 1 teaspoon

Copaiba . . . . 6 drops	Guaiacwood . . . . 5 drops
Sandalwood . . . . 5 drops	Tangerine . . . . 5 drops
Geranium . . . . 4 drops	Copaiba . . . . 5 drops
Carrier Oil . . . . 1 teaspoon	Carrier Oil . . . . 1 teaspoon

For the Shower

If you don't have time to enjoy a long soak in the bathtub, these body cleansers and scrubs are fantastic for the shower.

◎ Refreshing Sea Salt Scrub

1/2 cup sea salt
Water

Mix salt and water until pasty. Rub onto your body before you shower. After 1 minute, rinse.

◎ Lavishly Smooth Shower Gel

1/2 cup unscented shampoo
1/4 cup water
3/4 teaspoon salt
15 drops fragrance oil (e.g., kiwi extract, raspberry extract, strawberry
extract, coconut extract, vanilla extract, almond extract)
food coloring (optional)

Pour shampoo into a bowl and add the water. Stir until well mixed; add the salt, fragrance, and food coloring, if desired. Mix and match scents, or use one alone.

Deodorant

These formulas will keep you smelling fresh. Apply 10 drops of aloe vera onto each underarm, then combine one of the formulas listed next and rub in well. Finish by patting on cornstarch to dry off any remaining residue.

Make sure to remove any excess oil with a tissue to prevent clothing from becoming stained. Women, after you shave your underarms, wait 15 minutes before applying the deodorant in order to avoid any burning sensation.

Chamomile (Roman) . . 2 drops
Vanilla . . . . 2 drops
Spikenard . . . . 2 drops

Spikenard . . . . 2 drops
Lavender . . . . 2 drops
Vanilla . . . . 2 drops

Skin Care Creams

The skin gets taken for granted because of its ability to recover on its own from the minor burns, bruises, cuts, scrapes, and scratches that we receive in the course of our daily life.

◎ Body Lotion

3 tablespoons sunflower oil
2 tablespoons almond oil
2 tablespoons peanut oil
1 tablespoon olive oil
1 tablespoon wheat germ oil
6 drops perfume (optional)

Mix all oils. Add perfume, if desired. For larger quantities, it's okay to double or triple the ingredients. Smooth onto skin with a circular motion; blot excess with a tissue or towel.

◎ Skin Nutrient

2 tablespoons lanolin
1 tablespoon petroleum jelly
1 cup witch hazel
Perfume (optional)

Put lanolin and petroleum jelly into a small container. Stand the container in hot water until both ingredients have melted. Separately heat the witch hazel. Slowly add witch hazel to lanolin and petroleum jelly, stirring constantly. Allow the preparation to cool, then add several drops of perfume, if desired. For dry skin, use 1/2 cup witch hazel and 2 tablespoons of petroleum jelly.

◎ Rosewater Body Rub for Elbows and Knees

1/4 cup lanolin
1/4 cup safflower oil
1/2 cup rose water
5 to 10 drops red food coloring (optional)

In a food processor or blender, mix lanolin and safflower oil on low until well blended. Slowly blend in rose water and food coloring on high speed. Use a spatula to keep ingredients around the blades.

◎ Wintergreen Body Rub

This body rub is very soothing for tired muscles.

1/4 cup lanolin
1/4 cup safflower oil
2 tablespoons wintergreen oil
1/2 cup water

In a food processor or blender, mix lanolin, safflower oil, and wintergreen oil on low until well blended. Slowly blend in water on high speed. Use spatula to keep mixture around the blades.

Body Butters

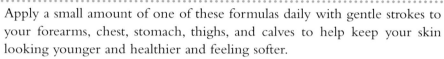

Apply a small amount of one of these formulas daily with gentle strokes to your forearms, chest, stomach, thighs, and calves to help keep your skin looking younger and healthier and feeling softer.

To prepare the formula, place the shea butter into a small, wide-mouthed glass jar. Put the jar into a small pot of water, and heat on a low flame. When the butter is melted, add the carrier oil, mix well, and remove from the heat. As the mixture cools, add the essential oils, and stir well.

Shea Butter . . . . 2 tablespoons Sesame . . . . 8 teaspoons Frankincense . . . . 20 drops Myrrh . . . . 8 drops Litsea Cubeba . . . . . . 7 drops	Shea Butter . . . . 2 tablespoons Sesame . . . . 8 teaspoons Ylang-Ylang . . . . 15 drops Myrrh . . . . 12 drops Orange . . . . 8 drops
Shea Butter . . . . 2 tablespoons Sesame . . . . 8 teaspoons Frankincense . . . . 12 drops Lemon . . . . 12 drops Patchouli . . . . 11 drops	Shea Butter . . . . 2 tablespoons Sesame . . . . 8 teaspoons Copaiba . . . . 15 drops Myrrh . . . . 11 drops Peppermint . . . . 9 drops
Shea Butter . . . . 2 tablespoons Sesame . . . . 8 teaspoons Sandalwood . . . . 15 drops Bois de Rose . . . . 10 drops Helichrysum . . . . 10 drops	Shea Butter . . . . 2 tablespoons Sesame . . . . 8 teaspoons Ylang-Ylang . . . . 15 drops Copaiba . . . . 10 drops Citronella . . . . 10 drops

Shea Butter	. . . . 2 tablespoons	Shea Butter	. . . . 2 tablespoons
Sesame	. . . . 8 teaspoons	Sesame	. . . . 8 teaspoons
Spearmint	. . . . 12 drops	Rosemary	. . . . 15 drops
Geranium	. . . . 12 drops	Elemi	. . . . 10 drops
Sandalwood	. . . . 11 drops	Bois de Rose	. . . . 10 drops

Shea Butter	. . . . 2 tablepoons	Shea Butter	. . . . 2 tablespoons
Sesame	. . . . 8 teaspoons	Sesame	. . . . 8 teaspoons
Lavender	. . . . 20 drops	Peru Balsam	. . . . 20 drops
Rose	. . . . 15 drops	Peppermint	. . . . 15 drops

Hair

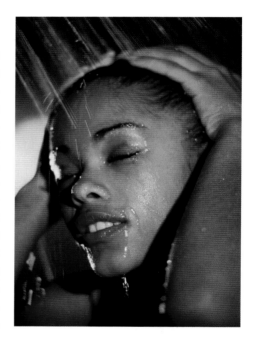

One of the first things we notice when we look at a person is the person's hair. Hair not only accentuates the appearance, it insulates the head from temperature variations, acts as a cushion to protect the skull, allows sweat to evaporate, and acts as a sensor when touched.

Each hair grows inside a tube-like follicle and at the base of each follicle is a hair bulb. This bulb is full of blood vessels that deliver oxygen and nourishment to the hair's root. The cells inside the bulb are alive. As they die, they are pushed upward to form the visible hair on the head.

Because the hair's appearance is determined by the condition of health inside the hair bulbs, your nutritional intake, circulatory system, and care of your scalp play important roles. Under the scalp are blood vessels, nerve endings, sebaceous glands, sweat glands, and a subcutaneous layer of fat cells. The sebaceous glands surround about half of each hair follicle. Their purpose is to lubricate the hair and scalp with an oily secretion called sebum. The sebaceous glands become more active during times of stress, physical activity, or alcohol consumption. For beautiful, healthy hair, treat yourself to these luxurious homemade shampoos, conditioners, and hot oil treatments.

Shampoos

As you shampoo, use your fingers to massage the shampoo into your scalp to cleanse and invigorate your hair from the roots to the tips. Rinse thoroughly, leaving behind no shampoo residue.

◎ Rosemary Chamomile Shampoo

1 1/2 cups boiling water
4 bags of chamomile tea
4 tablespoons pure soap flakes
1 1/2 tablespoons glycerin
5 drops of rosemary essential oil

Add boiling water to the teabags and let steep for 10 minutes. Remove the tea bags and add the soap flakes to the liquid. When the soap softens, stir in glycerin and rosemary essential oil until well mixed. Transfer mixture to a container and store in a cool, dark place.

◎ Lavender Ylang-Ylang Shampoo

3 1/2 ounces shampoo base
10 drops lavender essential oil
5 drops ylang-ylang essential oil

Thoroughly mix shampoo base and essential oils together. Transfer mixture to a container and store in a cool, dark place.

◎ Nettle Hair Tonic

3 cups water
1 handful stinging nettles

Boil water and nettles. Allow to cool in a screw-top bottle. Apply to towel-dried hair after shampooing.

Conditioners

If you have dry hair, you may want to work the conditioners through your hair completely; otherwise, just apply conditioner to the ends. For the best results, leave conditioner on for 1 to 3 minutes before rinsing, or longer for deep conditioners.

◎ Rich Conditioner

1 egg yolk
1/2 teaspoon olive oil
3/4 cup lukewarm water or herbal tea

Mix egg yolk, olive oil, and water or tea in a blender until emulsified. Transfer mixture to a container and use that day.

◎ Avocado Coconut Conditioner

1/2 an avocado
1/4 cup coconut milk
2 tablespoons jojoba oil

In a medium-size bowl, mash avocado and blend in coconut milk until thick and creamy. Add jojoba oil and mix again. Transfer mixture to a container and store in a cool, dark place.

◎ Deep Conditioner

1 small jar real mayonnaise
1/2 an avocado

In a medium-size bowl, mix enough mayonnaise and avocado with your hands to create a mixture with a minty green color. Smooth into hair from the scalp to the ends. Cover your hair with a shower cap or wrap your hair in plastic wrap for 20 minutes. For even deeper conditioning, place a hot, damp towel over the shower cap or plastic wrap.

If you have really long hair and need to deep-condition only the ends, halve the ingredients and apply conditioner to and wrap only the ends.

Hot Oil Treatments

For perfectly gleaming locks, try a hot oil treatment to infuse your hair with a radiant shine.

◎ Sandalwood Hot Oil Treatment

1/2 cup olive oil
1/2 cup boiling water
5 drops sandalwood essential oil

Pour olive oil into a bowl and add water and sandalwood oil. Whisk ingredients together until emulsified. Allow to cool slightly. Massage into hair. Cover hair with a shower cap and wrap your head in a hot towel. Leave treatment on for 1/2 hour and then shampoo and rinse.

◎ Rosemary Hot Oil Treatment

1/2 cup dried rosemary leaves
1/2 cup olive oil

Combine rosemary leaves and oil, then heat in a saucepan until warm. Remove rosemary leaves by straining the mixture. Use the strained oil to coat scalp and ends of hair. Cover hair with a shower cap and wrap head with a hot towel. Leave treatment on for 15 minutes and then shampoo and rinse.

Hair Care Creams

To prepare the formula, place the shea butter into a small, wide-mouthed glass jar. Put the jar into a pot of water, and heat on a low flame. When the shea butter is melted, add the carrier oil, mix well, and remove from the heat. As the mixture cools, add the essential oils and stir well.

Rub aloe vera juice and a small portion of the formula into the scalp once a day.

Shea Butter . . . . 2 tablespoons Jojoba . . . . 8 teaspoons Cedarwood (Atlas) . . . 20 drops Bay . . . . 10 drops Litsea Cubeba . . . . . . 10 drops	Shea Butter . . . . 2 tablespoons Jojoba . . . . 8 teaspoons Myrrh . . . . 15 drops Copaiba . . . . 13 drops Litsea Cubeba . . . . . . 12 drops
Shea Butter . . . . 2 tablespoons Jojoba . . . . 8 teaspoons Sandalwood . . . . 20 drops Palmarosa . . . . 13 drops Mandarin . . . . 7 drops	Shea Butter . . . . 2 tablespoons Jojoba . . . . 8 teaspoons Ylang-Ylang . . . . 15 drops Copaiba . . . . 15 drops Frankincense . . . . 10 drops
Shea Butter . . . . 2 tablespoons Jojoba . . . . 8 teaspoons Elemi . . . . 20 drops Lemon . . . . 12 drops Patchouli . . . . 8 drops	Shea Butter . . . . 2 tablespoons Jojoba . . . . 8 teaspoons Rosemary . . . . 15 drops Lavender . . . . 15 drops Myrrh . . . . 10 drops
Shea Butter . . . . 2 tablespoons Jojoba . . . . 8 teaspoons Cedarwood (Atlas) . . . 20 drops Myrrh . . . . 10 drops Spearmint . . . . 10 drops	Shea Butter . . . . 2 tablespoons Jojoba . . . . 8 teaspoons Ylang-Ylang . . . . 17 drops Lemon . . . . 17 drops Ginger . . . . 6 drops
Shea Butter . . . . 2 tablespoons Jojoba . . . . 8 teaspoons Lavender . . . . 20 drops Cedarwood (Atlas) . . . 20 drops	Shea Butter . . . . 2 tablespoons Jojoba . . . . 8 teaspoons Sandalwood . . . . 20 drops Bois de Rose . . . . 20 drops

Dry Scalp Treatments

Dry scalp or dandruff is dead skin that collects on the scalp. Skin cells are constantly dying and flaking off the scalp, but if the rate of production is increased and the scaly flakes remain, then they can be seen on the head. Normally, skin cells die and are replaced around once a month, but for people with dandruff, the process occurs about once every 2 weeks. A great remedy for itchy scalps and dandruff, these recipes will leave your hair feeling softer and more manageable and smelling wonderful.

◎ Dandruff Remover

1/2 cup water
1/2 cup white vinegar

Combine water and vinegar. Apply directly to the scalp before shampooing. Use twice a week.

◎ Ravishing Rosemary Hair Conditioner

Rosemary (*Rosmarinus officinalis*) is thought to stimulate hair growth.

1 teaspoon carrier oil (sweet almond or olive oil)
Rosemary essential oil

Slightly warm the carrier oil. Add 2 to 5 drops of rosemary essential oil and mix well. Dampen hair, and massage the mixture through hair and scalp. Wrap your head in a warm towel to deep-condition the hair. After 45 minutes, wash out and rinse with cool water. Keep out of eyes.

Hands and Feet

It's amazing how well a manicure and pedicure can relax you. Whether you do them yourself or go to a nail salon, soft hands and feet make you feel pampered and well cared for, as though you haven't had to work a day in your life. With the exercises that the *30-Day Revitalization Plan* requires, you'll especially need to take care of your feet, as increased movement can cause blisters and calluses and can toughen your feet, all of which can be fixed.

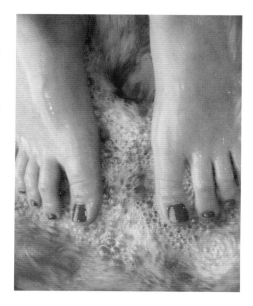

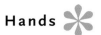
Smooth, soft hands and clean, healthy fingernails show the world that you take care of yourself—including the details. Well-cared for hands and fingernails can greatly improve the first impression you make, so you may want to take the extra time to pamper them before a first date, job interview, or other important occasion. Hand exfoliants will turn your rough hands into ones that anyone would want to hold, and hand creams will help maintain that softness. Fingernail treatments and cuticle softeners complete the look of well-groomed hands.

◎ Sugar Soft-Hand Exfoliant

2 tablespoons baby oil
3 tablespoons coarse sugar

Mix baby oil and sugar to form a paste. Rub gently onto hands. Rinse well with warm water and pat dry.

◎ Lemonade Hand Exfoliant

1 tablespoon lemon juice
1 teaspoon coarse sugar
1/2 teaspoon water

Mix lemon juice, sugar, and water together. Rub gently onto hands. Rinse with warm water and pat dry.

◎ Rose-Scented Hand Cream

1/3 cup glycerin
2/3 cup rose water
3 drops sandalwood essential oil

Shake glycerin, rose water, and oil together in a bottle. Massage gently onto hands. Store mixture in a cool, dark place.

◎ Extra Tough Hand Cream

2 tablespoons shaved beeswax
1/2 teaspoon carnuba wax
2 tablespoons jojoba oil
1 teaspoon aloe vera gel
10 drops vitamin E oil
3 drops sage essential oil

In a saucepan, melt the beeswax, carnuba wax, jojoba oil, and aloe vera gel. Remove from heat and beat until cool, adding the vitamin E oil before the mixture thickens. Continue beating until the mixture becomes creamy. Add sage essential oil, and continue beating until the cream has completely cooled. Transfer mixture to a container, and store in a cool, dark place for up to one week.

◎ Lemon Protective Hand Cream

This hand cream is a great sealant to protect your hands from hard work, and works wonders as an overnight hand cream too. It's also great for feet and elbows!

2 tablespoons glycerine
3 tablespoons fresh lemon juice
6 tablespoons water
1 teaspoon lemon extract
3 tablespoons lanolin
3 tablespoons safflower oil

In a food processor or blender, mix all ingredients on low until well blended. Increase speed to high, and blend for several minutes until mixture is creamy and ingredients are emulsified.

◎ Hand Cream for Chapped Hands

Large jar of petroleum jelly
Elderflowers

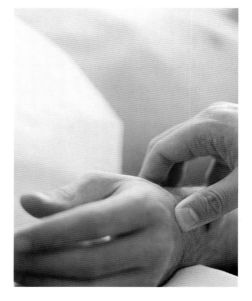

In a saucepan, dissolve the petroleum jelly. Do not boil. Gradually stir in as many elderflowers as possible, adding more as they become absorbed. Lower the heat and simmer for 45 minutes. Remove from heat and strain through a fine sieve. Pour into jars for storage.

◎ Liquid Hand Lotion

1 tablespoon glycerine
¹/₂ tablespoon rose water
¹/₂ tablespoon eau de cologne
    (optional)
Juice of one lemon

Mix glycerine, rose water, cologne, if desired, and lemon juice in a bottle. Shake well before applying to hands.

Nails

Before trimming your nails, soak them in warm, soapy water. This softens the nails, which makes them easier to cut. Then file them to follow the natural shape; most people's nails are either square or rounded. With a cuticle trimmer, trim hangnails or cracked cuticles. Then, with a flat-headed orange stick, push the cuticle back under the nail. Finally, moisturize, making sure to rub the softener thoroughly over the edges of the nail bed.

◎ Wheat Germ Hot Oil Strengthening Fingernail Treatment

1/4 cup wheat germ oil

Warm the wheat germ oil and soak fingernails in oil for about 5 minutes. Wipe off excess oil, and massage nails.

◎ Cuticle Softener

1 teaspoon olive oil
1 teaspoon jojoba oil
2 drops eucalyptus essential oil

In a small saucepan, mix oils together and then warm them over low heat. Rub gently into cuticles, using the tips of your fingers to massage in the oil.

◎ Nail Cleaner

2 teaspoons soap flakes
1 dash hydrogen peroxide
Small bowl of water

Dissolve soap flakes in water. Add peroxide. Soak fingertips in mixture for 5 minutes. Then clean nails with orange stick or scrub with nail brush.

◎ Nail Whitener

Citric acid
Water

In a screw-top bottle, mix 1 part citric acid with 12 parts water. Shake well and apply to discolored nails with a cotton ball.

Feet

Your feet are constantly working hard for you, and they often, as a result, do not look very pretty. However, when you take the time to care for your feet properly, they will not just look better; they will feel better too. The skin of the feet can get very rough, so using exfoliants and scrubs is an important first step. To relieve tired feel after a hard day, use some peppermint foot gel and an overnight treatment of banana foot lotion. You will be sure to be walking more energetically the next day, and your feet will be attractive even in sandals or flip-flops!

◎ Strawberry Foot Exfoliant

6 large strawberries
2 tablespoons olive oil
1 teaspoon coarse sugar

Mix strawberries, olive oil, and sugar together. Mash gently just until a paste is formed. Rub gently onto feet, rinse, and pat dry.

◎ Summer Sand Foot Scrub

2 tablespoons olive oil
2 tablespoons clean sand
3 drops rosemary essential oil

Mix all ingredients together until a paste is formed. Rub onto feet, rinse, and pat dry.

◎ Refreshing Peppermint Foot Gel

2 tablespoons aloe vera gel
1 teaspoon peppermint oil

Mix aloe vera and peppermint oil together and whisk until well blended. Gently rub mixture onto feet until absorbed.

◎ Banana Foot Lotion

1 banana, peeled and mashed
2 tablespoons honey
1 tablespoon lemon juice
1 tablespoon margarine

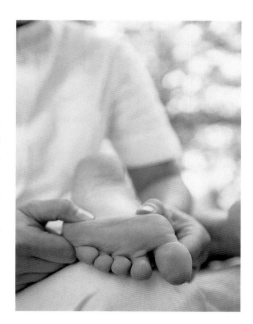

Mix banana, honey, lemon juice, and margarine together until a paste is formed. Gently rub mixture onto feet and leave on for 15 minutes. Rinse and pat dry. (For an overnight treatment, wear heavy socks over a thick coating of the mixture while you sleep.)

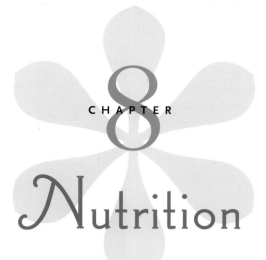

Nutrition

To create the body shape you want, you need to adopt eating habits that will help you keep the fat off. Most people who succeed in adopting a healthy, low-fat diet find their motivation in the desire for a better appearance. But there's a far better reason—your health and longevity! The diet that best protects you against heart disease, against adult-onset diabetes, and against colon, prostate, ovarian, and breast cancer is a low-fat one. It is a largely vegetarian diet low in saturated fat (less than 7 percent of daily calories), and cholesterol (200 mg or less per day), with low levels of sodium (1,800 mg or less per day), and plenty of foods rich in fiber.

The four basic food groups are a thing of the past. New research in nutrition shows that certain foods deserve much more emphasis than others in a healthy diet. A correctly balanced diet emphasizes complex carbohydrates (vegetables, fruits, rice, potatoes, yams, and grains—preferably whole grains). Next in emphasis come the protein foods (minus red meat). These are beans and legumes, white-meat poultry without the skin, fish, and egg whites. Then come low-fat dairy products, such as skim milk, low-fat or nonfat yogurt, and low-fat cottage cheese. Finally, in the smallest category of a healthy diet are the things you should eat sparingly, or not at all, including butter, oils, sweets and pastries, alcohol, red meat, and cheese. Red meat, cheese, and the skin of poultry are so high in fat and cholesterol that they do not belong with healthy low-fat protein sources.

Whether you're primarily concerned with your appearance, your health, or both, the most important single dietary guideline is to watch your fat consumption! Only 20 to 25 percent of your total daily calories should come from fat. Let's say you eat 1,500 calories a day: 1,500 times .25 equals 375, so you should eat no more than 375 calories a day from fat. There are 9 calories (to make the math easier, round up to 10) in 1 gram of fat; divide 375 by 10 and you get 37.5 grams. So to eat 25 percent of calories from fat with a daily intake of 1,500 calories, you are allowed 37.5 grams of fat each day.

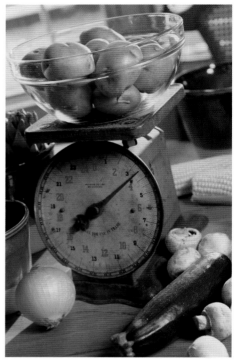

A more general range is from 300 to 500 calories a day from fat. If you're in the high end one day, cut back on the fat calories the next. Remember, your ultimate goal is a well-balanced diet that provides all the essential nutrients for optimum health.

Some people find it easier to control their fat intake with reference to individual foods. Food labeling requirements call for packagers of most prepared foods to state the total number of calories and the calories from fat. As long as you avoid food products that get more than 25 percent of their calories from fat, you'll be meeting the overall goal.

Cutting back on dietary fat can be tricky; different methods work for different people. Going "cold turkey"—eliminating fatty foods and restricting your total diet to no more than 25 percent of calories from fat—works best for many people. Others will find it easier to slowly reduce the frequency and amount of fatty foods. This tactic often ensures that fatty foods don't take on a forbidden status, which can make them harder to resist. Substituting nonfat varieties in place of their high-fat counterparts (e.g., nonfat frozen yogurt or sorbet in place of ice cream) is another strategy that works well. However you choose to do it, don't put it off. More and more evidence shows just how bad a high-fat diet is for your health, your heart, and your chances of living to a ripe old age.

Here is a list of some high-fat foods you should eliminate from your diet now. If you stop eating these foods, you will be cutting out the top ten sources of fat in the American diet.

- Whole and 2 percent low-fat milk (skim or 1 percent is better)

- Margarine and butter

- Shortening

- Mayonnaise (some nonfat varieties are tasty substitutes)

- Salad dressing (oil-free brands are good)

- Cheese (soy cheese alternatives still tend to be high in fat)

- Ground beef, even the leanest

- Egg yolks (the whites are fine, but eat no more than two yolks a week)

- Ice cream (plenty of nonfat alternatives are now on the market)

- Peanut butter

A low-fat diet is so important in reaching your fitness goals (as well as for your health!) that we'll give you some more tips on the subject in a separate section toward the end of this chapter. First, let's look at your other basic dietary requirements.

Protein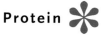

One of the most persistent dietary myths is that to build muscle, a person must load up on dietary protein. In fact, the typical American diet includes much more protein than people need, whether or not they are seeking to increase muscle mass. Getting too much protein can be dangerous. High-protein diets produce excess nitrogen in the blood. This leads to a high acid condition. The body's response is to neutralize the acidity by leaching calcium from the bones, then excreting it in the urine. This process, if carried out over a lifetime, can be a factor in causing osteoporosis. The typical American diet includes too much animal protein. Animal protein, especially beef, pork, egg yolks, poultry with the skin, and cheese, is accompanied by unhealthy levels of fat and cholesterol—bad news for your heart and your weight.

How much protein is enough? Active people should be eating no more than 1.5 to 2 grams of protein per kilogram (2.2 pounds) of body weight, per day, or about 20 to 25 percent of total daily calories. Good sources of lean protein are egg whites, fish, fat-free dairy products, beans and other legumes, and white-meat poultry minus the skin.

Because seafood is a recommended source of dietary protein, the three best sources are listed here, based on their percentage of calories from fat. They are cod, sole (flounder), and tuna (packed in water. However, there are reports that canned albacore tuna has higher levels of mercury, which can be harmful especially to children and pregnant women). All three are high in omega-3 fatty acids, which may help to reverse heart disease. Cod has the lowest percentage of calories from fat (7 percent), sole is second with 12 percent, and tuna is third with 16 percent of its calories from fat. Despite its higher percentage of fat calories, you can still eat salmon, as it is an excellent source of omega-3 fatty acids. So variety and moderation is the key when it comes to protein.

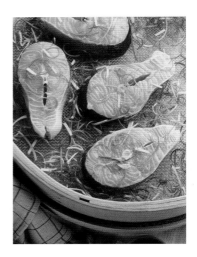

 Fiber

Getting plenty of fiber in your diet makes it easier to maintain a healthy (and shapely) body weight and helps prevent diabetes, colon cancer, and heart disease. People need about 25 to 35 grams of fiber from food sources each day. Fresh fruits and vegetables, legumes (beans, peas, lentils), and whole grains are excellent sources of fiber.

To make your shopping easier, here is a list of some good sources of dietary fiber:

- Bran cereals: 1/2 cup has 6–14 grams (depending on brand)
- Baked beans: 8 grams per 1/2 cup
- Kidney or lima beans: 7 grams per 1/2 cup
- Broccoli or brussels sprouts: 7 grams per cup
- Fresh corn: 7 grams per ear
- Apples: 4 grams each
- Sweet potatoes: 4 grams per medium-size sweet potato
- Brown rice: 3 grams per 2/3 cup serving
- Bananas: 3 grams each
- Oranges: 3 grams each
- Peaches: 3 grams each
- Whole wheat tortillas: 3 grams each
- Tomatoes: 2 grams each

If you eat a balanced diet from natural food sources, including fruits, grains, and vegetables, your fiber consumption is probably adequate. Unless you're having problems with regularity, there's no need to go out of your way to supplement your diet with fiber-rich foods such as bran. It is possible to eat too much fiber; fiber binds with calcium in the stomach, thereby reducing the amount of calcium that is absorbed. Women especially need plenty of calcium to guard against osteoporosis in their later years.

Phytochemicals

You may have heard or read about a group of compounds called phytochemicals. They are a variety of natural compounds recently discovered in fruits and vegetables. They have no nutritional value, but it is believed these compounds may work to help protect the body from disease.

Fruits and vegetables are the best sources of phytochemicals; it is not possible at this point to get the benefits of phytochemicals by taking supplements. Fruits and vegetables also contain vitamins, antioxidants, minerals, and fiber, all of which promote good health and help prevent disease.

Beta-carotene and vitamin C are antioxidant vitamins. Fortunately, beta-carotene substances are not destroyed by cooking, canning, freezing, or other processing of food.

Minerals

Minerals activate your body's enzymes, which are necessary for metabolism. They aid in the transfer of nerve impulses, muscle contraction, body growth and development, and water balance. Minerals are especially important for people who exercise, because they maintain the body's electrolyte (mineral) balance.

The major minerals are calcium, phosphorus, magnesium, and sulfur. Important electrolytes are sodium chloride and potassium. The trace minerals, needed in smaller quantities but still vital to health, are iron, zinc, iodide, copper, manganese, fluoride, chromium, selenium, and molybdenum.

If you eat a variety of wholesome foods, you don't have to worry about getting enough of these nutrients. (The one possible exception, especially for women, is calcium, which is discussed next.) The best way to meet your mineral needs is by eating a balanced diet. High-quality multi-mineral supplements, in moderation, will not hurt. However, taking some individual mineral supplements can greatly diminish the absorption and metabolism of other minerals. Again, this need not concern those who take calcium supplements to meet their daily needs.

✻ Calcium

Calcium is important in building teeth and strong bones and in preventing osteoporosis (loss of bone density) as we grow older. To make sure you don't join the millions of Americans with osteoporosis, get plenty of calcium in your diet.

The recommended daily allowances of calcium are: for individuals age 11 through 24, 1,200 mg; for individuals over 25 years, 800 mg; for women over 50 and men over 65, 1,500 to 1,800 mg.

Calcium requirements can be met through diet alone or through diet and supplements.

✻ Vitamins

Vitamins are found in all foods. They help regulate the metabolism and protect the body from disease. If you eat a wide variety of nutritious foods, you shouldn't have to worry about supplementing your diet with vitamin pills.

✻ Water

Water is found in fruits, vegetables, and liquids. It is the most essential nutrient of all. You can't survive more than a few days without it. It transports nutrients, regulates body heat, and aids in digestion. Drink plenty of water throughout the day, especially while you're working out!

✻ Low-Fat /Good Carbs

If your goal is to lose body fat, then cut down on your overall daily calorie intake, especially calories from fat.

If you want to maintain your current body weight, the number of calories you need to eat depends on how much exercise you get. But the appropriate generalized formula (see next page) will give you a rough idea of the calories you need to eat per day to maintain your current body weight.

Adult women: Multiply your current body weight by 10, then add your current body weight to that value.

Example: 130 pounds x 10 = 1,300
+ 130 = 1,430 calories per day
Adult men: Multiply your current body weight by 10, then add double your current body weight to that value.
Example: 180 pounds x 10 = 1,800
+ 360 = 2,160 calories per day

Make sure your diet always gives you at least 1,200 calories per day. Any number below that, and your body's metabolic rate (the rate at which you burn calories) will start to slow down. You don't want that to happen—you want your body to burn calories faster and more efficiently. To keep your metabolism revved up, eat about 55 percent of your total daily calories from carbohydrates (preferably complex carbohydrates—emphasize fruits and vegetables), eat 20 to 25 percent from fat (no more than 7 percent from saturated fat), and eat 20 to 25 percent from protein (vegetable and low-fat sources are best). When you eat this way, your body produces enough energy so that you have the stamina to exercise. After a short conditioning period, exercise itself produces energy.

There's a popular myth these days that if you eat a low-fat diet, you can eat all the carbohydrates you want and still not gain weight. Unfortunately, it's not true. If you eat too much in general (and don't burn enough calories through exercise), you won't lose weight, and you might gain weight.

Calories are units of energy that are used as fuel for your body. If you put more fuel in your body than your body can use, your body has a mechanism for storing this fuel—it's called fat. So even if you eat a high-carbohydrate, low-fat diet, the number of calories going in still must not exceed the number of calories going out, if you want to lose weight.

However, it certainly helps to eat a diet low in fat and high in complex carbohydrates. Fat in food is stored as body fat more easily than carbohydrates are. Simple carbohydrates, such as refined flour, many processed foods, sugars, sweets, and fruit juices, elevate blood glucose and insulin levels, and this process also stimulates fat storage. On the other hand, complex carbohydrates actually stimulate the cells of your body to burn calories faster. Complex carbohydrates include whole grains, brown rice, potatoes, vegetables, and beans.

Complex carbohydrates cannot add directly to body fat. In order for your body to store their energy, you have to chemically convert it to fat. This is not an easy task, and the conversion process "wastes" 23 percent of the calories contained in that food. When you eat fat, the task is much easier and only uses up 3 percent of the calories in that food.

Because there is more fiber in complex carbohydrates and fewer calories per gram (4 calories compared with 9 in a gram of fat), carbohydrates are more filling and have fewer calories. That means that if your diet is high in complex carbohydrates, you can get away with eating more in general! Remember, though, if you want to lose weight, not maintain it, you'll probably have to cut down on total calories, or exercise more.

If you want to be trim and fit, a good diet coupled with regular aerobic exercise, stretching for flexibility, and weight training is the name of the game. Consistent exercise is the key factor in teaching your body to be an efficient fat burner and not a fat storer.

Finally, be aware of "insulin resistance" and its relation to diet. The job of insulin is to transport sugar from the bloodstream into the cells, where it is needed for energy. Simply put, insulin resistance means that a person's insulin is not doing its job properly. If your insulin isn't effective, your pancreas will secrete more and more insulin. That can create problems—people with high insulin levels are at greater risk of developing high blood pressure, heart disease, and diabetes.

High insulin levels usually occur in people who are overweight. Because of their excess fat, the receptor sites on their body's cells don't recognize insulin very easily, and more insulin must be secreted in order for the hormone to do its job. How can you tell if you're insulin resistant? The best indicators are high triglyceride levels, low HDL levels (the good kind of cholesterol), and being overweight.

The bottom line: If you're overweight, you probably have some degree of insulin resistance. Exercise and lose weight, and your insulin levels should return to normal. Stay fat, and you have a good chance of becoming diabetic.

 ## Metabolism

"Metabolism" refers to the body's chemical and physiological processes that provide energy—energy to do everything from thinking and breathing to running a marathon.

Your metabolic rate is the speed at which your body burns calories. The higher your metabolic rate, the more efficiently you are getting energy to your cells, and the more calories you're burning. As we all know, burning more calories means you can eat more without gaining weight.

Metabolic rate is influenced by six factors. The good news is that most of them are under your control—that means you have the power to raise your metabolism, have more energy, and maintain a healthy and attractive body weight without depriving yourself of food. Let's look at the factors that determine your metabolic rate.

The ratio of lean to fat tissue in your body is the biggest factor in determining your metabolic rate. This ratio is commonly expressed in terms of your "percent body fat." See pages 148–149 for further discussion. The lower your percent body fat, the higher your ratio of lean to fat tissue, and the higher your metabolic rate. Lean tissue includes bone, muscle, organs, blood, and so on. We know all too well what fat is.

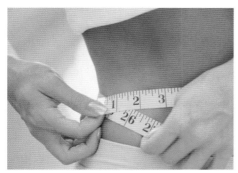

You can change your body composition by gaining lean muscle and bone mass, and by losing fat. Resistance training adds muscle and bone mass. Aerobic exercise and correct nutrition help decrease fat. The combination of resistance training, aerobic exercise, and proper eating dramatically affects body composition.

Reducing your percent body fat increases your metabolism because muscle tissue burns more calories just to maintain itself, even when at rest. Obese people have slow metabolism and thus tend to get fatter and fatter because their bodies aren't burning calories efficiently. If you've got a healthy ratio of muscle to fat, your internal engine will be revving at a higher speed both when you're active and when you're not. The result? More energy for all the activities in your life, and less tendency to put on weight.

Activity Level

Exercise temporarily boosts metabolic rate not just while you're exercising but for a while afterward. The longer and harder you exercise, the greater the temporary boost. You can burn a lot of calories during the period of that temporary boost!

Also, remember that muscle is active tissue; fat is inactive. More muscle means your body is generating more energy. When people tone and develop their muscles, they find that they naturally tend to become more active and use their muscles more in everyday life. The beautiful thing about this is that as your activity level increases, you maintain and build your muscles and reduce your body fat. If you do resistance exercise to build muscle, and also maintain a generally active lifestyle, you create a positive feedback loop that reinforces your increased metabolic rate, energizes you, and makes it easier to become more fit and stay strong and healthy.

If, on the other hand, you opt for a sedentary lifestyle, the result will be a negative feedback loop: as your activity level is reduced, you'll have less muscle mass and your metabolic rate also decreases. As a result, you need fewer calories to maintain your body weight. Most people don't decrease their caloric intake to match their declining needs. If you don't cut down on calories, your weight goes up and your percent body fat increases. Because fat is inactive tissue, that further slows down your metabolism, and you need still fewer calories. This self-reinforcing "vicious circle" makes overweight and sedentary people fatter and fatter. The way out is to convert from a sedentary to an active lifestyle, build muscle with resistance training, and get onto that positive feedback loop instead.

 ## Diet

What, how much, and when you eat are all important factors in determining your metabolic rate. In general, eating temporarily raises your metabolism. You've probably heard about the importance of breakfast—eating a healthy breakfast, containing complex carbohydrates and a low-fat source of protein, will kick-start your metabolism in the morning. But here's a more recent discovery that may go against what you've been told: eating small portions throughout the day keeps the metabolism revved up and can actually help you maintain a healthy body weight. Of course, this won't work if your snacks are cookies, potato chips, and ice cream. But "grazing" throughout the day on light, healthy foods is an excellent habit to get into. Try packing foods like baby carrots, pretzels, air-popped popcorn, bagels, apples, and nonfat yogurt into your lunch—and you don't need to wait until lunchtime to start eating them.

There are two eating habits to avoid if you want to raise your metabolism. First, you should know that hard-to-digest foods, most notably red meat, slow down the metabolism. Second, eating huge portions at one sitting clogs up the metabolic wheel and prevents it from turning very fast. Sumo wrestlers, who are trying to gain fat, do so by eating one huge meal every day for this reason.

 ## Age

As we get older, our resting metabolism tends to slow down. However, this won't happen to you nearly as soon or as quickly as it normally would if you're staying active and exercising regularly. The decrease in metabolic rate with age is primarily, if not entirely, due to the typical loss of muscle mass and the change in the fat-to-lean ratio. As we saw earlier, the less muscle mass you have, the fewer calories you burn even while resting.

To prevent loss of muscle mass as you age, you need to do some form of weight-bearing exercise. The most effective way by far is resistance training—lifting weights.

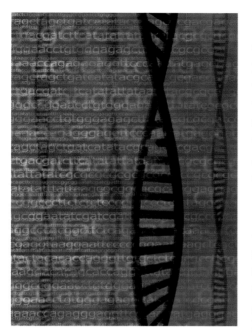

Hormones

Thyroid hormone, in particular, helps regulate metabolic rate. Those with hypoactive or hyperactive thyroids suffer reduced or increased metabolic rates. If you suspect a thyroid problem, see your doctor. Medications are available that can address these problems.

Genetics

Genetic predisposition does play a role in determining your metabolic rate, but its effect is relatively minor. Since you can't change your genes anyway, focus on the factors listed above that you can influence.

As we've seen, strength training helps you achieve and maintain a healthy body weight in two ways: Not only are you burning calories directly through the exercise activity itself, but you're simultaneously increasing your body's calorie-burning rate by adding muscle and raising your metabolism. Muscle burns more energy (calories) because it is active tissue.

Weight lifting builds muscle faster and better than any other form of exercise. The overall effect on your metabolism can be dramatic: training with weights three times a week increases the calories a person burns by about 15 percent. If you don't increase your caloric intake, your body will burn that extra 15 percent from its stored calories; in other words, you'll burn off body fat. Every pound of muscle added to the body burns about 35 extra calories per day, or about 3 to 4 pounds of fat per year.

Without exercise, during each decade the typical adult loses about 5 pounds of lean body weight (muscle), gains approximately 15 pounds of fat, and suffers a 5 percent drop in his or her resting metabolism. These numbers make it perfectly clear why everyone needs to exercise and should continue to do so throughout their entire lifetime.

◎ Soup for Fasting

3¹/₂ ounces celery root
3¹/₂ ounces parsley root
3¹/₂ ounces fennel root
1³/₄ ounces potatoes
1 ounce leeks
1 small carrot
1 quart water
2 bay leaves
4 juniper berries
4 peppercorns
Some grains sea salt
¹/₄ teaspoon yeast flakes

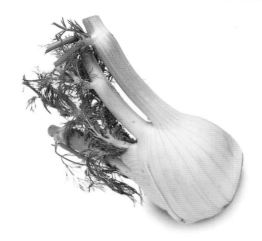

Peel and cut celery root, parsley root, fennel root, potatoes, leeks, and carrot; place in a saucepan in cold water. Add bay leaves, juniper berries, and peppercorns; bring to a boil, allowing to simmer over low heat for 20 to 30 minutes. Strain. Add salt and yeast flakes to season.

Makes 4 servings. Per serving: 44 calories, trace fat (trace saturated), 9 g carbohydrates, 2 g protein, 3 g fiber, 0 mg cholesterol, 56 mg sodium.

◎ Bircher Muesli

Dr. Max Bircher-Brenner (1867–1939), was a Swiss physician and specialist in nutrition, known for inventing the original Bircher muesli. The Bircher muesli, made with milk, grains, and fruit, is rich in calcium, fiber, vitamins, and minerals that provide nutrients beneficial to your enzyme metabolism.

This is the classic among the muesli varieties. It has a high fiber content, so it is especially good for the intestines. You can choose the nuts and fruit you want, and you can replace the oats with other flakes, wheat germ, or freshly ground grains (soaked overnight).

1 container low-fat yogurt   *1 teaspoon nuts, chopped*
2 to 3 tablespoons oats   *1 teaspoon honey*
1 small apple, shredded   *Fresh lemon juice to taste*

Mix all ingredients.

Makes 1 serving. Per serving: 340 calories, 7 g fat (3 g saturated), 57 g carbohydrates, 16 g protein, 6 g fiber, 14 mg cholesterol, 160 mg sodium.

◎ Thick Potato-Vegetable Soup

Vegetables of your choice, cubed
2 small potatoes with or without
  skin
1 quart cold water
3 teaspoons dried vegetable broth

Parsley to taste
Chives to taste
Lovage to taste
Yeast flakes to taste
1 tablespoon sour cream (optional)

Place vegetables and potatoes into water. Add vegetable broth. Bring to a boil. Reduce heat and simmer, covered, on low heat, 20 minutes. Purée the vegetables and season with parsley, chives, lovage, and yeast flakes. Add sour cream if desired.

Makes 2 servings. Nutrition varies depending on vegetables used.

Dr. Bircher-Brenner's Tips for Raw Food

For a plate of raw food, all ingredients need to be washed well, so that they can be taken up by the intestines under optimal conditions. You should cut the food as follows:

Grate: red beets, black radish, celery roots, carrots, kohlrabi, daikon, parsley root

Shred (or thinly slice): all varieties of cabbage and kale (white cabbage, red cabbage, Chinese cabbage, kohlrabi, etc.), fennel, cucumber, celery, endive, spinach, radish (or leave whole), zucchini

Slice somewhat larger: peppers, endive, chicory

Slice: tomatoes

Do not cut or tear: Boston lettuce, cress

During a single meal, it's best not to eat more than three kinds of vegetables. Season your raw food with a dressing made from high-grade kernel, germ, or seed oil, or use yogurt, lemon, fresh herbs (chives, parsley, basil, dill), a bit of onion, raw garlic, yeast flakes, and spices (no salt).

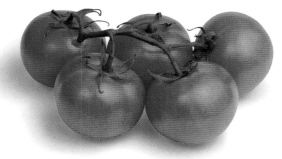

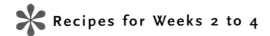
Recipes for Weeks 2 to 4

Soups

◎ **Cold Dilled Tomato Soup**

Chill out. Dill out. And enjoy this creative, sure-to-please soup. It features tomato juice, sour cream, and sassy seasonings: red pepper flakes, onions, ginger, curry, and lemon peel.

3 cups low-sodium tomato juice
1 celery stalk, chopped
1 medium onion, chopped
1/4 teaspoon red pepper flakes
1/2 teaspoon curry powder

1/4 teaspoon ginger
1 teaspoon grated lemon peel
1 cup nonfat sour cream
2 tablespoons snipped fresh dill
*   or chives*

In a 3-quart pot, bring 1 cup tomato juice to a boil. Add the celery, onion, and pepper flakes, and simmer for 10 minutes. Remove from the heat. Stir in the curry, ginger, lemon peel, and the remaining 2 cups tomato juice. Transfer the mixture to a blender and purée. Chill for 45 minutes.

Stir in the sour cream. Top each serving with dill or chives.

Makes 4 servings. Per serving: 103 calories, 1 g fat (1 g saturated), 20 g carbohydrates, 5 g protein, 2 g fiber, 6 mg cholesterol, 74 mg sodium.

◎ **Fast Gazpacho**

Hailing from Spain, gazpacho is an intriguing chilled soup of tomatoes, cucumbers, and other summertime vegetables. This version, which gets its zest from garlic and dried chili, is ready in the whirl of a blender's blade.

2 cans (15 ounces each) diced
*   tomatoes*
1 1/2 cups reduced-sodium tomato
*   juice*
1 medium cucumber, chopped
1 green sweet pepper, chopped
1 medium onion, chopped

1 mild dried chili pepper, seeded
*   and chopped*
4 cloves garlic, chopped
2 teaspoons red wine vinegar
2 teaspoons olive oil
2 cups croutons, for garnish

Combine the tomatoes, tomato juice, cucumber, sweet pepper, onion, chili pepper, garlic, vinegar, and olive oil in a blender. Process the mixture until the vegetables are partially puréed. Chill the soup until cold, 30 to 40 minutes. Top each serving with croutons.

Makes 4 servings. Per serving: 146 calories, 4 g fat (1 g saturated), 26 g carbohydrates, 5 g protein, 4 g fiber, 0 mg cholesterol, 279 mg sodium.

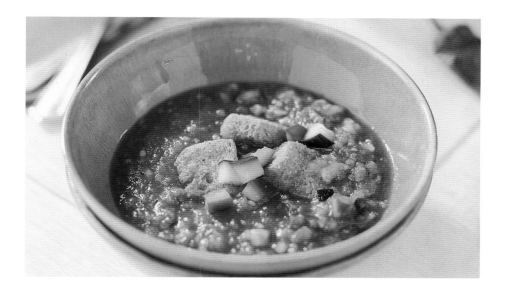

Quick cooking tips: Ancho peppers, which are dried poblano peppers, give this recipe just the right zip. If you can't find them, simply use ¹/₄ to ¹/₂ of a minced, seeded cayenne pepper. Peel the cucumber only if it is waxed.

◎ Celery-Leek Chowder

Dressed up with ham and paprika, this creamy chowder gets a light cheese flavor from ricotta.

1 teaspoon olive oil
3 leeks, white part only, sliced
2 ounces finely diced deli smoked ham
2 large potatoes, peeled and diced
3 cups fat-free beef broth
1 celery stalk, sliced

1 teaspoon white wine vinegar
¹/₂ teaspoon ground celery seeds
¹/₄ teaspoon white pepper
1 cup nonfat ricotta cheese
Paprika

Warm the oil in a 4-quart pot over medium–high heat for 1 minute. Add the leeks and ham; cook until the leeks are wilted, 3 to 5 minutes.

Stir in the potatoes, broth, celery, vinegar, celery seeds, and pepper. Cover the pot, and bring the mixture to a boil. Reduce the heat, and simmer for 15 minutes. Stir in the ricotta. Serve garnished with paprika.

Makes 6 servings. Per serving: 158 calories, 5 g fat (2 g saturated), 19 g carbohydrates, 11 g protein, 2 g fiber, 19 mg cholesterol, 471 mg sodium.

Quick cooking tip: After stirring in the ricotta, take care not to let the soup boil.

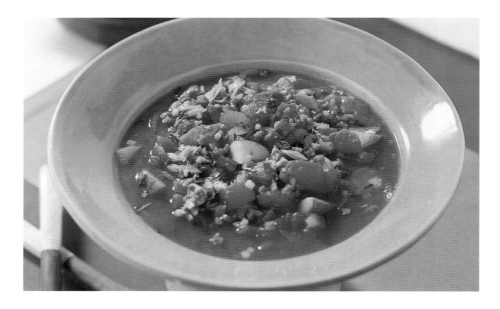

◎ Easy Manhattan-Style Clam Chowder

Tomato clam chowder aficionados: This chunky version is brimming with clams, tomatoes, potatoes, and bacon, and is ready to serve in less than 20 minutes.

4 ounces Canadian bacon, diced
1 large Spanish onion, chopped
1 stalk celery, thinly sliced
1 can (10 ounces) clam juice
1 can (15 ounces) whole tomatoes,
*   cut up*

2 medium red potatoes, chopped
2 bay leaves
¹/₄ teaspoon lemon pepper
1 can (6 ounces) minced clams
*   with juice*
¹/₄ cup snipped fresh parsley

Sauté the bacon in a 4-quart pot until lightly browned. Add the onion and celery, and sauté until the onion is transparent, about 3 minutes.

Stir in the clam juice, tomatoes, potatoes, bay leaves, and lemon pepper. Cover the pot, and bring the mixture to a boil. Reduce the heat, and simmer until the potatoes are tender, 12 to 15 minutes.

Stir in the clams and simmer the soup for 5 minutes more. Discard the bay leaves. Top each serving with parsley.

Makes 4 servings. Per serving: 230 calories, 3 g fat (1 g saturated), 31 g carbohydrates, 20 g protein, 3 g fiber, 43 mg cholesterol, 877 mg sodium.

Quick cooking tip: If you use fresh minced clams, keep the cooking time short, 5 to 10 minutes, or the clams will be tough.

⊚ Puerto Principe Chicken Chowder

Fusion cuisine is hot, and so is this Caribbean goodie, which sports Spanish and Cuban influences. Look to sofrito sauce, hot pepper sauce, and sunflower seeds for mouth–watering sizzle.

1 teaspoon olive oil
³/4 pound boneless, skinless chicken breasts, cut into ¹/2–inch cubes
1 onion, chopped
1 can (14 ounce) fat-free chicken broth
1 can (15 ounces) pigeon peas, rinsed and drained

1 pound tomatoes, chopped
2 cups packed torn chard leaves
2 tablespoons sofrito sauce
1 teaspoon Louisiana hot pepper sauce
¹/4 cup sunflower seeds, toasted

Warm the oil in a 4-quart pot over medium-high heat for 1 minute. Add the chicken, and sauté the pieces until they are lightly browned, about 5 minutes. Add the onion, and sauté until translucent, about 3 minutes.

Stir in the broth, peas, and tomatoes. Cover the pot, and bring the mixture to a boil. Reduce the heat, and simmer for 10 minutes. Stir in the chard and sofrito, and cook, uncovered, for 1 minute.

Stir in the hot-pepper sauce. Top each serving with sunflower seeds.

Makes 4 servings. Per serving: 343 calories, 8 g fat (1 g saturated), 37 g carbohydrates, 32 g protein, 10 g fiber, 49 mg cholesterol, 760 mg sodium.

Quick cooking tip: Pigeon peas come in either green or yellow and can be found in the international section of many supermarkets.

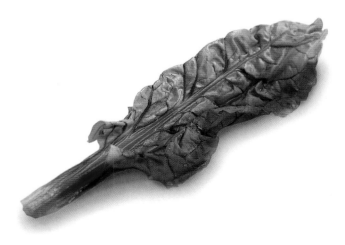

◎ Zucchini Soup Margherita

Refreshing and light, this soup, which is brimming with mozzarella and basil, takes its name from a pizza specialty of Naples, Italy. According to legend, the cheese pizza was created to honor a Queen Margherita.

2 teaspoons olive oil
1 cup zucchini, halved and sliced
1 medium onion, chopped
4 cloves garlic, chopped
2 cans (14 ounces each) fat-free
*   chicken broth*
8 ounces plum tomatoes, sliced

1/4 teaspoon freshly ground black
*   pepper*
1 teaspoon balsamic vinegar
1/2 cup shredded part-skim
*   mozzarella cheese*
1/2 cup snipped fresh basil

Warm the oil in a 4-quart pot over medium-high heat for 1 minute. Add the zucchini, onion, and garlic, and sauté until the vegetables start to brown, 3 to 5 minutes. Stir in the broth, tomatoes, pepper, and vinegar.

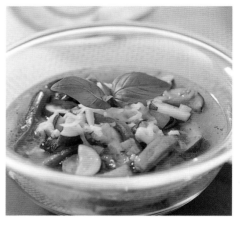

Cover the pot, and bring the mixture to a boil. Reduce the heat, and simmer for 10 minutes. Serve garnished with mozzarella and basil.

Makes 4 servings. Per serving: 147 calories, 10 g fat (2 g saturated), 11 g carbohydrates, 6 g protein, 2 g fiber, 8 mg cholesterol, 515 mg sodium.

◎ Asparagus Soup

Can a soup be light, creamy, elegant, easy, and brimming with asparagus, the harbinger of spring, all at once? Absolutely. Check out this beguiling dish to be sure.

1 pound asparagus
2 teaspoons canola oil
1 medium Spanish onion, chopped
1 medium potato, cut into
*   1/2-inch cubes*

3 cups low-sodium vegetable broth
1/4 teaspoon white pepper
1 cup 2 percent milk
1/2 teaspoon ground savory
1/4 cup snipped fresh parsley

Cut off the asparagus tips. Cut the stalks into 1/2-inch slices, discarding the woody bases. Blanch the tips and stalks for 3 minutes; plunge them into cold

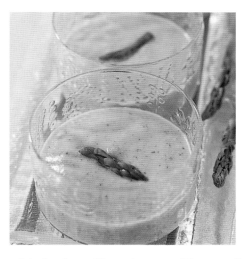

water and drain them. Reserve the tips.

Warm the oil in a 4-quart pot over medium–high heat for 1 minute. Add onion and sauté until translucent. Stir in the potato, broth, asparagus stalks, and pepper. Cover the pot, and bring the mixture to a boil. Reduce heat, and simmer until potatoes and asparagus are tender, about 12 minutes. Using a handheld immersion blender, purée the mixture.

Stir in the milk and savory. Heat until the soup is hot throughout (do not boil), about 3 minutes. Top each serving with parsley and asparagus tips.

Makes 6 servings. Per serving: 92 calories, 3 g fat (1 g saturated), 11 g carbohydrates, 6 g protein, 2 g fiber, 3 mg cholesterol, 413 mg sodium.

Quick cooking tip: The easiest way to remove an asparagus's woody base is to snap it off. If the stalk is tough, remove the outer layer with a vegetable peeler.

◎ Broccoli Bisque

Cooking time is short, so this soup has plenty of bright and fresh broccoli color and flavor. Nonfat sour cream adds body without fat.

1 can (14 ounces) fat-free chicken broth
1 small potato, finely chopped
1 small onion, finely chopped
1/2 teaspoon reduced–sodium soy sauce
2 cups broccoli florets
1/2 cup nonfat sour cream
1/2 cup 1 percent milk
1/4 teaspoon fennel seeds, toasted and crushed

In a 4-quart pot, combine the broth, potato, onion, and soy sauce. Cover the pot, and bring the mixture to a boil. Reduce the heat, and simmer until the potato is tender, about 10 minutes.

Add the broccoli, and simmer until the broccoli is tender, 5 to 7 minutes. Using a handheld immersion blender, purée the mixture, adding the sour cream, milk, and fennel. Heat the soup until it's hot throughout; do not boil.

Makes 4 servings. Per serving: 91 calories, 1 g fat (1 g saturated), 16 g carbohydrates, 5 g protein, 1 g fiber, 4 mg cholesterol, 296 mg sodium.

Quick cooking tip: To toast fennel seeds, place them in a small, nonstick skillet. Warm them over medium heat until lightly browned, 3 to 5 minutes, shaking the pan occasionally.

◎ Carrot Soup with Madeira

In this tamed version of a fiery Indian soup, curry provides a bit of nip that is balanced by smooth and flavorful Madeira.

*2 cans (15 ounces each) reduced-
    sodium vegetable broth*
1 pound carrots, thinly sliced
*1 pound potatoes, peeled and cut
    into 1/2-inch cubes*

2 medium onions, chopped
1 teaspoon curry powder
1/2 teaspoon thyme
1 cup 1 percent milk
1/2 cup Madeira

Combine the broth, carrots, potatoes, onions, curry, and thyme in a 4-quart pot. Cover the pot, and bring the mixture to a boil. Reduce the heat, and simmer until the potatoes and carrots are very tender, 15 to 20 minutes.

Using a handheld immersion blender, purée the vegetables, stirring in the milk a little at a time. Stir in the Madeira. Warm the soup until it is hot throughout.

Makes 4 servings. Per serving: 278 calories, 4 g fat (2 g saturated), 44 g carbohydrates, 13 g protein, 7 g fiber, 10 mg cholesterol, 787 mg sodium.

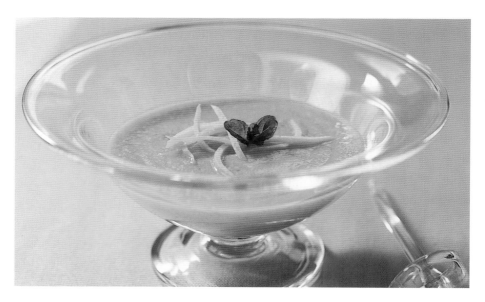

Quick cooking tip: A food processor will make short work of chopping the vegetables for this recipe.

Variation: You may substitute fat-free chicken broth for the vegetable broth, and sherry for the Madeira.

◎ Fresh Tomato-Corn Soup

In summer, when fresh vegetables and herbs are at their peak, create a sensation with this lively vegetarian soup. It comes together in a snap and takes less than 15 minutes to cook.

2 teaspoons olive oil
1 cup chopped red onion
4 cloves garlic, minced
1 can (14 ounces) low-sodium vegetable broth
2 cups diced zucchini

1 pound fresh tomatoes, chopped
1 1/2 cups frozen corn
1/2 teaspoon crushed red pepper flakes
1/4 cup snipped fresh basil leaves
2 tablespoons bacon bits

Warm the oil in a 4-quart pot over medium-high heat for 1 minute. Add the onion and garlic, and sauté until the onion is translucent, about 3 minutes.

Stir in the broth, zucchini, tomatoes, corn, and red pepper flakes. Cover the pot, and bring the mixture to a boil. Reduce the heat, and simmer until the zucchini is tender, about 10 minutes.

Stir in the basil. Top each serving with bacon bits.

Makes 4 servings. Per serving: 157 calories, 5 g fat (1 g saturated), 25 g carbohydrates, 7 g protein, 4 g fiber, 2 mg cholesterol, 369 mg sodium.

Quick cooking tip: Keep the cooking time short so the tomatoes and zucchini retain their fresh flavor.

◎ Hearty Parsnip-Turnip Soup

Because cooking time is short, the root veggies—parsnips, carrots, and turnips—in this soup taste flavorful yet mild. Dill and thyme provide just the right seasoning.

2 cans (14 ounces each) fat-free chicken broth
1 parsnip, diced
1 turnip, diced
1 yellow summer squash, diced
1 carrot, diced
1 potato, peeled and diced

1 onion, chopped
1/2 teaspoon thyme leaves
1/4 teaspoon freshly ground black pepper
1/4 teaspoon dill weed
1/4 teaspoon paprika, for garnish

Combine the broth, parsnip, turnip, squash, carrot, potato, onion, thyme, pepper, and dill weed in a 4-quart pot. Cover the pot, and bring the mixture to a boil. Reduce the heat, and simmer until the vegetables are tender, about 12 minutes. Transfer half the vegetables to a bowl; cover with foil to keep them warm.

Using a handheld immersion blender, purée the vegetables remaining in the pot. Return the reserved vegetables to the pot. Serve garnished with paprika.

Makes 4 servings. Per serving: 76 calories, trace fat (trace saturated), 17 g carbohydrates, 3 g protein, 4 g fiber, 0 mg cholesterol, 252 mg sodium.

◎ Portobello Mushroom Soup

For mushroom aficionados, here's a splendid soup that's thick and dark with tons of substantial portobello mushrooms. For mellowness, there's a splash of dry sherry, and for bright color, each serving is topped with snipped chives.

2 teaspoons butter
6 ounces small portobello mushrooms, sliced
1 large onion, chopped
2 cups fat-free chicken broth
1 large potato, peeled and shredded
2 bay leaves

1/4 teaspoon white pepper
1 cup 2 percent milk
1 tablespoon dry sherry
1/4 cup snipped fresh chives
Reserve 4 attractive mushroom slices for a garnish.

Melt the butter in a 4-quart pot over medium-high heat. Add the mushrooms and onion, and sauté until the onion is translucent. Stir in the broth, potato, and bay leaves. Cover the pot, and bring the mixture to a boil. Reduce the heat, and simmer for 15 minutes. Discard the bay leaves. Stir in the pepper.

Using a handheld immersion blender, purée the mixture. Stir in the milk and sherry. Heat the soup until it is hot throughout (do not boil), about 5 minutes. Top each serving with chives and the reserved mushroom slices.

Makes 4 servings. Per serving: 110 calories, 4 g fat (2 g saturated), 12 g carbohydrates, 7 g protein, 2 g fiber, 10 mg cholesterol, 442 mg sodium.

Quick cooking tip: To clean mushrooms, wipe them with a damp paper towel or rinse them quickly under cool running water. Never soak mushrooms; their flavor will be diluted.

◎ Shallot Watercress Soup

Six ingredients—that's all it takes to make this sensational soup, which show-cases piquant shallots and watercress. In each spoonful, a caper or two pro-vides an intriguing burst of flavor.

2 teaspoons butter
8 shallots, thinly sliced
1 medium potato, finely chopped
2 cans (14 ounces each) fat-free
* chicken broth*

¹/₂ bunch (about 2 ounces)
* watercress, leaves only*
2 teaspoons capers, rinsed
* and drained*

Melt the butter in a 4-quart pot over medium-high heat. Add the shallots, and cook them until they are translucent, about 3 minutes. Add the potato and 1/2 cup broth, and cook until the potato is tender, about 10 minutes.

Using a handheld immersion blender, purée the mixture. Stir in the remain-ing broth, and heat the soup until it is hot throughout, 3 to 5 minutes. Stir in the watercress, and heat for 1 minute more. Add the capers and serve immediately.

Makes 4 servings. Per serving: 101 calories, 3 g fat (2 g saturated), 13 g carbohydrates, 6 g protein, 1 g fiber, 5 mg cholesterol, 705 mg sodium.

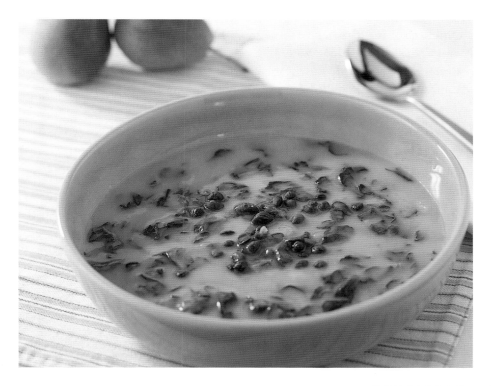

◎ Tomato and Leek Soup

Here's a marvelous tomato soup that's very low in calories and fat. Beef broth and a measure of sherry are the secret flavor ingredients.

1 teaspoon olive oil
2 large leeks, white part only,
    thinly sliced
2 celery stalks, thinly sliced
2 cans (14 ounces each) fat-free
    beef broth
1 can (28 ounces) whole plum
    tomatoes, cut up

1 tablespoon brown sugar
1/4 teaspoon lemon pepper
2 tablespoons dry sherry
2 bay leaves
2 teaspoons dried dill weed

Warm the oil in a 4-quart pot over medium-high heat for 1 minute. Add the leeks and celery, and sauté until the leeks are translucent and the celery is tender, about 5 minutes. Stir in the broth, tomatoes, sugar, pepper, sherry, and bay leaves.

Cover the pot and bring the mixture to a boil. Reduce the heat, and simmer the soup for 30 minutes. Discard the bay leaves. Stir in the dill.

Makes 8 servings. Per serving: 56 calories, 1 g fat (trace saturated), 10 g carbohydrates, 3 g protein, 2 g fiber, 0 mg cholesterol, 347 mg sodium.

Quick cooking tips: Have some fresh dill on hand? Garnish each serving with a small sprig—along with a slice of lemon. For a vegetarian soup, substitute vegetable broth for the beef variety. Prefer a silky smooth tomato soup? After discarding the bay leaves, purée the soup, in batches, in a blender.

Salads & Sides
. . . .

◎ Roasted Chioggia Beets with Feta & Raspberry Vinegar

Chioggia beets give tangy feta cheese a sweet accent. Use imported sheep's milk cheese to get the best flavor.

1/2 cup raspberry vinegar
3 tablespoons honey
1 medium shallot, minced
kosher salt
coarsely cracked black pepper
1/4 cup grapeseed oil

8 small beets, washed and trimmed
1 tablespoon unsalted butter, cut
    into small bits
4 ounces feta cheese, thinly sliced
1 handful spicy baby greens, such
    as mizuna, for garnish

Preheat the oven to 350°F. In a medium bowl, whisk together 1/4 cup of raspberry vinegar, 1 1/2 tablespoons of the honey, the shallot, 1/2 teaspoon

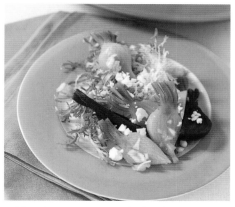

of salt and $1/2$ teaspoon of pepper. Whisk in the grapeseed oil until emulsified.

Arrange the beets so they fit snugly in a single layer in a deep baking dish. Add enough water to barely cover the beets and add the remaining $1/4$ cup of vinegar and $11/2$ tablespoons of honey and the butter. Season with salt and pepper. Cover with foil and bake for 50 to 60 minutes, or until the beets are tender when pierced with a knife. Let cool slightly.

Drain and peel the beets and slice them $1/4$-inch thick. Add them to the honey dressing and let marinate for up to 4 hours.

To serve, arrange half the beet slices on 8 small plates and cover with the feta. Top with the remaining beet slices and drizzle each serving with about 1 tablespoon of the dressing. Garnish with the greens and serve.

Makes 8 servings. Per serving: 174 calories, 11 g fat (4 g saturated), 16 g carbohydrates, 4 g protein, 3 g fiber, 17 mg cholesterol, 368 mg sodium.

◎ Crispy Bacon & Avocado Salad

This color- and texture-rich salad makes a delicious light supper or lunchtime dish or an accompaniment for a picnic or barbecue. Use bottled balsamic dressing for convenience, or whip up a batch from your favorite recipe.

4 ounces thick-slice bacon
1 tablespoon olive oil
2 slices bread, cubed
1 garlic clove, crushed
12 cups mixed salad greens
4 ounces cherry tomatoes, halved
1 ripe avocado, pitted, peeled, and sliced

12 black olives, halved and pitted
1 yellow pepper, seeded and diced
4 hard-cooked eggs, shelled and quartered lengthwise
1/3 cup bottled balsamic vinaigrette dressing

Fry the bacon in a skillet until crisp, drain on paper towels, and cut into cubes. Clean the skillet, add the oil, and place over medium heat. Add the bread cubes and garlic and cook until the croutons are golden, 2 to 3 minutes. Drain well on paper towels.

Arrange the salad greens, tomatoes, avocado slices, olives, and diced pepper on a large serving platter. Sprinkle the bacon and croutons over the salad. Arrange the eggs on top. Drizzle with the vinaigrette just before serving.

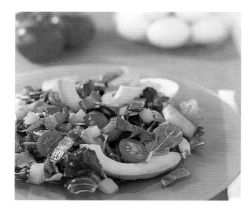

Makes 6 servings. Per serving: 354 calories, 30 g fat (8 g saturated), 15 g carbohydrates, 9 g protein, 5 g fiber, 154 mg cholesterol, 301 mg sodium.

◎ BLT Salad

The flavors of the perfect BLT sandwich are here in breadless form.

8 cups torn romaine lettuce leaves
1/4 pound slab bacon, diced into
    1/2-inch pieces
1 tablespoon olive oil
1 pint cherry tomatoes, halved

1 clove garlic, crushed through
    a press
1/2 teaspoon freshly ground pepper
2 tablespoons red-wine vinegar

Place lettuce in salad bowl. Cook bacon in large skillet until crisp; remove to bowl. Discard all but 1 tablespoon fat from pan. Add olive oil; heat over medium-high heat. Add tomatoes; sauté 1 minute. Add garlic and pepper; sauté 30 seconds. Add vinegar; stir to coat. Pour over lettuce; toss to coat.

Makes 4 servings. Per serving: 215 calories, 20 g fat (7 g saturated fat), 6 g carbohydrates, 5 g protein, 3 g fiber, 19 mg cholesterol, 220 mg sodium.

◎ Juicy Summer Salad

How do you put the "crunch" into ripe melon? Use jicama! This amazing root vegetable is a staple in Mexican cuisine and is celebrated for its juicy and crunchy qualities. Its consistency is similar to a cross between a potato and an apple.

1/2 medium jicama, peeled and
    cut in julienne strips
1/2 medium cantaloupe, cut into
    1/2-inch cubes
2 tablespoons chopped fresh mint

1 teaspoon grated lime rind
3 tablespoons lime juice
1 teaspoon honey
1/4 teaspoon salt

Combine the jicama, melon, mint, lime rind and juice, honey, and salt in a glass or plastic bowl. Toss to coat.

Makes 6 servings. Per serving: 41 calories, trace fat (0 g saturated), 10 g carbohydrates, 1 g protein, 3 g fiber, 0 mg cholesterol, 103 mg sodium.

◎ Tuna and White Bean Salad

4 ounces mesclun salad mix
2 (8-ounce) cans imported tuna in oil, drained
1 (19-ounce) can cannellini beans, drained and rinsed
2 plum tomatoes, chopped
1/2 cup chopped red onion
1 Kirby cucumber, chopped

2 tablespoons torn fresh Italian parsley leaves
salt and freshly ground black pepper to taste
extra-virgin olive oil for drizzling
1 lemon, cut into wedges, for serving

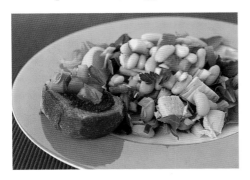

Arrange mesclun on 4 plates. Top with tuna, beans, tomatoes, onion, cucumber, and parsley. Sprinkle with salt and pepper. Drizzle with oil and serve with lemon wedges.

Makes 4 servings. Per serving: 381 calories, 11 g fat (2 g saturated), 35 g carbohydrates, 36 g protein, 8 g fiber, 15 mg cholesterol, 462 mg sodium.

◎ Caribbean Stewed Vegetables

The colors and flavors of this hearty dish are as lively as the islands themselves. It tastes even better if cooked a day ahead of serving. Try it with jerked chicken and cooked rice or fresh crusty bread.

2 tablespoons vegetable oil
2 cups chopped onions
3 cups chopped cabbage
1/4 teaspoon cayenne pepper or 1 fresh chile, minced and seeded for a milder flavor
1 tablespoon grated peeled fresh ginger root
3 cups peeled sweet potatoes chooped into 1/2-inch cubes

2 cups undrained chopped tomatoes, fresh or canned
2 cups sliced okra, fresh or frozen
3 tablespoons fresh lime juice
2 tablespoons chopped fresh cilantro
salt to taste
1 cup chopped peanuts
plus (optional) sprigs for garnish

Heat the oil in a Dutch oven over medium heat and add the onions. Sauté until softened, 4 or 5 minutes. Add the cabbage and the cayenne or chile and sauté, stirring often, until the onions are translucent, about 8 minutes.

Add the ginger and 2 cups water, cover, and heat to boiling. Stir in the sweet

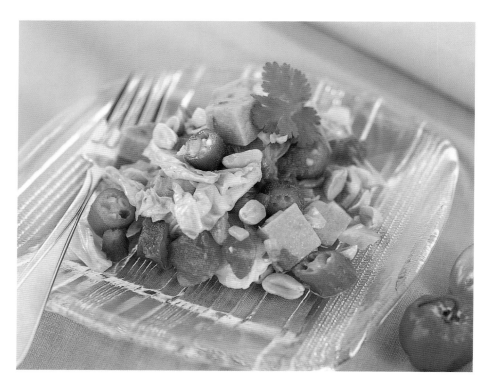

potatoes, sprinkle with salt, and simmer until the potatoes are barely tender, 5 or 6 minutes. Add the tomatoes, okra, and lime juice. Simmer until the vegetables are tender, about 15 minutes. Stir in the chopped cilantro and salt to taste.

To serve: Sprinkle the stew with chopped peanuts. Top with a few sprigs of cilantro, if you like. Serve the stew on rice or with fresh crusty bread.

Makes 12 servings. Per serving: 163 calories, 9 g fat (1 g saturated), 20 g carbohydrates, 5 g protein, 4 g fiber, 0 mg cholesterol, 61 mg sodium.

◎ Slivered Cucumber & Chicken Salad

Because of the simplicity of the salad, it is important to use juicy chicken.

3 to 4 Kirby cucumbers, peeled and julienned
1 large cooked chicken breast half, skinned, boned, and julienned

Dressing
2 tablespoons rice vinegar
1 tablespoon reduced sodium soy sauce
1/2 teaspoon dry yellow mustard or dry wasabi
1/2 teaspoon salt
1 teaspoon toasted sesame seeds

Combine cucumbers and chicken in a bowl. Mix dressing ingredients in a cup and drizzle on top. Toss to coat. Cover and marinate in refrigerator 30 minutes to 1 hour. Serve cold, sprinkled with sesame seeds.

Makes 2 servings. Per serving: 127 calories, 2 g fat (1 g saturated), 11 g carbohydrates, 17 g protein, 3 g fiber, 34 mg cholesterol, 923 mg sodium.

◎ Roasted Asparagus with Orange Sauce

Surprise your guests with this unusual but delicious combination!

2 (1-pound) bunches asparagus, ends trimmed
2 tablespoons olive oil

1 teaspoon grated orange zest
2 tablespoons fresh orange juice
salt and freshly ground pepper

Place oven rack 4 inches from heat source. Preheat broiler. Line a large shallow roasting pan with a sheet of foil.

Spread asparagus in a straight line in prepared pan; sprinkle with oil, orange zest and juice, salt, and pepper. Toss to coat. (Keep spears in a straight line.) Broil 4 minutes; turn spears. Roast 3 to 5 minutes longer, until asparagus is tender.

Makes 6 servings. Per serving: 77 calories, 5 g fat (1 g saturated), 8 g carbohydrates, 4 g protein, 3 g fiber, 0 mg cholesterol, 51 mg sodium.

◎ Steamed Vegetables

2 cups water
Vegetables (carrots, broccoli, Brussels sprouts, spinach, green beans, peas, cauliflower)

Seasoning (pepper, lemon juice, garlic, dill)

Boil water. Place vegetables in steamer tray over water. Cover. Steam for 4 minutes. Remove. Season vegetables with choice of seasoning.

Makes 4 servings. Nutrition varies with vegetables used.

◎ Greek Salad

1/2 head romaine lettuce
1/2 red bell pepper, diced
1/2 yellow bell pepper, diced
1/2 green bell pepper, diced

1/2 cucumber, skinned and sliced
1/8 cup feta cheese
Oil and vinegar

Rinse and spin lettuce. Place lettuce in a large bowl; add peppers and cucumber. Top with cheese. Dress salad with oil and vinegar and toss.

Makes 4 servings. Per serving: 67 calories, 5 g fat (1 g saturated), 6 g carbohydrates, 2 g protein, 2 g fiber, 4 mg cholesterol, 57 mg sodium.

◎ Spinach and Mandarin Orange Salad

1 bunch spinach	*1/4 cup walnuts*
1 can mandarin oranges	*Raspberry vinaigrette*

Rinse and spin spinach. Place spinach in a large bowl. Drain mandarin oranges and add to spinach. Add walnuts. Dress with vinaigrette and toss.

Makes 4 servings. Per serving: 157 calories, 10 g fat (1 g saturated), 17 g carbohydrates, 4 g protein, 6 g fiber, 0 mg cholesterol, 67 mg sodium.

Fish

◎ Cajun Salmon

This special and spicy entrée takes mere minutes to prepare. Serve with baked potatoes and asparagus.

1/2 cup white wine	*1 teaspoon olive oil*
1 pound salmon fillet	*1 teaspoon Cajun seasoning*

Soak a medium-size clay pot and lid in water for 10 to 15 minutes. Drain the pot and lid. Line the bottom of the pot with parchment paper. Pour in the wine. Arrange the salmon in the pot. Rub with olive oil and Cajun seasoning.

Cover the pot, and place in a cold oven. Set oven to 400°F, and cook until the salmon is done throughout and flakes easily when probed with a fork, 30 to 40 minutes.

Makes 4 servings. Per serving: 222 calories, 11 g fat (2 g saturated), 1 g carbohydrates, 24 g protein, 0 g fiber, 70 mg cholesterol, 55 mg sodium.

Quick cooking tip: Have salmon steaks but no fillet? Follow the same recipe; it'll work just as nicely.

◎ Alaskan Salmon Salad Sandwiches

These are lunchtime fare but fancy enough for little tea sandwiches. The tangy yogurt and lemon juice in the dressing brightens the mixture more than mayonnaise could.

1 (15 1/2-ounce) can Alaskan salmon	*1/3 cup chopped celery*
	1 tablespoon lemon juice
1/3 cup plain nonfat yogurt	*freshly ground pepper to taste*
1/3 cup chopped scallions	*6 pita loaves*

Drain the salmon and place in a large bowl. Separate into flakes using a fork. Stir in the yogurt, scallions, celery, lemon juice, and pepper and mix well.

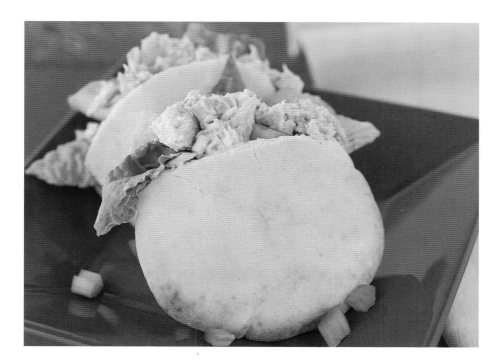

Cut a slice off of a pita edge so you can open it. Place the slice at the bottom of the pocket to help absorb the juices from the filling. Repeat with the remaining pitas.

To serve, spoon the salad into the pitas.

Makes 6 servings. Per serving: 211 calories, 7 g fat (1 g saturated), 18 g carbohydrates, 19 g protein, 1 g fiber, 46 mg cholesterol, 202 mg sodium.

◎ Cod Fillets with Lemon and Thyme

Lemon predominates in this delectable fish dish, which can be served with baked potatoes and green peas or a tossed salad. Cod, a lean and firm-fleshed fish, is a close cousin to haddock and pollock.

1/2 cup dry white wine	*1/2 teaspoon thyme leaves*
2 bay leaves	*1 leek, white part only, sliced*
1 pound cod fillet	*4 cloves garlic, minced*
Juice of 1 lemon	*1/2 lemon, thinly sliced*
1/4 teaspoon white pepper	

Soak a medium-size clay pot and lid in water for 10 to 15 minutes. Drain the pot and lid. Line the pot with parchment paper. Pour in the wine and add the bay leaves. Add the cod, skin side down. Pour the lemon juice over the cod. Season with the pepper and thyme. Top with the leek, garlic, and lemon slices.

Cover the pot, and place in a cold oven. Set oven to 400°F, and cook until the cod is done throughout and flakes easily when probed with a fork, 30 to 40 minutes. Discard the bay leaves.

Makes 4 servings. Per serving: 140 calories, 1 g fat (trace saturated), 9 g carbohydrates, 21 g protein, 3 g fiber, 42 mg cholesterol, 88 mg sodium.

Quick cooking tip: To squeeze the most juice from a lemon, roll it on a work surface, pressing down firmly, then juice.

◎ Baked Cod with Seasoned Tomatoes

Cod is a white, very mild fish. The slightly assertive flavors of mustard and onion in this recipe give it some welcome pep.

1 can (14 ounces) stewed tomatoes	*1 teaspoon yellow mustard seeds*
2 teaspoons Worcestershire sauce	*1 onion, thinly sliced*
1 pound cod fillets	*1 lemon, sliced*

Soak a medium-size clay pot and lid in water for 10 to 15 minutes. Drain the pot and lid. Combine the tomatoes and Worcestershire sauce in the pot. Add the cod fillets. Top with the mustard seeds, onion, and lemon.

Cover the pot, and place in a cold oven. Set oven to 375°F, and cook until the cod is done and flakes easily when probed with a fork, 50 to 60 minutes.

Makes 4 servings. Per serving: 142 calories, 1 g fat (trace saturated), 13 g carbohydrates, 22 g protein, 3 g fiber, 42 mg cholesterol, 472 mg sodium.

Quick cooking tips: Before cooking the cod, use needle-nose pliers to remove fine bones. When the cod is done, it will flake apart easily and appear opaque from top to bottom.

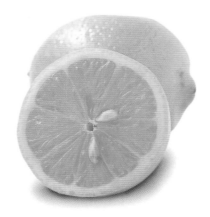

◎ Lime Flounder with Mandarin Salsa

Luscious mandarin oranges, lively cilantro, and tangy lime make this refreshing salsa and tropical fish entrée sing. It's elegant enough for company, fast enough for weeknight dinners, and guaranteed to please.

1/4 cup white wine
1/4 cup lime juice
1 pound flounder fillets
Dash white pepper
1/4 teaspoon ground celery seed
1 shallot, thinly sliced
1/2 cucumber, seeded and diced

1 can (11 ounces) mandarin
*   oranges, drained*
1 tablespoon chopped fresh chives
1 teaspoon olive oil
1 tablespoon cider vinegar
Dash of ground red pepper
2 teaspoons chopped fresh cilantro

Soak a medium-size clay pot and lid in water for 10 to 15 minutes. Drain the pot and lid.

Place parchment paper in the bottom of the pot. Pour in the wine and lime juice. Add the flounder. Season with the white pepper and celery seed; top with the shallots.

Cover the pot, and place in a cold oven. Set oven to 375°F and cook until the fish flakes easily when probed with the tip of a knife, 30 minutes.

While the flounder is cooking, combine the cucumber, oranges, chives, oil, vinegar, red pepper, and cilantro in a small bowl. Chill for 15 to 20 minutes. Serve with the flounder.

Makes 4 servings. Per serving: 166 calories, 3 g fat (1 g saturated), 11 g carbohydrates, 22 g protein, 1 g fiber, 54 mg cholesterol, 99 mg sodium.

Quick cooking tip: Shallots are closely related to onions. Use the two interchangeably, if you wish.

◎ Grilled Trout with Horseradish Crust

Enjoy the crunch of a crust without the carbs!

2 skinless trout fillets
1 tablespoon olive oil plus extra
*   for greasing the pan*
1 slice whole-wheat bread, ground
*   into small, coarse crumbs*
2 teaspoons creamed horseradish
1 tablespoon chopped fresh parsley
grated rind of 1/2 lemon

For the Dressing
1 teaspoon Dijon mustard
juice of 1/2 lemon
salt to taste
freshly ground pepper to taste
2 tablespoons virgin olive oil
1 cup mixed crisp salad leaves

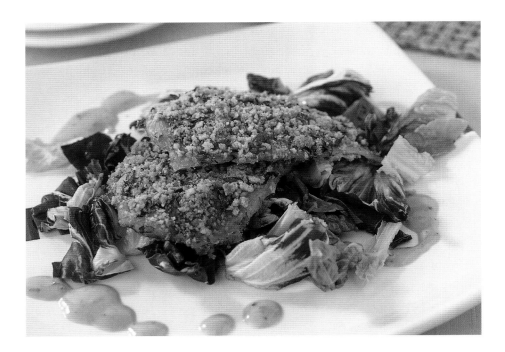

Preheat the broiler. Brush a broiler pan with oil. Sprinkle the trout fillets with salt and pepper.

In a bowl, mix together the bread, horseradish, parsley, 1 tablespoon olive oil, and the lemon rind. Spread this mixture over the trout fillets and place under the grill for 5 minutes to cook.

For the dressing: Mix the mustard and lemon juice together in a bowl. Add a little salt and pepper and whisk in the oil very slowly. Mix the salad leaves with a little of the dressing and place on a large dinner plate. Drizzle the remaining dressing around the outside of the plate. Place the crusted trout on top of the salad leaves and serve warm.

Makes 2 servings. Per serving: 351 calories, 26 g fat (4 g saturated), 13 g carbohydrates, 19 g protein, 4 g fiber, 46 mg cholesterol, 195 mg sodium.

◉ Mahi-Mahi with Persimmons

Get psyched for a mouth-watering experience. This exotic dish calls for mahi-mahi, a firm, flavorful, somewhat fatty fish that also goes by the name dorado, and persimmons, the national fruit of Japan.

1 pound mahi-mahi fillets
1/2 cup white grape juice
1/4 teaspoon allspice

1/4 cup fresh cilantro leaves
1 small onion, sliced
1 persimmon, sliced

Soak a medium-size clay pot and lid in water for 10 to 15 minutes. Drain the pot and lid. Line the pot with parchment paper. Arrange the mahi-mahi in the pot. Pour in the grape juice and season with the allspice. Top with the cilantro, onion, and persimmon.

Cover the pot, and place in a cold oven. Set oven to 400°F, and cook until the mahi-mahi is done throughout and flakes easily when probed with a fork, 40 to 45 minutes.

Makes 4 servings. Per serving: 112 calories, 2 g fat (trace saturated), 8 g carbohydrates, 18 g protein, 2 g fiber, 23 mg cholesterol, 74 mg sodium.

Quick cooking tip: The Japanese persimmon (also called a Hachiya) is the most widely available variety in the United States. Use it when completely ripe and quite soft; its flavor will be tangy-sweet. When underripe, the Hachiya is extremely astringent.

◎ Lemon-Orange Roughy

This lively fish entrée is unusually tart and tangy, thanks to lemon slices and orange juice. Sesame seeds provide a rich mellowness. Be sure to use toasted seeds; they have the richest flavor.

6 sprigs fresh lemon thyme
1 pound orange roughy fillets
1/2 cup orange juice
1/4 teaspoon lemon pepper

1 shallot, chopped
1 lemon, sliced
2 teaspoons toasted sesame seeds,
 for garnish

Soak a medium-size clay pot and lid in water for 10 to 15 minutes. Drain the pot and lid. Arrange the lemon thyme in the bottom of the pot.

Arrange the orange roughy over the thyme. Season with the lemon pepper and shallots. Top with the lemon slices.

Cover the pot, and place in a cold oven. Set oven to 400°F, and cook until the orange roughy is done throughout and flakes easily when probed with a fork, 35 to 45 minutes.

Garnish with sesame seeds and serve immediately.

Makes 4 servings. Per serving: 112 calories, 2 g fat (trace saturated), 8 g carbohydrates, 18 g protein, 7 g fiber, 23 mg cholesterol, 74 mg sodium.

Quick cooking tip: Most orange roughy, which hails from New Zealand, arrives at the market frozen. If you purchase thawed fillets, do not refreeze them. The process of thawing, refreezing, and thawing will lower the quality.

◎ Perch with Duck Sauce and Pineapple

Here's an unforgettably tasty combination of sweet (pineapple and apple juice) and savory (scallions and tomatillos) that gives perch a fresh flavor.

1/2 cup apple juice
4 teaspoons duck sauce
1 pound perch fillets
2 scallions, sliced in strips

2 tomatillos, thinly sliced
2 pineapple rings
Chinese chili sauce (optional)

Soak a medium-size clay pot and lid in water for 10 to 15 minutes. Drain the pot and lid. Line the pot with parchment paper. Pour in the apple juice. Spread the duck sauce over the perch. Arrange the perch in the pot. Top with the scallions, tomatillos, and pineapple rings.

Cover the pot, and place in a cold oven. Set oven to 400°F, and cook until the perch is done throughout and flakes easily when pierced with a fork, 40 to 45 minutes. Serve immediately with a small dab of the Chinese chili sauce, if desired.

Makes 4 servings. Per serving: 153 calories, 2 g fat (trace saturated), 12 g carbohydrates, 23 g protein, 1 g fiber, 102 mg cholesterol, 159 mg sodium.

Quick cooking tip: Use Chinese chili sauce sparingly; it's hot stuff!

◎ Rainbow Trout with Orange

Farm-raised trout and fresh oranges play a delightful duet in this flavorful entrée. You'll win accolades, guaranteed.

1 pound rainbow trout fillets
1/2 cup clam juice
1/4 teaspoon lemon pepper

6 sprigs lemon thyme
2 oranges, thinly sliced

Soak a medium-size clay pot and lid in water for 10 to 15 minutes. Drain the pot and lid. Line pot with parchment paper. Arrange the trout in the pot. Pour in the clam juice. Season with the lemon pepper. Top with the thyme sprigs and orange slices from 1 orange.

Cover the pot, and place in a cold oven. Set oven to 400°F, and cook until the trout is done and flakes easily when probed with a fork, about 45 minutes. Discard the thyme sprigs. Serve with the fresh orange slices.

Makes 4 servings. Per serving: 177 calories, 6 g fat (2 g saturated), 5 g carbohydrates, 24 g protein, 1 g fiber, 67 mg cholesterol, 150 mg sodium.

Quick cooking tip: If you can't find lemon thyme in your market, use the standard variety.

◎ Scallops Edam

Haul in some well-earned compliments with this extra-easy dish. The tender sea scallops play well with creamy Edam cheese and its subtle smoky flavors.

1/2 cup clam juice
1/2 cup dry vermouth
6 cloves garlic, crushed
1 teaspoon olive oil
1/4 teaspoon white pepper

1/4 teaspoon dried tarragon leaves
1 pound sea scallops
1/2 cup shredded Edam cheese
Parsley sprigs

Soak a medium-size clay pot and lid in water for 10 to 15 minutes. Meanwhile, combine the clam juice, vermouth, garlic, oil, pepper, and tarragon in a small bowl. Drain the clay pot and lid. Line the pot with parchment paper. Arrange the scallops in the pot and pour in the clam juice mixture.

Cover the pot, and place in a cold oven. Set oven to 400°F, and cook until done and opaque, 35 to 45 minutes. Transfer to a serving dish. Top with the Edam and garnish with the parsley.

Makes 4 servings. Per serving: 203 calories, 6 g fat (3 g saturated), 8 g carbohydrates, 23 g protein, 0 g fiber, 50 mg cholesterol, 432 mg sodium.

Quick cooking tip: Halve or quarter large scallops so all pieces are a uniform size for even cooking.

◎ Baked Fish and Vegetable Packets

This recipe is fast, simple, and guaranteed to be a hit!

6 large romaine leaves
1 medium carrot, shredded
1 1/2 cups shredded coleslaw mix
or a mix of shredded red and
green cabbage and carrots
2 teaspoons balsamic vinegar

1 1/2 pounds cod or halibut filets,
cut into 6 square pieces (they
don't have to be exact, they just
shouldn't be strips)
salt and freshly ground pepper
2 tablespoons butter

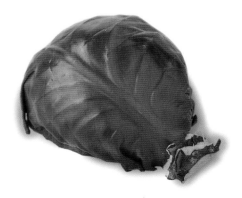

Preheat oven to 400°F. Blanch romaine leaves in boiling water 1 minute; drain in colander and place in bowl of ice and water until cold. Drain; place on work surface.

Pile 1/4 cup coleslaw mix near root end of romaine leaves. Drizzle with vinegar. Top with a piece of fish. Sprinkle with salt and pepper.

Grease a 2-quart shallow baking dish with some of the butter; dot the remainder over the fish. Fold stem end of romaine up over the fish; fold sides over. Roll up, egg-roll fashion. Place seam side down in prepared dish. Cover with foil; bake until fish is cooked through, 25 to 30 minutes.

Makes 6 servings. Per serving: 138 calories, 5 g fat (3 g saturated), 3 g carbohydrates, 21 g protein, 1 g fiber, 52 mg cholesterol, 127 mg sodium.

◎ Simply Monkfish

Poor man's lobster, as monkfish is often called, just got better in this extra-easy-to-prepare dish. It's succulent. It's delicious, thanks to Asian fish sauce, a dab of butter, and fresh chives. And it's fit for a feast—on any weeknight or weekend.

1/4 cup clam juice
1/4 cup dry white wine
1/2 teaspoon Asian fish sauce
2 bay leaves

1 pound monkfish fillets,
   membranes removed
2 teaspoons whipped butter
1/2 cup minced fresh chives

Soak a medium-size clay pot and lid in water for 10 to 15 minutes. Meanwhile, combine the clam juice, wine, fish sauce, and bay leaves in a small bowl. Drain the clay pot and lid. Line the pot with parchment paper. Arrange the monkfish in the pot. Pour in the clam juice mixture. Dot the monkfish with the butter. Top with the chives.

Cover the pot, and place in a cold oven. Set oven to 400°F, and cook until the fish is cooked throughout and flakes easily when probed with a fork, about 45 minutes.

Makes 4 servings. Per serving: 113 calories, 3 g fat (1 g saturated), 1 g carbohydrates, 17 g protein, 0 g fiber, 33 mg cholesterol, 79 mg sodium.

Quick cooking tip: Removing monkfish's grayish membrane is fairly easy. Simply lift it with your fingers and, using scissors, snip any places where it clings to the white flesh.

◎ Curried Beef & Potatoes

It's back to the basics with this recipe: meat and potatoes, but with a very fresh spin!

12 ounces top round beef steak

8 ounces potatoes, peeled, halved, and thinly sliced

1/2 cup beef broth

2 teapoons cornstarch

1/4 teaspoon salt

nonstick cooking spray

3/4 cup chopped onion

3/4 cup chopped green or red bell pepper

1 tablespoon vegetable oil

1 teaspoon curry powder

1 medium tomato, coarsely chopped

Partially freeze the meat. Thinly slice across the grain into bite-sized strips and set aside.

Cook the potatoes in boiling water until tender, about 8 minutes. Drain and set aside.

Combine the beef broth, cornstarch, and salt. Set aside.

Grease a wok or large skillet with cooking spray. Heat over medium-high heat. Add the onion and stir-fry 2 minutes. Add the bell pepper and stir-fry

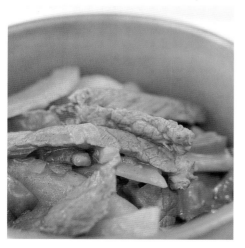

until the vegetables are crisp and tender, about 2 minutes. Remove to a bowl.

Add the oil to the hot wok. Add the beef and curry powder. Stir-fry until cooked to the desired doneness, 2 to 3 minutes. Push beef from center of the wok. Stir broth mixture to recombine and add to center of wok. Heat to boiling, stirring until thickened. Stir in onion mixture, potatoes, and tomato. Cook, stirring, until heated through.

Makes 4 servings. Per serving: 263 calories, 12 g fat (3 g saturated), 18 g carbohydrates, 21 g protein, 3 g fiber, 50 mg cholesterol, 294 mg sodium.

◎ Thai Pork Chops

These juicy, spicy pork chops are easy to coat and quick to cook. There will be seasoning mix left over for your next batch or for cooking chicken or fish.

Thai Seasoning
18 pieces of low-sodium sesame-
* flavored Melba toast*
1 tablespoon garlic powder
1 tablespoon ground ginger
1 teaspoon sugar

¹/2 teaspoon cayenne pepper
4 lean center-cut loin pork chops,
* ¹/2-inch thick*
1 tablespoon low-sodium soy sauce
nonstick cooking spray

Place the Melba toast in a food processor, and process until finely crushed. Combine the crushed Melba toast and remaining ingredients in a zip-top heavy-duty plastic bag, seal bag, and shake well. Store tightly sealed, shake well before each use. Use as a coating mix for pork or poultry.

Preheat the oven to 450°F. Grease a baking sheet with cooking spray.

Trim the fat from the pork chops, and brush pork with soy sauce. Place ¹/3 cup Thai Seasoning in a large zip-top heavy-duty plastic bag. Add chops, seal bag, and shake to coat. Place chops on the prepared baking sheet and bake until cooked through, about 15 minutes.

Makes 4 servings. Per serving: 205 calories, 5 g fat (2 g saturated), 14 g carbohydrates, 24 g protein, 1 g fiber, 62 mg cholesterol, 218 mg sodium.

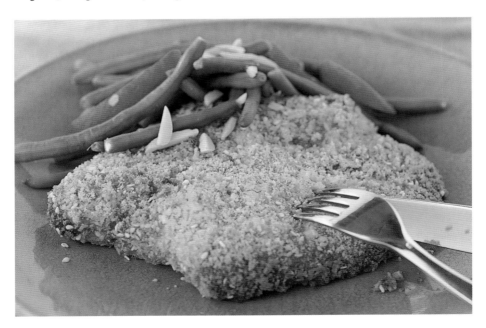

◎ Jamaican Jerk Pork

This trendy entrée gets its flavorful, hot zing from a rub with eight spices, including pungent cloves and nippy peppers.

2 cups fat-free beef broth or homemade stock	1/4 teaspoon powdered ginger
2 teaspoons dried minced onions	1/4 teaspoon allspice
1 teaspoon dried thyme	1/4 teaspoon cloves
1 teaspoon garlic powder	1 pound pork tenderloin
1 teaspoon crushed red pepper flakes	3 tablespoons cold water
1/4 teaspoon cinnamon	2 tablespoons cornstarch

Pour the broth into a pressure cooker. Place a rack or trivet in the bottom of the cooker.

In a small bowl, combine the onions, thyme, garlic, red pepper flakes, cinnamon, ginger, allspice, and cloves. Rub the spice mixture into all sides of the pork. Place the pork on the rack in the cooker.

Place the lid on the cooker, lock it into position, and place the pressure regulator on the vent pipe if you are using a first-generation cooker. Over medium-high or high heat, bring the cooker up to pressure. Then lower the heat, adjusting it as necessary to maintain pressure (regulator should rock gently), and cook the mixture for 35 minutes.

Let the pressure drop naturally for 15 minutes; then quick-release any remaining pressure (under cold running water if you're using a first-generation cooker). Carefully remove the pressure regulator and lid. Transfer the pork to a platter, leaving the broth in the cooker; keep the pork warm.

In a small cup, whisk together the cold water and cornstarch. Stir the cornstarch into the broth, and cook the gravy, uncovered, until it's slightly thickened and hot. Slice the pork and serve it with the gravy.

Makes 4 servings. Per serving: 166 calories, 4 g fat (2 g saturated), 5 g carbohydrates, 25 g protein, 1 g fiber, 74 mg cholesterol, 449 mg sodium.

Quick cooking tip: Some supermarkets carry jerk seasoning. If yours does, give the prepared combo a try.

◎ Egg Noodles with Chicken & Vegetables

6 ounces dried Chinese egg noodles
8 ounces chicken breast
1 tablespoon oil
1 medium carrot, peeled and
    julienned
4 ounces green beans, trimmed

and cut in half lengthwise
1 cup julienned daikon radish
2 tablespoons soy sauce
1 tablespoon oyster sauce
1 julienned chile
2 sprigs fresh cilantro, leaves only

Soak the noodles in boiling water until softened, about 1 minute. Drain in a colander and rinse well with cold water. Squeeze off excess water. Slice the chicken breast into thin pieces.

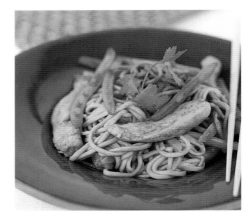

Heat the oil in a wok over medium-high heat and add the chicken pieces and vegetables. Stir-fry until the chicken is almost cooked through. Add the noodles and heat through. Add the soy sauce and the oyster sauce and stir-fry until the chicken and noodles are coated. Let cook 2 minutes, until heated through and the chicken is cooked.

Turn out the noodle mixture onto a serving plate and garnish with the slices of chile and cilantro leaves. Serve hot.

Makes 8 first-course servings. Per serving: 140 calories, 3 g fat (trace saturated), 18 g carbohydrates, 10 g protein, 2 g fiber, 37 mg cholesterol, 301 mg sodium.

◎ Greek Chicken Sandwiches

Who says hummus is just for vegetables? This great chicken dish proves otherwise.

1/4 cup plain Greek yogurt
2 tablespoons hummus (homemade
    or store-bought chickpea dip)
1 teaspoon ground cumin
1 teaspoon ground coriander
1/2 teaspoon turmeric
3 tablespoons fresh lime juice
1 tablespoon chopped fresh mint
pinch of salt

4 boneless, skinless chicken breast
    halves, cut into thin strips
2 tablespoons Basil Oil (recipe
    follows) for serving
4 white pita bread pockets
mixed salad greens
sliced tomatoes
sliced yellow bell pepper

Mix together the yogurt and hummus in a bowl, cover, and refrigerate.

In a shallow bowl blend together the cumin, coriander, turmeric, lime juice, mint, and salt. Add the chicken to the spice mixture, mix well to coat, cover,

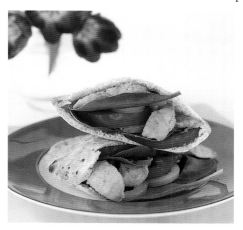

and leave to marinate in a cool place for at least 30 minutes, stirring occasionally.

Heat the Basil Oil in a large skillet over medium heat and fry the chicken until cooked through, 8 to 10 minutes, stirring occasionally, until golden.

Toast the pita pockets on each side until golden brown. Cut in half crossways, open up, and fill with the chicken mixture. Add salad leaves, tomato slices, and yellow bell pepper slices. Top with a generous spoonful of the hummus–yogurt mixture and serve immediately.

Makes 4 servings. Per serving: 295 calories, 10 g fat (2 g saturated), 20 g carbohydrates, 31 g protein, 1 g fiber, 69 mg cholesterol, 329 mg sodium.

◎ Basil Oil

*1/4 cup loosely packed fresh
    basil leaves*
1/2 cup olive oil

salt to taste
freshly ground pepper to taste

Combine the basil and oil in a blender and season with salt and pepper. Purée until the oil is finely flecked with the basil.

Makes 1/2 cup. Per serving: 120 calories, 14 g fat, trace carbohydrates, 0 g protein.

◎ Grilled Turkey & Tomato Burgers

Fire up the barbecue and get ready for these vegetable-packed, tasty turkey burgers.

1 egg white
1/4 cup fine dry breadcrumbs
1/4 cup finely shredded carrot
1/4 cup finely chopped onion
1/4 cup finely chopped green pepper
1/2 teaspoon salt

1/8 teaspoon pepper
1 pound ground turkey
*2 tablespoons grated Parmesan
    cheese*
nonstick cooking spray
1 medium tomato, sliced

In a large bowl combine the egg white and breadcrumbs. (If using beef, 2 tablespoons water.) Stir in the carrot, onion, green pepper, salt, and pepper. Add the ground meat and Parmesan cheese and mix well. Shape meat mixture into four 3/4-inch-thick patties.

Prepare an outdoor grill for barbecue. When the coals are ready, grease a cold grill rack with nonstick cooking spray and place the rack on a grill. Grill the burgers over medium coals for 7 minutes. Turn and grill 8 to 11 minutes or until no pink remains. Place 1 tomato slice on each burger and grill 1 minute longer.

Makes 4 servings. Per serving: 227 calories, 11 g fat (3 g saturated), 9 g carbohydrates, 23 g protein, 1 g fiber, 92 mg cholesterol, 519 mg sodium.

◎ Honey Turkey Fajitas

You can substitute chicken breast or pork tenderloin for the turkey. These margarita-inspired seasonings go well with many meats.

1 pound (uncooked) turkey breast
juice and grated rind of 1 lime
juice of 1 orange
1 red chili pepper, finely diced
2 tablespoons tequila
2 tablespoons olive oil

1 tablespoon strong-flavored honey
1 teaspoon chopped fresh cilantro
salt and pepper to taste
8 warm flour tortillas
1 (8-ounce) container crème fraîche
or sour cream for serving

Cut the turkey into strips no longer than your little finger. Place in a large bowl and add the lime juice and grated rind, orange juice, chili, tequila, oil, honey, and 1 teaspoon cilantro. Mix well. Cover and marinate in the refrigerator for 4 to 6 hours.

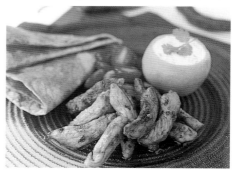

When ready to serve, heat a heavy, nonstick skillet. Drain the turkey, reserving the marinade. Add the turkey to the skillet and cook rapidly to brown quickly. Add the marinade and heat to boiling, over medium-high heat, while stirring the turkey. Cook until the turkey is glazed and the marinade has sizzled away. Season with salt and pepper.

Sprinkle the tortillas with a little water and heat for 30 seconds in another skillet. Place a little turkey on each tortilla, fold up and serve with a little crème fraîche and chopped cilantro.

Makes 8 servings. Per serving: 288 calories, 15 g fat (5 g saturated), 20 g carbohydrates, 16 g protein, 1 g fiber, 49 mg cholesterol, 201 mg sodium.

◎ Spicy Orange Beef with Broccoli

This recipe adds a little extra flavor to a favorite dish!

1 pound thinly sliced beef top round

1/2 cup chopped green onions

1/4 cup roasted-garlic teriyaki sauce

2 tablespoons grated orange zest

2 tablespoons dry sherry

1 tablespoon rice-wine vinegar

1 tablespoon plus 1 teaspoon cornstarch

4 tablespoons peanut or vegetable oil

1/2 teaspoon crushed red-pepper flakes

2 cups broccoli florets, halved lengthwise if large

1/2 teaspoon salt

1/4 teaspoon sugar

4 tablespoons water

Cut beef slices into 2-inch-wide strips. Combine beef, onions, sauce, zest, sherry, vinegar, and 1 tablespoon cornstarch in a plastic food-storage bag. Squeeze to mix and coat beef evenly with marinade. Let stand 10 minutes.

To finish: Heat 2 tablespoons oil in wok over high heat. Add pepper flakes; stir-fry 30 seconds. Add broccoli; stir-fry 2 minutes. Sprinkle with salt and sugar; toss to coat. Add 2 tablespoons water; cover and steam 2 minutes, stirring once. Scrape out into a bowl.

Heat remaining 2 tablespoons oil in wok over high heat. Add beef and marinade; stir-fry until beef is cooked and browned, 1 to 2 minutes. Add broccoli and juices; stir-fry until hot, 1 to 2 minutes. Mix remaining 1 teaspoon cornstarch with remaining 2 tablespoons water; pour around edges of wok so it goes into liquid. Stir-fry until juices are thickened and shiny, about 2 minutes.

Makes 6 servings. Per serving: 231 calories, 14 g fat (4 g saturated), 7 g carbohydrates, 18 g protein, 1 g fiber, 45 mg cholesterol, 699 mg sodium.

◎ Skillet Salsa Beef

Just because you're eating good carbs doesn't mean you have to miss out. Enjoy this fantastic good-carb spin on tacos!

1 pound flank steak, thinly sliced across the grain

2 tablespoons balsamic vinegar

1 teaspoon dried oregano leaves

1/2 teaspoon garlic powder

5 tablespoons corn oil or other vegetable oil

2 stalks celery, thinly sliced on the diagonal

1 cup hot salsa fresca

2 (8-inch) corn tortillas

1/4 cup tender cilantro sprigs

Combine beef, vinegar, oregano, and garlic powder in medium bowl; stir to mix.

Heat 1 tablespoon oil in large nonstick skillet over medium-high heat. Add celery; sauté 1 minute. Add steak mixture; sauté until browned, about 3 minutes. Add salsa; mix well. Cover and simmer 5 minutes.

While steak mixture cooks, stack tortillas on cutting board and cut with pizza wheel into 1/2-inch wide strips. Heat remaining oil in medium skillet; fry tortilla strips until crisp. Drain on paper towels.

Spoon steak mixture onto serving dish; sprinkle with tortilla strips and cilantro.

Makes 4 servings. Per serving: 448 calories, 31 g fat (7 g saturated), 12 g carbohydrates, 31 g protein, 2 g fiber, 71 mg cholesterol, 397 mg sodium.

◎ Gorgonzola Cheeseburgers on Crostini

A fabulous modern spin on a classic food!

8 ounces ground sirloin or chuck
salt to taste
freshly ground pepper to taste
8 thin slices pancetta
4 ounces Gorgonzola cheese cut
*   into 4 (3/4-inch-thick) slices*

4 slices Italian bread
1 large garlic clove, sliced in half
8 basil leaves, shredded
1/2 cup chopped tomato
1/4 cup chopped red onion
extra-virgin olive oil for drizzling

Preheat the broiler or prepare an outdoor grill for barbecuing. Shape the meat into 4 patties and season on both sides with salt and pepper. Wrap each hamburger in 2 slices of pancetta.

Broil the burgers about 5 inches from the heat source or grill the burgers over a medium-hot fire for about 4 minutes, or until the pancetta is nicely

browned. Flip the burgers and top them with the Gorgonzola. Grill for about 4 minutes longer, or until nicely browned on the second side and cooked through.

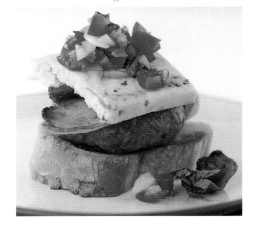

Meanwhile, rub the cut sides of the garlic over the bread and grill the bread on both sides until lightly toasted. Combine the basil, tomato, and onion in a small bowl and sprinkle with salt and pepper. Toss to mix.

To serve: Place one crostini on a serving plate. Top with the basil mixture and drizzle with oil. Set the burgers on top and serve at once.

Makes 4 servings. Per serving: 440 calories, 30 g fat (12 g saturated), 14 g carbohydrates, 27 g protein, 1 g fiber, 85 mg cholesterol, 1,153 mg sodium.

◎ Stir-Fried Sesame Lamb

The wonderful marinade and the tasty sauce give this lamb recipe an extra boost.

1 pound boneless lean lamb from
    the leg or center-cut chops,
    slightly frozen

8 ounces sliced mushrooms
2 tablespoons toasted sesame seeds

Marinade
2 teaspoons cornstarch
1/2 teaspoon sugar
2 tablespoons soy sauce
1 tablespoon water
1 bunch large green onions
1/4 cup peanut oil
2 garlic cloves, thinly sliced
1 (8-ounce) can bamboo shoots,
    drained and rinsed

Sauce
1 tablespoon soy sauce
1 tablespoon dry sherry
1 tablespoon dark sesame oil
1 teaspoon distilled white vinegar

Cut lamb into 2- x 1- x 1/8–inch slivers. Place in bowl. Add marinade ingredients; toss with your hands to incorporate marinade into meat. Set aside. Mix sauce ingredients in small bowl; set aside.

Line up green onions on cutting board with root ends even; trim off root ends in one chop. Trim off dried green portions. With paring knife, quarter each onion lengthwise; line up and cut crosswise into 1-inch pieces.

Heat wok or large nonstick skillet over high heat. Add oil; when hot but not smoking, add garlic and lamb; stir-fry until lamb pieces are dark brown and firm enough to separate. Add green onions; stir-fry 1 minute. Add bamboo shoots and mushrooms; stir-fry 1 minute.

Stir sauce and pour around edges of lamb. Stir-fry until sauce thickens and forms a shiny glaze on lamb mixture. Scrape out onto warm platter; sprinkle with sesame seeds.

Makes 4 servings. Per Serving: 445 calories, 34 g fat (8 g saturated), 9 g carbohydrates, 26 g protein, 2 g fiber, 76 mg cholesterol, 850 mg sodium.

Warm Fresh Fruit Delight

This delicate, refreshing dessert focuses on five favorite fruits: apples, pears, oranges, grapes, and nectarines. If juicy nectarines are elusive, try frozen peaches instead. The seasoning in this dish is subtle; if you want something spicier, add lemon juice and a dash of mace.

2 cups white grapes

2 nectarines, peeled and sliced

2 Anjou pears, peeled and cubed

2 Golden Delicious apples, peeled and cubed

2 oranges, peeled and sectioned

1 stick cinnamon

1/4 teaspoon ground nutmeg

1 cup orange juice

2 cups low-fat vanilla yogurt, frozen low-fat vanilla yogurt, or orange sherbet

Soak a medium-size clay pot and lid in water for 10 to 15 minutes. Drain the pot and lid.

Combine the grapes, nectarines, pears, apples, oranges, cinnamon, nutmeg, and orange juice in the pot. Toss gently to mix. Cover the pot, and place in a cold oven. Set oven to 375°F, and cook for 30 minutes.

Discard the cinnamon; stir to mix. Let cool, covered, for 5 minutes. Serve immediately topped with the yogurt, frozen yogurt, or sherbet.

Makes 6 servings. Per serving: 211 calories, 2 g fat (1 g saturated), 47 g carbohydrates, 6 g protein, 5 g fiber, 4 mg cholesterol, 55 mg sodium.

Quick cooking tip: Serve within 30 minutes of cooking; otherwise, the fruit will begin to darken.

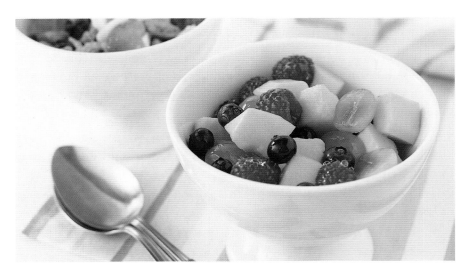

◎ Apple-Plum Crisp

Most fruit crisps have soft tops. Not this one. Fresh from the oven, the top is crisp and crunchy, thanks to egg white and almond slices. Macintosh apples form the sweet, fruity base. Prefer apple slices that are a little less sweet and hold their shape when cooked? Then try the Golden Delicious or Granny Smith variety.

6 Macintosh apples, peeled
*   and sliced*
3 plums, peeled and sliced
Juice of 1/2 lemon
1 cup quick oats
1 cup packed dark brown sugar

1 teaspoon ground cinnamon
1/4 teaspoon ground ginger
1/4 cup almond slices
2 tablespoons canola oil
1 egg white, lightly beaten

Soak a medium-size clay pot and lid in water for 10 to 15 minutes. Drain the pot and lid. Line the bottom of the pot with parchment paper. Arrange the apples and plums in the pot. Sprinkle the lemon juice over the fruit.

Cover the pot, and place in a cold oven. Set oven to 375°F, and cook for 40 minutes.

While the fruit is cooking, combine the oats, sugar, cinnamon, ginger, almonds, oil, and egg white, beating with a fork until well mixed. The mixture will be crumbly. Sprinkle over the fruit. Bake, uncovered, until the topping is puffed and golden brown, about 20 minutes. Serve with low-fat vanilla yogurt or nonfat whipped topping.

Makes 6 servings. Per serving: 374 calories, 10 g fat (1 g saturated), 69 g carbohydrates, 7 g protein, 8 g fiber, 0 mg cholesterol, 21 mg sodium.

Quick cooking tips: For a more pronounced flavor, toast the almonds before adding them to the topping. Regular oats can be substituted for the quick oats.

◎ Ginger-Poached Pears

There's nothing shy about these pears. During cooking, they soak up the sensational flavors of rum, cinnamon, and crystallized ginger and become subtly sweet yet slightly spicy. Serve them warm or at room temperature, and top each half with a dollop of your favorite lemon sherbet.

4 Bosc pears, peeled, cored,
*   and halved*
3 cups unsweetened apple juice
1/4 cup light rum

1 teaspoon chopped crystallized
*   ginger*
1 cinnamon stick
1 lemon, sliced

Soak a medium-size clay pot and lid in water for 10 to 15 minutes. Drain the pot and lid. Arrange the pears in the pot. Combine the juice, rum, and ginger, and pour the mixture over the pears. Add the cinnamon. Arrange the lemon slices over the pears.

Cover the pot, and place in a cold oven. Set oven to 375°F, and cook the pears for 1 hour. Remove the pot from the oven and place it on a towel or pot holders to cool. Serve the pears and poaching liquid warm or at room temperature, discarding the cinnamon stick and lemon slices.

Makes 4 servings. Per serving: 226 calories, 1 g fat (trace saturated), 51 g carbohydrates, 1 g protein, 6 g fiber, 0 mg cholesterol, 7 mg sodium.

Quick cooking tip: For best results, use slightly underripe pears.

◎ Pear-Strawberry Crisp

This sweet treat takes advantage of three luscious fruits: apples, pears, and strawberries. But you could use all apples or all pears plus berries of your choice. Optional crystallized ginger adds spicy bite for diners who like a little zing in their desserts.

3 Gala apples, peeled and sliced
3 Bosc pears, peeled and sliced
3 cups fresh, or frozen and thawed, unsweetened whole strawberries
1 cup white grape juice
2 tablespoons quick tapioca
1/2 cup unbleached flour

1/2 cup whole wheat flour
1 cup sugar
1 tablespoon canola oil
1 egg white, slightly beaten
1 teaspoon baking powder
2 teaspoons minced crystallized ginger (optional)

Soak a medium-size clay pot and lid in water for 10 to 15 minutes. Drain the pot and lid. Line the bottom of the pot with parchment paper. Combine the apples, pears, strawberries, grape juice, and tapioca in a large bowl, tossing gently to mix thoroughly. Pour into the pot.

Cover the pot, and place in a cold oven. Set oven to 375°F, and cook for 40 minutes.

While the fruit is baking, combine the unbleached flour, whole wheat flour, sugar, oil, egg white, baking powder, and crystallized ginger, if you use it. After the 40 minutes are up, sprinkle over the fruit. Bake, uncovered, until the topping is puffed and golden brown, about 25 to 30 minutes. Serve with low-fat vanilla yogurt or nonfat whipped topping.

Makes 6 servings. Per serving: 369 calories, 4 g fat (trace saturated), 85 g carbohydrates, 4 g protein, 7 g fiber, 0 mg cholesterol, 12 mg sodium.

Quick cooking tip: Crystallized ginger is hard and sticky. To mince it, use a heavy, sharp chef's knife or sharp kitchen scissors.

◎ Mixed Fruit Compote

Most cooks have a favorite dried fruit compote recipe. This one's a tasty combination that's ideal for breakfast, brunch, or dessert. Dry white wine, orange peel, cinnamon, and cloves tone down the dried fruit's sweetness.

3 cups unsweetened apple juice
1 package (8 ounces) mixed dried fruit
3/4 cup raisins
1 orange, sectioned and chopped
3 strips (about 2 x 3 inches each)
   orange zest

1/2 cup dry, fruity white wine,
   such as Riesling
1 stick cinnamon
2 whole cloves

Soak a medium-size clay pot and lid in water for 10 to 15 minutes. Drain the lid and pot. Pour the juice into the pot. Stir in the dried fruit, raisins, orange, orange zest, wine, cinnamon, and cloves.

Cover the pot, and place in a cold oven. Set oven to 375°F, and cook the fruit for 1 hour. Remove the pot from the oven and place it on a towel or pot holders to cool. Serve the fruit and poaching liquid warm or at room temperature, discarding the cinnamon stick and orange zest.

Makes 4 servings. Per serving: 476 calories, 1 g fat (trace saturated), 119 g carbohydrates, 4 g protein, 8 g fiber, 0 mg cholesterol, 53 mg sodium.

Quick cooking tip: When cutting orange zest, take care not to cut deeply into the white part (pith); it tastes bitter.

◎ Mocha Bread Pudding

Hooked on chocolaty-coffee flavors? Then you'll adore this pudding. It's satisfyingly rich-tasting but low in fat. Like most bread puddings, this one is best when made with a hearty country-style bread.

4 tablespoons cocoa
1 cup hot coffee
1 egg
1/4 cup fat-free egg substitute
2 cups 1 percent milk
1 cup skim milk
1/2 cup sugar

1 teaspoon vanilla
6 slices dry firm white bread,
   cubed
1/2 teaspoon ground cinnamon
Nonfat whipped topping
   (optional)

Whisk the cocoa into the coffee in a small bowl or a 2-cup measure. Let cool. Soak a medium-size clay pot and lid in water for 10 to 15 minutes.

While the coffee is cooling and the pot soaking, lightly beat the egg and egg substitute in a medium-size bowl. Stir in the coffee mixture, low-fat milk, skim milk, sugar, and vanilla.

Drain the pot and lid. Line the pot with parchment paper. Arrange the bread in the pot. Pour in the milk mixture. Using the back of a spoon, press the bread down to moisten all pieces. Sprinkle the cinnamon over the bread.

Cover the pot, and place in a cold oven. Set oven to 375°F, and cook until a knife inserted in the center comes out clean, 45 to 60 minutes. Let cool to room temperature. Serve with whipped topping, if desired.

Makes 6 servings. Per serving: 262 calories, 6 g fat (3 g saturated), 42 g carbohydrates, 13 g protein, 3 g fiber, 49 mg cholesterol, 281 mg sodium.

Quick cooking tip: Stored in a covered container in the refrigerator, the pudding will keep for 2 to 3 days.

◎ Chocolate-Cappuccino Dream Creams

A sweet finish to a meal makes everyone leave the table in a good mood. Most of the preparation can be done ahead of time, so you'll have to leave the table only to put it together.

3/4 cup heavy cream
1 tablespoon sugar
1 (8-ounce) container crème fraîche
1 tablespoon strong espresso coffee
6 amaretti cookies, roughly crushed
2 ounces bittersweet chocolate, grated

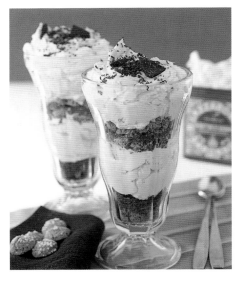

Pour the cream into a large bowl and add the sugar. Whip until it just begins to hold its shape, and then fold in the crème fraîche and coffee.

Add a layer of amaretti crumbs to 4 small elegant stemmed glasses. Sprinkle with one-third of the chocolate. Cover with half of the cream mixture and repeat the layers, finishing with grated chocolate. Set on a serving plate and serve at once.

Makes 4 servings. Per serving: 435 calories, 38 g fat (23 g saturated), 25 g carbohydrates, 5 g protein, 3 g fiber, 86 mg cholesterol, 152 mg sodium.

The Plan

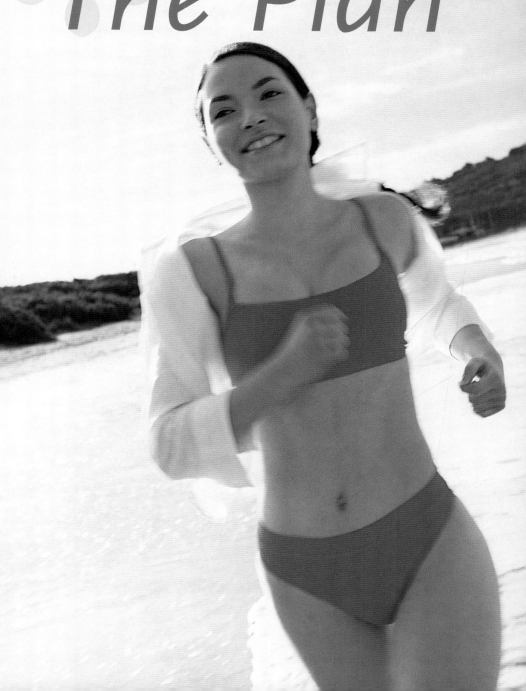

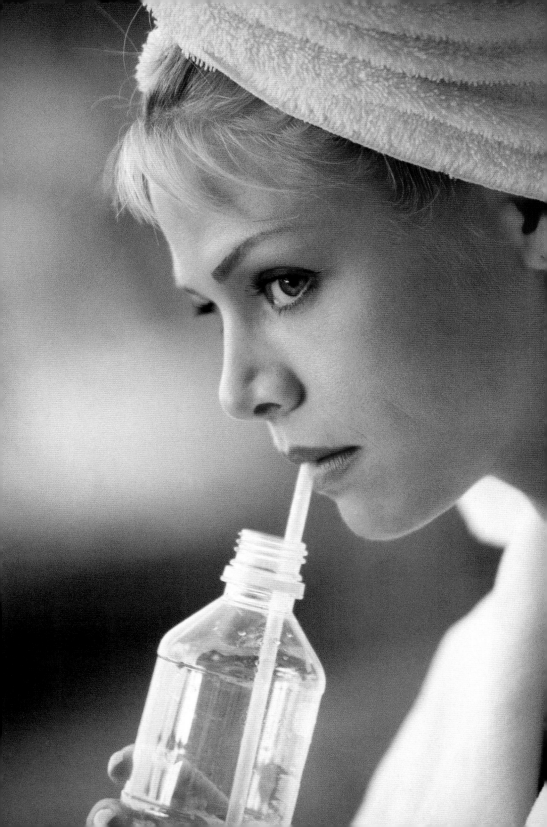

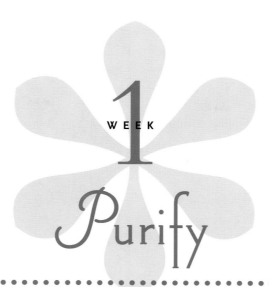

WEEK

1

Purify

. . . .

Warning: Before beginning the *30-Day Revitalization Plan* you should consult with a qualified health care professional, especially if you have any existing medical conditions, are taking any medications, are pregnant, or nursing.

Read carefully to find out what you need to know for the week.

The focus of Week 1 is to purify your body—inside and out, from head to toe—of accumulated, harmful toxins that have disrupted your system, affecting your energy level, slowing down your metabolism, and disturbing your blood and oxygen circulation. While the cleansing of your intestines, liver and gallbladder, kidneys, and skin will be felt and seen immediately after you implement your food regimen, spa treatments, and hair and skin care, you still need to purify your lungs, so exercise is vital.

Detox

During a week of purification, all five organs of elimination (including the liver and gallbladder) need to be stimulated at the same time. This is accomplished by fasting or partial fasting, whereby you consume certain foods or beverages, or both, that have tissue-cleansing, diuretic, and purifying properties. In addition, further measures of purification are used.

Meditation

Meditation, like exercise, is something that you cannot just jump in to, but rather have to incorporate into your life gradually. With practice, your body will be able to maintain meditative postures for longer periods of time, and

your mind will eventually be conditioned to sustain concentration
for extended sessions, compared
with the average of 30 seconds. But
for this week, you will ease into the
discipline by meditating 5 minutes
each day in a quiet space.

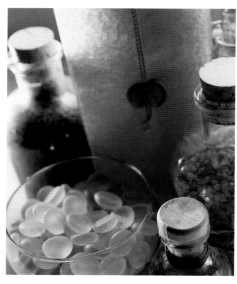

 ## Aromatherapy

As you begin a rigorous detoxification cure and a new exercise
regimen, it is natural to experience
both mental and physical stress and
anxiety. Aromatherapy will relax
you, reenergize you, and help you
prepare your body and mind for the tasks at hand. Each day the aromatherapy portion of the *30-Day Revitalization Plan* addresses a different
theme, but you are free to choose the actual formula, depending on what
aromas appeal to you.

 ## Exercise

Because you will be focused this week on purifying your body, it is best to
begin exercising with aerobic activities that are beneficial to the body as a
whole. Strength training, body toning, and endurance building will come in
subsequent weeks after your body is purified and adjusts to its increased
energy and movement. The plan for this week is to accompany an aerobic
exercise with a breathing exercise.

As part of the detox process, you will need to purify your breathing; thus,
it is essential to purify your lungs through exercise. Inhaling and exhaling
deeply will loosen impurities in the breathing passages. The best means of
detoxification for the lungs is to increase the depth of your breathing at least
once a day until you are almost out of breath. This increases the oxygen content in your blood and other body fluids, leads to an excretion of hormones,
and thus elevates your mood and stimulates blood circulation and digestion.

When exercising this week, overdress to induce perspiration, and wear
clothing made from natural fibers. Don't forget to wash off the perspiration
afterward with warm water followed by a cold rinse to close your pores and
strengthen your resistance. If you take a walk, walk briskly, which will induce
deeper breathing and lead to an increase of oxygen in the tissue. If you feel

weak on liquid-fast days, then reduce your exercises, but don't eliminate all physical activity. And don't be alarmed: highly odorous perspiration is a sign of intensive elimination of waste products. Be sure to hydrate yourself constantly before, during, and after each exercise session.

Home Spa

During this week of detox and purification, it's just as important to cleanse your skin as your internal organs. So every day this week, you will need to dry-brush your skin and complete the specified daily purifying spa treatment. Also, each day, you will perform spa treatments on a specific area of your body (hair, arms, legs, skin, hands, and feet) to help revitalize your appearance.

Dry-Brush Massage

To dry-brush your skin, massage your skin by brushing it with a loofah glove. Dry-brushing has many benefits: Not only will it stimulate the metabolism and the ability of your skin to eliminate toxins, but it will energize the involuntary nervous system and increase the flow of blood and help you slough off dead skin cells. You can use a body brush instead of a loofah glove.

1. Starting with your right foot, brush your entire body with a dry loofah glove, using a circular motion and always in the direction of the heart.

2. Brush for 2 to 3 minutes, until your skin turns slightly red.

3. Afterward, rub your body with a good skin oil.

This dry-brushing massage also can be done in water while taking a bath. Finish off your bath by taking a cold shower, and then rest. When you do this, a wonderful feeling of well-being will set in. Your body will get warm, and you will feel refreshed and rejuvenated.

Body Care

As you purify your body this week, you will also want to cleanse your hair and skin, so there are some deep-conditioning and cleansing treatments worked into your week. Use the Rosemary Chamomile Shampoo (see page 249) for fantastic results. Several key things to remember: Always be sure to rinse all product out of your hair. This will instantly restore shine and body that had been hidden behind product residue. As for your skin, exfoliate it every day, and never leave the house without wearing sunscreen. Although your attention will be on the purification plan, there is no reason not to begin the face-building exercises that will tone your facial muscles. It's never too early to begin working on your face, especially because the face-building exercises are effective but take time before results are noticeable. They require only 5 to 10 minutes a day and will make a huge difference in the long run.

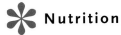

Nutrition

Regard every meal (even though it might consist only of liquids) as a true meal, and sit down at a nicely set table. Sip your fasting drink with a spoon, or drink it slowly.

If possible, rest for an hour each day after the midday meal; this rest period stimulates the liver. Place a hot-water bottle against your stomach. When you are lying down, the blood supply in your liver increases by 40 percent.

Don't drink any alcohol during these seven days. Limit your use of tobacco. If you can't or don't want to do without coffee, you may drink a cup in the morning, but without milk or sugar.

During the entire fast, make sure you drink a lot of liquid. Specific recipes are found in Chapter 8, Nutrition.

Day 1

7-Day Cure: Day of Fasting

Fasting days are days for drinking. You may drink more than the amounts indicated for the fast. Drinking is also helpful if you are feeling hungry.

Meditation

For today's session, begin with one of the Basic Relaxation Exercises (see page 29), followed by the Awareness Breath (see page 32), and for your meditation technique, use the Alignment meditation (see page 35).

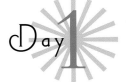

Aromatherapy

With the *30-Day Revitalization Plan*, it's imperative to learn to value hard work and to value yourself. So begin the program with an aromatherapy application formula for Appreciation, and follow the instructions (see page 115).

Exercise

Breathing Exercise

Sing for 10 minutes. Singing is an excellent breathing exercise because it supports exhaling and the cleansing of the lungs. The increased expulsion of carbon dioxide is one of the reasons singers rarely suffer from depression.

Aerobic Exercise

Go for a fast bicycle ride, at least 20 minutes long.

Stretching

To avoid pain and injury from your bicycle ride, be sure to do the following stretches for warming up before and cooling down after the bicycle ride (see pages 173–183).

1. Neck Turn	14. Figure Four Stretch
2. Neck Tilt with Slight Extension	15. Lying Hamstring Stretch
3. Deltoid Stretch	16. Cat Stretch
4. Rotator Cuff Stretch	17. Back Arch
5. Middle Chest Stretch	18. Lying Back Extension
6. Squatting Chest Stretch	19. Pelvic Tilt
7. External Rotation Stretch	20. One Leg Stretch
8. Internal Rotation Stretch	21. T-Stretch
9. Wrist Extension Stretch	22. Straight Leg Stretch
10. Wrist Flexion Stretch	23. Half-Kneeling Shin Stretch
11. Open Hand Stretch	24. Outer Ankle Stretch
12. Closed Hand Stretch	25. Inner Ankle Stretch
13. Figure-4 Stretch	

Home Spa

Dry-Brush Massage (see page 313).

Purifying Sauna

The hot air in the sauna (140°F to 194°F) enlarges the blood vessels, and blood flows to the surface. By way of the wide-open pores, perspiration laden with toxins flows out. During the following shower, pores close again, the blood vessels contract, and the blood receeds into deeper layers. Besides having a diaphoretic (having the power to increase sweating) effect, during this process vascular muscles also are trained. At a single visit to the sauna, about 6¹/₂ ounces of sweat are secreted and, along with it, many toxins and water that has collected in the tissue (or edema). The lost fluids will be replaced by fat tissue, which is rich in water.

The sauna has numerous additional benefits: it improves the blood circulation throughout the entire body; levels out blood pressure that is either too high or too low; strengthens the body's defense mechanisms against infections; moistens the breathing passages and increases the elimination of mucus; relaxes muscles; beautifies, rejuvenates, and moisturizes the skin; has a positive effect on the involuntary nervous system and the hormonal system; supports weight reduction; relaxes; and fosters peace of mind.

Hair
Refresh your hair with Rich Conditioner, Sandalwood Hot Oil Treatment, and Hair Care Cream (see pages 249, 250, and 251).

Face-Building Exercises (see page 242)

Nutrition: Dr. Otto Buchinger's Recommend Day of Fasting

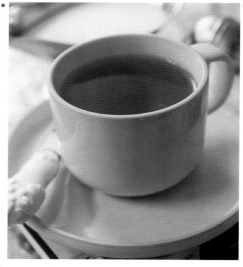

◎ Morning
1 cup of lukewarm water mixed with 1 teaspoon of Epsom or Glauber's salt in small gulps on an empty stomach to cleanse your intestines (to improve the taste, add a few drops of lemon). Afterward, have a cup of unsweetened peppermint tea. You will soon need to empty your bowels, so stay near a bathroom.

However, if you have too frequent bowel movements or even diarrhea, then restrict your cleansing measures by drinking a glass of buttermilk, whey, or sauerkraut juice on an empty stomach.

◎ Breakfast
2 cups of herbal tea (rosemary, peppermint, mallow, or ginseng) or diluted black tea; add a teaspoon of honey, if desired

◎ Mid-Morning
2 glasses of mineral water or 2 cups of fruit or herbal tea

◎ Lunch

1 cup Soup for Fasting or ¹/₂ cup of fresh vegetable juice mixed with ¹/₂ cup of hot or cold mineral water

◎ Afternoon

2 cups of herbal or fruit tea with lemon or half a teaspoon of honey, or both

◎ Dinner

¹/₂ cup of fruit or vegetable juice diluted with ¹/₂ cup of mineral water or vegetable broth

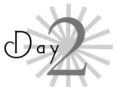

7-Day Cure: Day of Fasting

If you find yourself experiencing circulatory problems, brew yourself a cup of black tea and add half a teaspoon of honey. However, don't drink this too late at night, or you might not be able to sleep. A glass of buttermilk is helpful for alleviating dizziness and weakness.

Meditation

Relax with the Tension/Release Exercise (see page 30), followed by the Counting Breath (see page 33), and for your meditation technique, try the Basic Zazen Meditation (see page 36).

Aromatherapy

Select a diffuser formula for Improvement (see page 117).

Exercise

Detox Breathing Exercise

Do the Basic Breathing Technique for 10 minutes. Sit up straight in a chair and relax. Exhale as long as you can (count slowly in your mind), and then inhale automatically. Feel how your stomach rises and falls. Always inhale through your nose. To support exhaling, you also can exhale while making a "fff" sound or a slight whistling noise. Repeat several times.

Aerobic Exercise

Go for a 25-minute jog. Run until you are out of breath, then change to fast-paced walking, then run again, then walk, then run, then walk, and so on.

Stretching

To avoid injury from your jog, be sure to do the following stretches for warming up before and cooling down after your jog (see pages 173–183).

1. Deltoid Stretch
2. Middle Chest Stretch
3. Sitting Twist (on floor)
4. Knee to Opposite Chest Stretch
5. Hamstring Stretch to Bench
6. Ankle Reach
7. One Leg Stretch
8. T-Stretch
9. Lunge Against Wall
10. Side Lunge
11. Calf Stretch on a Step
12. Inner Calf Stretch
13. Outer Calf Stretch
14. Standing Shin Stretch
15. Inner Ankle Stretch
16. Outer Ankle Stretch

Home Spa

Dry-Brush Massage (see page 313).

Hot and Cold Body Compresses Method 1
Hot and cold body compresses are a milder form of sauna for in-between times.

1. Dip a bath towel into hot water, wring it out, and wrap it around your body.

2. Now wrap a dry towel and a blanket around the wet towel.

3. Thus wrapped, go to bed and cover yourself with another blanket.

4. Stay in bed until you start to perspire heavily.

5. Because many toxins are excreted by means of the skin, take a warm shower afterward and finish with a cold rinse of water.

Arms
Pamper your arms with a body butter (see page 247) followed by the Rosewater Body Rub for Elbows and Knees (see page 246).

Face-Building Exercises (see page 242).

Nutrition

Repeat diet from Day 1 (see page 316).

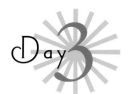

Day 3

7-Day Cure: Partial Fast

A Day of Uncooked Food, Devised by Dr. Bircher-Brenner

A partial fast is based on mainly monodiets, whereby intake of food is restricted to the consumption of a few foods—for the most part, vegetarian

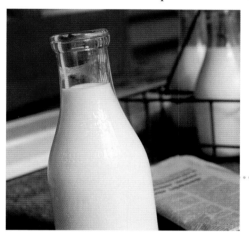

food and milk products. Mono-diets are great for healthy people as preventive purification and detox-ification measures, but they also are recommended for individuals suffering from obesity, digestive and skin problems, or unfavorable blood counts.

Meditation

Begin with the Progressive Relaxation Exercise I (see page 30), then do the Standing Breath (see page 33), and for your meditation technique, use the Thought meditation (see page 39).

Aromatherapy

Select a mist spray formula for the aromatherapy Introspection (see page 118).

Exercise

Detox Breathing Exercise

Do the Lion Exercise. The Lion Exercise is a cleansing breathing exercise derived from yoga. It got its name because while doing it, you will resemble a yawning lion. The exercise has proven to be an excellent prevention against tonsillitis and a sore throat, and also is helpful in their beginning stages. If you do this exercise three times a day, you will be fairly well protected against illness. At the same time, you will be cleansing your bronchi as well.

You must always do this exercise outdoors in fresh air so try it on your way to work, at lunch, and on your way home. Here is how it is performed:

1. Stand or sit up straight.

2. Exhale vigorously and for a long duration in the following manner.

3. Stretch your head and neck forward (your back has to remain straight).

4. Open your mouth as wide as possible.

5. Stick out your tongue as far as you can. If you feel embarrassed about being seen, try it while taking a solitary walk.

6. Wait until you have exhaled completely, and put your tongue back in your mouth; then inhale through your nose.

7. Roll up your tongue, and press it firmly to the back of your palate.

8. At the same time, push your chin downward as far as possible.

9. Exhale and repeat the exercise several times. When doing the lion exercise, make sure you don't stretch your jaw muscles too much!

Aerobic Exercise

Play a game of tennis. You will pump more oxygen into your body if you move your upper torso and your arms. If you really aren't a tennis player, try running up and down stairs quickly for 30 minutes to loosen the mucus that has accumulated in your lungs.

Stretching Exercises

Because you will be working so many different muscles during your tennis game, it's really important to complete all of the following stretches for warming up before and cooling down after your tennis game (see pages 173–183).

1. Neck Turn	13. Knee to Opposite Chest Stretch
2. Neck Tilt with Slight Extension	14. Knee to Chest Stretch
3. Deltoid Stretch	15. Sitting Twist (on floor)
4. Arm over Head Stretch	16. Ankle Reach
5. Rotator Cuff Stretch	17. One Leg Stretch
6. Front Press Out	18. Lunge Against Wall
7. Middle Chest Stretch	19. Side Lunge
8. Lower Chest Stretch	20. Straight Leg Stretch
9. Wrist Extension Stretch	21. Bent Knee Calf Stretch
10. Wrist Flexion Stretch	22. Side of Leg Stretch
11. Bottom of Wrist Stretch	23. Calf Stretch on a Step
12. Top of Wrist Stretch	

Dry-Brush Massage (see page 313).

Bath with Rising Temperatures

Bathing with rising temperatures leads to a gradual warming of the body, until you will finally break out into a sweat. A note of caution: If you don't feel well (weakness, dizziness, feeling of oppression), interrupt the bath immediately and refresh your body with cool water. This is the process:

1. If you feel like it, drink a perspiration-producing tea from elderberry flowers beforehand.

2. Lie in a bathtub with water at a temperature of about 98.6°F.

3. Slowly let very hot water flow into the tub until the water becomes so hot that you can barely stand it (between 98.6°F and 107.6°F, depending on what you are used to).

4. Stay in the bathtub for 15 minutes. You can gradually increase the duration of the bath each time from 5 to 15 minutes.

5. For a cooling effect, put a cold washcloth on your forehead.

6. Get up carefully, and take a warm shower to remove toxins eliminated with the perspiration. Finish with a cool-to-cold shower.

7. Rest afterward, well covered, for at least 15 minutes.

It is best to take this bath every two days during a cure of purification because, aside from relaxation, it also promotes sleep.

Legs

Beautify your legs with a body butter (see page 247) and follow with the Rosewater Body Rub for Elbows and Knees (see page 246).

Hair

For extra oomph, apply a Hair Care Cream (see page 251).

Face-Building Exercises (see page 242).

Nutrition

Today's diet is based on fresh vegetarian food ("refreshing food for life," according to Dr. Bircher-Brenner), consisting of raw fruits and vegetables and muesli. This is especially useful for curing obesity, and for all digestive problems, such as constipation, intestinal infections, and so forth. Because of the high content of fiber and pectin in whole wheat, vegetables, and fruits, these foods are better for digestion than other foods. What's more, you are chewing for a longer time and using more saliva, and thus you are satiated sooner and eat less.

◎ Morning

1 cup of lukewarm water mixed with 1 teaspoon of Epsom or Glauber's salt in small gulps on an empty stomach to cleanse your intestines (To improve the taste, add a few drops of lemon). Afterward, have a cup of unsweetened peppermint tea. You will soon need to empty your bowels, so stay near a bathroom.

However, if you have too frequent bowel movements or even diarrhea, then restrict your cleansing measures by drinking a glass of buttermilk, whey, or sauerkraut juice on an empty stomach.

◎ Breakfast

1 cup Bircher Muesli
1 pint of tea (rose hip tea is especially effective) or mineral water

◎ Mid-Morning

1 pint of mineral water or tea made from birch leaves, nettle, or juniper berries to cleanse the blood and eliminate water from the tissues

◎ Lunch

1 plate of raw (or slightly cooked) vegetables and fruit with a light dressing: (Raw plants contain natural antibiotics, vital mineral salts, vitamins, and enzymes.)
1 pint of tea or mineral water

◎ Afternoon

1 pint of tea or mineral water.

◎ Dinner

Same as lunch; use a different mix of vegetables and fruit for variety.

Day 4

7-Day Cure: Partial Fast

Today, the partial fast continues. If you start to feel restless, move around a lot and don't forget to drink lots of fluids. Also, be sure to vary your fruits and vegetables from meal to meal so you don't get bored and tempted to stray.

Meditation

Begin with the Progressive Relaxation Exercise II (see page 31), followed by the Yogi Complete Breath (see page 34), and then use the meditation technique for Mind Expansion (see page 39).

Aromatherapy

Choose an aromatherapy application formula for the theme Loving Yourself (see page 120).

Exercise

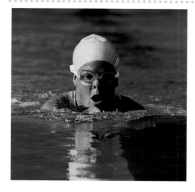

Detox Breathing Exercise

Do the Basic Breathing Technique for 10 minutes. Sit up straight in a chair and relax. Exhale as long as you can (count slowly in your mind), and then inhale automatically. Feel how your stomach rises and falls. Always inhale through your nose. To support exhaling, you also can exhale while making a "fff" sound or a slight whistling noise. Repeat several times.

Aerobic Exercise

Go for a 35-minute swim. It's okay to vary your strokes; just make sure that you're constantly moving.

Stretching

Although swimming causes very little nerve damage, and on its own strengthens and stretches the entire body, be sure to perform these stretches beforehand to have a more enjoyable and beneficial swim (see page 173–183)

1. Open Mouth Stretch
2. Jaw Protrusion Stretch
3. Neck Tilt
4. Neck Turn
5. Neck Tilt with Slight Extension
6. Deltoid Stretch
7. Arm over Head Stretch
8. Rotator Cuff Stretch
9. Shoulder Blade Squeeze
10. Front Press Out
11. Lower Chest Stretch
12. Upper Chest Stretch
13. Wrist Extension Stretch
14. Wrist Flexion Stretch
15. One Leg Stretch
16. Lunge Against Wall
17. Side Lunge
18. Standing Shin Stretch
19. Straight Leg Stretch
20. Outer Ankle Stretch
21. Inner Ankle Stretch
22. Knee to Chest Stretch
23. Supine Groin Stretch

Dry-Brush Massage (see page 313).

Water Treatment with Kneipp's Gushes

The gushes can be warm, cold, or alternate between warm and cold, but the final gush should be cold. The stream of water has to be uniform, and you shouldn't use a shower head.

If you use alternating cold and warm gushes, direct the warm stream of water to a part of your body until it feels warm and relaxed; afterward, use a stream of cold water for the same place for 15 seconds to 1 minute. Always start the Kneipp's gushes with your right arm. Be sure the bathroom where you perform the treatment is well heated. After the procedure, rub yourself dry with a towel until your skin turns slightly red and your body is warm. You also can just brush off the wetness with your hands, and then go to bed.

1. Alternating hot and cold showers cleanse the blood, detoxify, invigorate your circulatory system, and are helpful in cases of muscular strains, colds, and infections.

2. For a gush for the arms, direct the stream of water to the outside of your right arm, starting at the back of your hand and going up to your shoulder; then direct the water to the inside of your arm, from the shoulder down to your palm. Do the same with your left arm.

3. For a gush for the legs, direct the stream of water to your right leg, starting at the front of your right foot and proceeding to the knee, then going downward along the back of your leg to the sole of your foot. Follow the same procedure with your left leg.

4. For a gush for the face, circle the stream of water over your face.

Face

Rejuvenate your face with the Walnut Scrub (see page 232); choose one Facial Sauna formula (see page 233); use Rosewater Toner (see page 234); apply Cold Cream (see page 235); and use the Carrot and Honey Mask (see page 235), or if you feel your skin needs extra attention, choose either Face Mask for Balancing Oily Skin, Face Mask for Improving Skin Texture, or Face Pack for Normal, Dry, or Sensitive Skin (see page 237).

Nutrition

Repeat the Dr. Bircher-Brenner diet from Day 3, but give your body a rest and skip the morning intestinal cleanser.

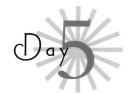

Day 5

7-Day Cure: Partial Fast

This is the last day of the partial fast. Keep in mind the benefits that the past 4 days of fasting and partial fasting have had on your body—eliminating toxins from your intestines, kidneys, and liver. Also remember the four basic eating rules: take small bites, chew all food for a long time to produce saliva, enjoy every bite, and stop eating when you feel full.

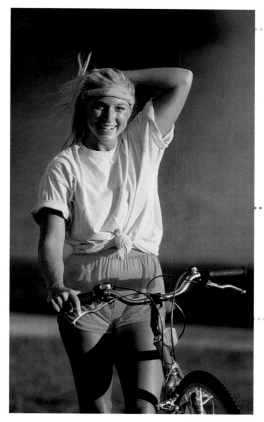

Meditation

Relax with the Tension/Release Exercise (see page 30); then perform the Awareness Breath (see page 32); and for your meditative technique, select an Energy meditation, either Contacting Universal Energy or Illumination meditation (see pages 40–41).

Aromatherapy

Further your meditative experience with one of the aromatherapy diffuser formulas for the theme Meditation (see page 123).

Exercise

Detox Breathing Exercise
Sing for 15 minutes.

Aerobic Exercise
Go for a fast, 35-minute bicycle ride.

Stretching

To avoid pain and injury from your bicycle ride, be sure to do the following stretches for warming up before and cooling down after your bike ride (see pages 173–183).

1. Neck Turn	13. Figure-4 Stretch
2. Neck Tilt with Slight Extension	14. Lying Hamstring Stretch
3. Deltoid Stretch	15. Cat Stretch
4. Rotator Cuff Stretch	16. Back Arch
5. Middle Chest Stretch	17. Lying Back Extension
6. Squatting Chest Stretch	18. Pelvic Tilt
7. External Rotation Stretch	19. One Leg Stretch
8. Internal Rotation Stretch	20. T-Stretch
9. Wrist Extension Stretch	21. Straight Leg Stretch
10. Wrist Flexion Stretch	22. Half-Kneeling Shin Stretch
11. Open Hand Stretch	23. Outer Ankle Stretch
12. Closed Hand Stretch	24. Inner Ankle Stretch

Home Spa

Dry-Brush Massage (see page 313).

Treading Water

1. Fill the bathtub with cold water so that the water reaches between your knees and ankles, just up to your fibula.

2. Tread in place in the water.

3. Alternating, lift one leg and then the other out of the water.

4. If you are becoming too cold, get out of the bathtub and run around a bit.

5. If you go to sleep right after treading water, you will have a restful sleep.

Body

Indulge your body with the Body Lotion (see page 246) and your choice of body butters (see page 247).

Face-Building Exercises (see page 242).

Nutrition

Repeat the Dr. Bircher-Brenner diet from Days 3 and 4, but do include the morning intestinal cleanser.

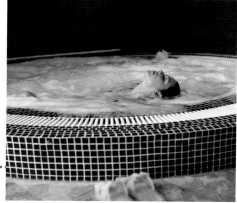

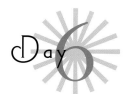

Day 6

7-Day Cure: Day of Buildup

The days of buildup are used to get your body acquainted with normal food once more. The intestines, in particular, must gradually get accustomed to having more food come in from the outside. Remember, as soon as you feel satiated, stop eating. Eat slowly and chew thoroughly so you will feel satiated sooner. Also drink a lot of liquid.

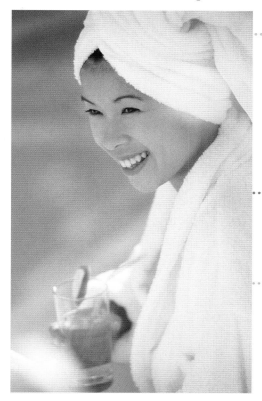

Meditation

Begin with the Progressive Relaxation I (see page 30), then do the Yogi Complete Breath (see page 34); for your meditation, choose the mantra among the Mantra meditations (see page 43) that most appeals to you.

Aromatherapy

Explore Motives for Our Actions with one of the mist spray formulas (see page 125).

Exercise

Detox Breathing Exercise
Do the Basic Breathing Technique for 10 minutes. Sit up straight in a chair and relax. Exhale as long as you can (count slowly in your mind), and then inhale automatically. Feel how your stomach rises and falls. Always inhale through your nose. To support exhaling, you also can exhale while making a "fff" sound or a slight whistling noise. Repeat several times.

Aerobic Exercise
Go for a jog, as you did on Day 2, but today increase the length of time you jog.

To avoid injury from your jog, be sure to do the following stretches for warming up before and cooling down after your jog (see pages 173–183).

1. Deltoid Stretch	9. Lunge Against Wall
2. Middle Chest Stretch	10. Side Lunge
3. Sitting Twist (on floor)	11. Calf Stretch on a Step
4. Knee to Opposite Chest Stretch	12. Inner Calf Stretch
5. Hamstring Stretch to Bench	13. Outer Calf Stretch
6. Ankle Reach	14. Standing Shin Stretch
7. One Leg Stretch	15. Inner Ankle Stretch
8. T-Stretch	16. Outer Ankle Stretch

Home Spa

Dry-Brush Massage (see page 313).

Bath with Rising Temperatures

Take another bath with rising temperatures; it's an excellent way to purify your skin (see page 321).

Hair and Skin Care

Hands

Indulge your hands with the Sugar Soft Hand Exfoliant (see page 253), Rose Scented Hand Cream (see page 253), and Wheat Germ Hot Oil Strengthening Fingernail Treatment (see page 255).

Face-Building Exercises (see page 242).

Nutrition

On a buildup day, you can eat bread and rolls, linseed oil, soaked prunes or figs, cooked vegetables or vegetable soup, raw food in easy-to-digest salads and vegetable dishes, buttermilk, yogurt, curdled milk, low-fat milk, or low-fat quark or baker's cheese, butter, soft-boiled eggs, lean ham, or turkey breast. You should still avoid legumes and all types of cooked cabbage, fatty foods, red meat, sausages, organ meats, sweets, and stimulants such as coffee or depressants such as alcohol.

◎ **Morning**

To clean out your intestines, have an enema or continue with 1 cup of luke-warm water mixed with 1 teaspoon of Epsom or Glauber's salt in small gulps on an empty stomach. To improve the taste, add a few drops of lemon. Afterward, have a cup of unsweetened peppermint tea. You will soon need to empty your bowels, so stay near a bathroom.

◎ Breakfast

1 slice of whole wheat bread or 2 slices of crisp bread with some butter
1 apple
2 cups of herbal or black tea

◎ Lunch

Thick Potato–Vegetable Soup
1 small container of yogurt with 1 teaspoon of buckthorn juice
Herbal tea

◎ Dinner

2 slices of crisp bread with a little butter
Quark or baker's cheesewith herbs
1 glass of buttermilk with 1 teaspoon of linseed oil
Herbal tea

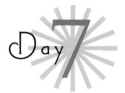

$\mathcal{D}$ay 7

7-Day Cure: Day of Buildup

A second day of buildup is necessary to ease your body back into eating regular foods. You don't want to overburden the intestines now, because cramps,

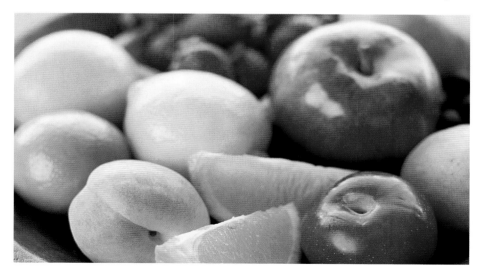

stomach trouble, or malaise could be the outcome. Furthermore, your hard-won results of purification could quickly disappear. However, if you are in tune with your body, you won't be craving heavy meals after 5 days of reduced food intake.

Because tomorrow you will begin strength training, you want to build up stamina and energy, and you don't want to delay your progress by advancing too quickly.

Meditation

Start with one of the Basic Relaxation Exercises (see page 29), then perform the Standing Breath (see page 33), and finish up your first week with the Goodness meditation (see page 49).

Aromatherapy

Evaluate your first week of the *30-Day Revitalization Plan* with one of the application formulas for Reflection (see page 127).

Exercise

Detox Breathing Exercise
Do the Lion Exercise.

Aerobic Exercise
Let your body rest from high-impact activities, but go for a brisk walk to keep up your blood circulation.

Stretching

Although you won't be doing high-impact aerobic activity, it's still extremely important to stretch, as follows (see pages 173–183).

1. Deltoid Stretch	9. Lunge Against Wall
2. Middle Chest Stretch	10. Side Lunge
3. Sitting Twist (on floor)	11. Calf Stretch on a Step
4. Knee to Opposite Chest Stretch	12. Inner Calf Stretch
5. Hamstring Stretch to Bench	13. Outer Calf Stretch
6. Ankle Reach	14. Standing Shin Stretch
7. One Leg Stretch	15. Inner Ankle Stretch
8. T-Stretch	16. Outer Ankle Stretch

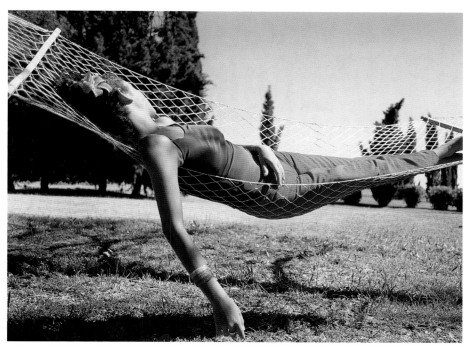

Spa

. . . . ◎

Dry-Brush Massage (see page 313).

Hot and Cold Body Compresses Method 2

This version of the body compress has proven to be an excellent remedy in cases of insomnia and fever, in addition to an excellent purifier.

1. Warm up by taking a sunbath or a hot bath.

2. Dip a large bath towel in cold water, and wrap it around you.

3. Wrap a blanket around the towel and, thus wrapped, go to bed and cover yourself with another blanket.

4. Soon you will become warm, which will make you very sleepy, so it's best to use this in the evening.

Feet

Treat your feet well with the luxurious Strawberry Foot Exfoliant (see page 256).

Nutrition

. . . . ◎

◎ **Breakfast**

1 cup Bircher Muesli

2 cups of herbal tea

◎ Lunch

1 plate of raw, easy-to-digest salads and vegetables

Potatoes with skin or potatoes with cumin

Lean ham or turkey breast

Herbal tea

◎ Dinner

2 slices of whole wheat bread or rolls with a little bit of butter and some quark or baker's cheese or quark with fresh herbs

Or 1 soft-boiled egg

Or 1 small container yogurt with 1 teaspoon linseed oil

Herbal tea

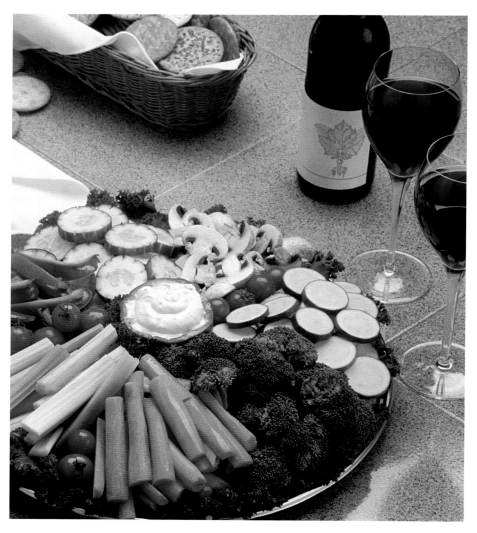

2
Strengthen

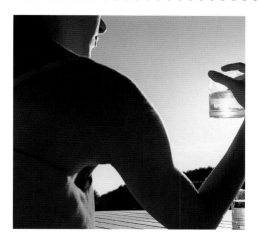

This week you will begin to strengthen your core and your muscles through the addition of yoga and weight-training exercises to the *30-Day Revitalization Plan*. You will also continue to reinvigorate your mind through meditation, relax with aromatherapy, and rejuvenate your hair, skin, hands, and feet with natural spa treatments, as well as enjoy a balanced diet of super-nutritious recipes.

Meditation

Now that you've built up some meditative stamina, you should be able to hold the more simple postures for longer periods of time, and the more advanced postures for some length of time. Each day, meditate for 10 minutes in a quiet place, but add incense (see page 25) to your meditation routine to further enhance your experience.

Aromatherapy

Because strength-building exercises can be intense, it is particularly important that you be relaxed. In addition to helping you prepare your body and mind for the tasks at hand, aromatherapy will help you unwind. Each day the aromatherapy portion of the *30-Day Revitalization Plan* will address a different theme, but you are free to choose the actual formula, depending on what aromas appeal to you.

Exercise

In addition to four aerobic workouts this week, you will also be incorporating five yoga practice sessions into your program. The aerobic exercise will help strengthen your heart, while the yoga exercises will help improve your flexibility and stamina. Before each yoga session, be sure to do the Yoga Warm-Ups (see page 154). Depending on your fitness level, you might want to repeat a practice session from the previous day and build up through the week.

Stretching

To prevent muscle injury, it is extremely important to stretch before and after any exercise activity. The stretching routines presented each day will stretch the muscles that you will be using for either aerobic or weight-training exercises.

Weight Training

The weight-training exercises will help strengthen your muscles as well as increase the efficiency of your metabolism.

Home Spa

Hair and Skin Care

This week, indulge your hair with the wonderful Lavender Ylang-Ylang Shampoo (see page 249). Continue to use daily the Strawberry Night Cream (see page 238), the Strawberry Facial Cream (see page 238), the Deodorant (see page 245), and the Liquid Hand Lotion (see page 254).

Food and Nutrition

The daily menu suggestions (see Chapter 8 for specific recipes) offer a wide array of flavors that are healthy and will ensure that you get all of the necessary nutrients for a balanced diet. Supplement each recipe suggestion with a steamed vegetable of your choice and a green salad. Dress the salad with olive oil and vinegar or a low-fat bottled salad dressing.

Remember, as your activities increase, you need to fuel yourself adequately. Snack on fresh veggies or a piece of fruit when you are hungry.

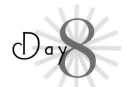

Day 8

Meditation

For today's session, begin with the Progressive Relaxation Exercise II (see page 31), followed by the Counting Breath (see page 33), and for your meditation technique, choose either the Meditation of Gratitude 1 or 2 (see pages 50–51).

Aromatherapy

To stay invigorated and energized, select an aromatherapy diffuser formula for Mood Uplifting and follow the instructions (see page 129).

Exercise

Get your heart going and your blood pumping with a 30-minute jog, either outdoors or on a treadmill. Run until you are out of breath, then change to fast-paced walking, then run again, then walk, then run, then walk, and so on. Then switch gears to yoga first with the Yoga Warm-Ups (see page 154) followed by Yoga Practice Session One (see page 155).

Stretching

To avoid injury from your jog, be sure to do the following stretches before and after your workout (see pages 173–183).

1. Deltoid Stretch	9. Lunge Against Wall
2. Middle Chest Stretch	10. Side Lunge
3. Sitting Twist (on floor)	11. Calf Stretch on a Step
4. Knee to Opposite Chest Stretch	12. Inner Calf Stretch
5. Hamstring Stretch to Bench	13. Outer Calf Stretch
6. Ankle Reach	14. Standing Shin Stretch
7. One Leg Stretch	15. Inner Ankle Stretch
8. T-Stretch	16. Outer Ankle Stretch

Home Spa

Hair

Focus on your hair today with the Avocado Coconut Conditioner (see page 250), Dandruff Remover (see page 252), and Hair Care Cream (see page 251).

Face-Building Exercises (see page 242).

Nutrition

◎ **Breakfast**

2 egg-white omelet

1 piece of fresh fruit

1 piece of toast

◎ **Lunch**

Easy Manhattan-Style Clam Chowder

◎ **Dinner**

Baked Cod with Seasoned Tomatoes

Steamed vegetable of your choice

Green salad

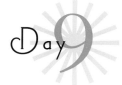

Day 9

Meditation

For today's session, begin with the Progressive Relaxation Exercise I (see page 30), followed by the Awareness Breath (see page 32), and for your meditation technique, choose a Healing meditation (see page 51).

Aromatherapy

Unwind with an aromatherapy mist spray formula for Relaxing and follow the instructions (see page 130).

Exercise

Go for a fast, 35-minute bicycle ride then unwind with yoga: first Yoga Warm-Ups (see page 154), then Yoga Practice Session Two (see page 156).

Stretching

To avoid pain and injury from your bicycle ride, be sure to do the following stretches before and after your workout (see pages 173–183).

1. Neck Turn	13. Figure-4 Stretch
2. Neck Tilt with Slight Extension	14. Lying Hamstring Stretch
3. Deltoid Stretch	15. Cat Stretch
4. Rotator Cuff Stretch	16. Back Arch
5. Middle Chest Stretch	17. Lying Back Extension
6. Squatting Chest Stretch	18. Pelvic Tilt
7. External Rotation Stretch	19. One Leg Stretch
8. Internal Rotation Stretch	20. T-Stretch
9. Wrist Extension Stretch	21. Straight Leg Stretch
10. Wrist Flexion Stretch	22. Half-Kneeling Shin Stretch
11. Open Hand Stretch	23. Outer Ankle Stretch
12. Closed Hand Stretch	24. Inner Ankle Stretch

Home Spa

Arms
Today, pay extra, loving attention to your arms. First apply the Rosewater Body Rub for Elbows and Knees (see page 246), and then follow up with your choice of body butters (see page 247).

Face-Building Exercises (see page 242).

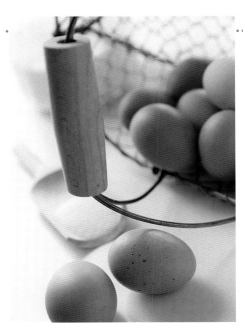

Nutrition

◎ **Breakfast**
1 hard-boiled egg
1 piece of fresh fruit
1/2 cup of granola

◎ **Lunch**
Puerto Principe Chicken Chowder

◎ **Dinner**
Lime Flounder with Mandarin
 Salsa
Steamed vegetables of your choice
Green salad

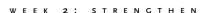

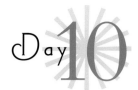

$\mathcal{D}ay\ 10$

Meditation

For today's session, begin with the Tension Release Exercise (see page 30), followed by the Yogi Complete Breath (see page 34), and for your meditation technique, choose a Water Meditation (see page 62).

Aromatherapy

To beat the workout blues, select an aromatherapy application formula for Surrender Your Stress and follow the instructions (see page 130).

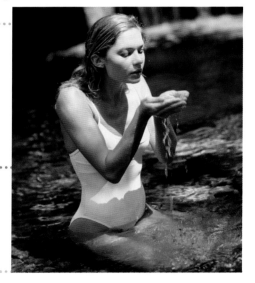

Exercise

Although most of your exercise program today will be devoted to weight training, it's important to get your heart going, so start your workout today with a brisk, 20-minute walk.

Stretching

Walking Stretches

Be sure to stretch before and after your workout (see pages 173–183).

1. Deltoid Stretch	9. Lunge Against Wall
2. Middle Chest Stretch	10. Side Lunge
3. Sitting Twist (on floor)	11. Calf Stretch on a Step
4. Knee to Opposite Chest Stretch	12. Inner Calf Stretch
5. Hamstring Stretch to Bench	13. Outer Calf Stretch
6. Ankle Reach	14. Standing Shin Stretch
7. One Leg Stretch	15. Inner Ankle Stretch
8. T-Stretch	16. Outer Ankle Stretch

Weight-Lifting Stretches

1. Neck Turn
2. Neck Tilt with Slight Extension
3. Reach Stretch
4. Rotator Cuff Stretch
5. Arm over Head Stretch
6. Middle Chest Stretch
7. Tall Stretch
8. One Leg Stretch
9. T-Stretch
10. Bent Knee Calf Stretch
11. Standing Shin Stretch
12. Straight Leg Stretch
13. Supine Groin Stretch
14. Knee to Chest Stretch
15. Cat Stretch
16. Back Arch

Weight Training: Weekly Workout 1

Legs
Knee Extension
Leg Curl
Adduction

Chest
Bench Press, Flat Bench
Fly on Incline Bench

Back
Lat Pull-Down
Seated Row

Shoulders
Bar Press (2 sets only)
Lateral Raise (2 sets only)

Biceps
Bar Curl

Triceps
Kickback

Forearms
Reverse Curl

Abs
Tailbone Lift
Crunch
Pelvic Tilt
Curl-Up—Center

Home Spa

Legs
Today, pay extra, loving attention to your legs. First apply the Rosewater Body Rub for Elbows and Knees (see page 246), and then follow up with your choice of body butters (see page 247).

Hair
Give your hair an extra boost with the Hair Care Cream (see page 251).

Face-Building Exercises (see page 242).

Nutrition

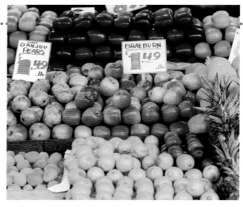

◎ Breakfast
2 scrambled egg whites
1 piece of fresh fruit

◎ Lunch
Cold Dilled Tomato Soup

◎ Dinner
Cajun Salmon
Steamed vegetables of your choice
Green salad
Apple Plum Crisp or Pear Strawberry Crisp

Day 11

Meditation

For today's session, begin with one of the Basic Relaxation Exercises (see page 29), followed by the Awareness Breath (see page 32), and for your meditation technique, select a Walking Meditation (see page 69).

Aromatherapy

Enjoy all that you have accomplished in the past 11 days, and select an aromatherapy diffuser formula for Appreciation and follow the instructions (see page 115).

Exercise

Take a break from aerobic exercise today and perform Yoga Practice Session Three (see page 157), preceded by Yoga Warm-Ups (see page 154).

Home Spa

Face
Pamper your face today. First, apply an Oatmeal Scrub (see page 232); then choose one Facial Sauna formula (see page 233). Next use the Strawberry Refresher (see page 234), followed by the Peaches-and-Cream Complexion Mask (see page 236), or, if you feel your skin needs extra attention, choose either Face Mask for Balancing Oily Skin, Face Mask for Improving Skin Texture, or Face Pack for Normal, Dry, or Sensitive Skin (see page 237).

Nutrition

◎ **Breakfast**

$1/2$ cup Bircher Muesli
1 piece of fresh fruit

◎ **Lunch**

Zucchini Soup Margherita

◎ **Dinner**

Cod Fillets with Lemon and Thyme
Steamed vegetables of your choice
Green salad

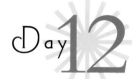

Day 12

Meditation

For today's session, begin with the Progressive Relaxation Exercise I (see page 30), followed by the Counting Breath (see page 33), and for your meditation technique, select a Seeing and Listening exercise (see page 71).

Aromatherapy

Muster up enthusiasm with an aromatherapy mist spray formula for Improvement, and follow the instructions (see page 117).

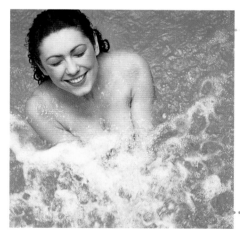

Exercise

Go for a 35-minute swim. It's okay to vary your strokes; just make sure that you're constantly moving. Unwind after your swim with Yoga Practice Session Four (see page 157). Before your yoga, be sure to perform the Yoga Warm-Ups (see page 154).

Stretching

While swimming causes very little nerve damage and on its own strengthens and stretches the entire body, be sure to perform these stretches before and after your swim to have a more enjoyable and beneficial swim (see page 173–183).

1. Open Mouth Stretch
2. Jaw Protrusion Stretch
3. Neck Tilt
4. Neck Turn
5. Neck Tilt with Slight Extension
6. Deltoid Stretch
7. Arm over Head Stretch
8. Rotator Cuff Stretch
9. Shoulder Blade Squeeze
10. Front Press Out
11. Lower Chest Stretch
12. Upper Chest Stretch
13. Wrist Extension Stretc
14. Wrist Flexion Stretch
15. One Leg Stretch
16. Lunge Against Wall
17. Side Lunge
18. Standing Shin Stretch
19. Straight Leg Stretch
20. Outer Ankle Stretch
21. Inner Ankle Stretch
22. Knee to Chest Stretch
23. Supine Groin Stretch

Home Spa

Body

Care for your body with a Milk Bath (see page 244) or, if you prefer a shower, the Refreshing Sea Salt Scrub (see page 245), followed by the Skin Nutrient (see page 246).

Face-Building Exercises (see page 241).

Nutrition

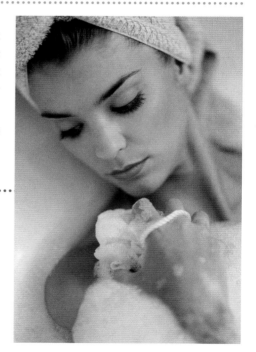

◎ Breakfast

2 scrambled egg whites
1 piece of fresh fruit
1 piece of toast

◎ Lunch

Alaskan Salmon Salad Sandwiches

◎ Dinner

Jamaican Jerk Pork
Steamed vegetables of your choice
1 small baked potato
Green salad

Day 13

Meditation

For today's session, begin with the Tension Release Exercise (see page 30), followed by the Standing Breath (see page 33), and for your meditation technique, use Seeking Wisdom (see page 73).

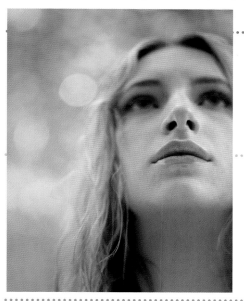

Aromatherapy

Consider all that you have accomplished with an aromatherapy application formula for Introspection, and follow the instructions (see page 118).

Exercise

Although most of your exercise program today will be devoted to weight training, it's important to get your heart going, so start your workout today with a brisk, 20-minute walk.

Stretching

Be sure to stretch before and after your workout (see pages 173–183).

Walking Stretches

1. Deltoid Stretch
2. Middle Chest Stretch
3. Sitting Twist (on floor)
4. Knee to Opposite Chest Stretch
5. Hamstring Stretch to Bench
6. Ankle Reach
7. One Leg Stretch
8. T Stretch
9. Lunge Against Wall
10. Side Lunge
11. Calf Stretch on a Step
12. Inner Calf Stretch
13. Outer Calf Stretch
14. Standing Shin Stretch
15. Inner Ankle Stretch
16. Outer Ankle Stretch

Weight-Lifting Stretches

1. Neck Turn
2. Neck Tilt with Slight Extension
3. Reach Stretch
4. Rotator Cuff Stretch
5. Arm over Head Stretch
6. Middle Chest Stretch
7. Tall Stretch
8. One Leg Stretch
9. T-Stretch
10. Bent Knee Calf Stretch
11. Standing Shin Stretch
12. Straight Leg Stretch
13. Supine Groin Stretch
14. Knee to Chest Stretch
15. Cat Stretch
16. Back Arch

Weight Training: Weekly Workout 2

Legs
  Hip Extension or Knee Extension

Dip
  Squat (2 sets only)
  Calf Raise

Chest
  Incline Bench Press
  Decline Dumbbell Press

Back
  Dead Lift
  One-Arm Row

Shoulders
  Rear Delt Raise (2 sets only)
  Front Shoulder Raise
  (2 sets only)

Biceps
  Hammer Curl

Triceps
  Reverse-Grip Bench Press

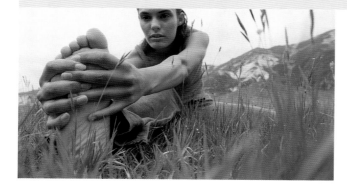

Home Spa

Hands
Pamper your hands with the Lemonade Hand Exfoliant (see page 253), followed by the Extra Tough Hand Cream (see page 253), and finish up with Cuticle Softener (see page 255).

Face-Building Exercises (see page 242).

Nutrition

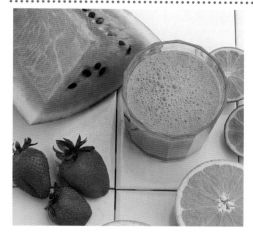

◎ **Breakfast**
1 hard boiled egg
1 piece of fresh fruit
$1/2$ cup of granola

◎ **Lunch**
Fast Gazpacho

◎ **Dinner**
Mahi-Mahi with Persimmons
Steamed vegetables of your choice
$1/2$ cup brown rice
Green salad
Ginger-Poached Pears

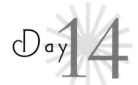

Day 14

Meditation
For today's session, begin with the Progressive Relaxation Exercise II (see page 31), followed by the Awareness Breath (see page 32), and for your meditation technique, use Managing Pain meditation (see page 56).

Aromatherapy
Consider all that you have accomplished with an aromatherapy diffuser formula for Loving Yourself, and follow the instructions (see page 120).

Exercise
Take it easy today with the Yoga Warm-Ups (see page 154) and then Yoga Practice Sessions Four and Five (see pages 157–158).

Home Spa

Feet

Treat your feet with the Summer Sand Foot Scrub (see page 256).

Nutrition

◎ **Breakfast**

$1/2$ cup Bircher Muesli

1 piece of fruit

◎ **Lunch**

Asparagus Soup

◎ **Dinner**

Grilled Trout with Horseradish Crust

Steamed vegetables of your choice

Green salad

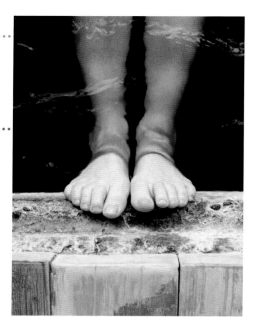

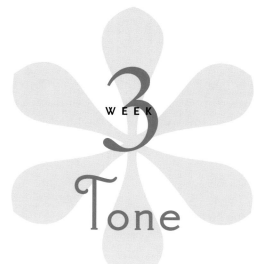

WEEK

3

Tone

• •

In addition to building strength, this week you will work on toning your body by continuing with yoga and weight-training exercises. You will also keep up with meditation, aromatherapy, spa treatments, and a balanced diet of super-nutritious recipes to reinvigorate your mind, relax, and rejuvenate your hair, skin, hands, and feet.

Meditation

As this week progresses, meditation should become easier for you. You should be able to hold the more simple postures for longer periods of time, and the more advanced postures for a greater length of time. Each day, meditate for 10 to 15 minutes in a quiet place, but this week, work on creating a home altar to further enhance your experience.

Aromatherapy

Since you are well into the *30-Day Revitalization Plan* at this point, it is particularly important that you relax. Aromatherapy will help you unwind mentally and physically. Each day the aromatherapy portion of the *30-Day Revitalization Plan* will address a different theme, but choose a formula that contains aromas that appeal to you.

Exercise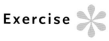

This week you will continue with four days of aerobic exercise, five yoga practice sessions, and two days of weight-training exercises. Depending on your fitness level, you might want to repeat a practice session from the previous day and build up through the week.

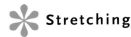

Stretching

To prevent muscle injury, it is extremely important to stretch before and after any exercise activity. The stretching routines presented each day will stretch the muscles that you will be using for either your aerobic or weight-training exercises.

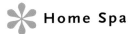

Home Spa

Pamper your hair this week with Rosemary Chamomile Shampoo (see page 249) followed by the Nettle Hair Tonic (see page 249). Continue to use daily the Strawberry Night Cream (see page 238), the Strawberry Facial Cream (see page 238), the Deodorant (see page 245), and the Liquid Hand Lotion (see page 254).

Nutrition

The daily menu suggestions (see Chapter 8 for specific recipes) offer a wide array of flavors that are healthy and will ensure that you get all of the necessary nutrients for a balanced diet. Supplement each recipe suggestion with a steamed vegetable of your choice and a green salad. Dress the salad with olive oil and vinegar or a low-fat bottled dressing.

Remember, as your activities increase, you need to fuel yourself adequetly. Snack on fresh veggies or a piece of fruit when you are hungry.

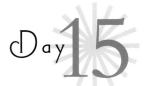

Meditation

For today's session, begin with one of the Basic Relaxation Exercises (see page 29), followed by the Counting Breath (see page 33), and for your meditation technique, use the meditation for dealing with Trauma and Shock (see page 57).

Aromatherapy

To relax and ponder your achievements, select an aromatherapy mist spray formula for Meditation and follow the instructions (see page 124).

Exercise

Get your heart going and your blood pumping with a 30-minute jog, either outdoors or on a treadmill. Run until you are out of breath, then change to fast-paced walking, then run again, then walk, then run, then walk, and so on. Then switch gears to yoga with first the Yoga Warm-Ups (see page 154) followed by Yoga Practice Session Six (see page 158).

Stretching

To avoid injury from your jog, be sure and do the following stretches before and after your workout (see pages 173–183).

1. Deltoid Stretch	9. Lunge Against Wall
2. Middle Chest Stretch	10. Side Lunge
3. Sitting Twist (on floor)	11. Calf Stretch on a Step
4. Knee to Opposite Chest Stretch	12. Inner Calf Stretch
5. Hamstring Stretch to Bench	13. Outer Calf Stretch
6. Ankle Reach	14. Standing Shin Stretch
7. One Leg Stretch	15. Inner Ankle Stretch
8. T-Stretch	16. Outer Ankle Stretch

Home Spa

Hair

Focus on your hair today first by using the Deep Conditioner (see page 250), followed by the Rosemary Hot Oil Treatment (see page 250), and finishing up with Hair Care Cream (see page 251).

Face-Building Exercises (see page 242).

Nutrition

◎ Breakfast
2 egg-white omelet
1 piece of fresh fruit
1 piece of toast

◎ Lunch
Crispy Bacon & Avocado Salad

◎ Dinner
Lemon-Orange Roughy
Steamed vegetables of your choice
Green Salad
1/2 cup brown rice

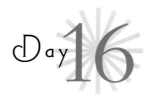

Day 16

Meditation

For today's session, begin with the Tension Release Exercise (see page 30), followed by the Yogi Complete Breath (see page 34), and for your meditation technique, use the meditation Transforming Feelings (see page 58).

Aromatherapy

To stay invigorated and energized, select an aromatherapy application formula for Motives for Our Actions and follow the instructions (see page 125).

Exercise

Go for a fast, 35-minute bicycle ride; then unwind with yoga: first Yoga Warm-Ups (see page 154), then Yoga Practice Session Seven (see page 159).

Stretching

To avoid pain and injury from your bicycle ride, be sure to do the following stretches before and after your workout (see pages 173–183).

1. Neck Turn	13. Figure-4 Stretch
2. Neck Tilt with Slight Extension	14. Lying Hamstring Stretch
3. Deltoid Stretch	15. Cat Stretch
4. Rotator Cuff Stretch	16. Back Arch
5. Middle Chest Stretch	17. Lying Back Extension
6. Squatting Chest Stretch	18. Pelvic Tilt
7. External Rotation Stretch	19. One Leg Stretch
8. Internal Rotation Stretch	20. T-Stretch
9. Wrist Extension Stretch	21. Straight Leg Stretch
10. Wrist Flexion Stretch	22. Half-Kneeling Shin Stretch
11. Open Hand Stretch	23. Outer Ankle Stretch
12. Closed Hand Stretch	24. Inner Ankle Stretch

Home Spa

Arms

Today, pay extra, loving attention to your arms. First apply the Rosewater Body Rub for Elbows and Knees (see page 246), and then follow up with your choice of body butters (see page 247).

Face-Building Exercises (see page 242).

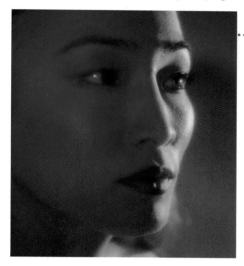

Nutrition

◎ **Breakfast**
1 hard-boiled egg
1 piece of fresh fruit
$^1/2$ cup granola

◎ **Lunch**
Broccoli Bisque

◎ **Dinner**
Perch with Duck Sauce and Pineapple
Steamed vegetables of your choice
Green salad
1 small baked potato

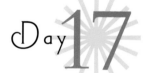

Day 17

Meditation

For today's session, begin with the Progressive Relaxation Exercise I (see page 30), followed by the Standing Breath (see page 33), and for your meditation technique, use the Kabbalah (see page 58).

Aromatherapy

To marvel over your achievements of the past three weeks, select an aromatherapy diffuser formula for Reflection, and follow the instructions (see page 127).

Exercise

Although most of your exercise program today will be devoted to weight training, it's important to get your heart going, so start your workout today with a brisk, 20-minute walk.

Stretching

Be sure to stretch before and after your workout (see pages 173–183).

Walking Stretches

1. Deltoid Stretch
2. Middle Chest Stretch
3. Sitting Twist (on floor)
4. Knee to Opposite Chest Stretch
5. Hamstring Stretch to Bench
6. Ankle Reach
7. One Leg Stretch
8. T-Stretch
9. Lunge Against Wall
10. Side Lunge
11. Calf Stretch on a Step
12. Inner Calf Stretch
13. Outer Calf Stretch
14. Standing Shin Stretch
15. Inner Ankle Stretch
16. Outer Ankle Stretch

Weight-Lifting Stretches

1. Neck Turn
2. Neck Tilt with Slight Extension
3. Reach Stretch
4. Rotator Cuff Stretch
5. Arm over Head Stretch
6. Middle Chest Stretch
7. Tall Stretch
8. One Leg Stretch
9. T-Stretch
10. Bent Knee Calf Stretch
11. Standing Shin Stretch
12. Straight Leg Stretch
13. Supine Groin Stretch
14. Knee to Chest Stretch
15. Cat Stretch
16. Back Arch

Weight Training: Weekly Workout 3

Legs
Lunge
Leg Curl
Adduction

Chest
Dumbbell Press, Flat Bench
Decline Bar Press

Back
Lat Pull-Down, Back,
    Close Grip
One-Arm Low-Pulley
    Cable Row

Shoulders
One-Arm Dumbbell Press
    on Incline
One-Arm Rear Delt Raise

Biceps
Standard Dumbbell Curl

Triceps
French Press—Black Eye

Abs
Side Curl-Up
Combined Trunk Curl/Pelvic Tilt

Home Spa

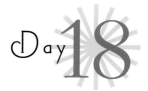

Legs

Today, pay extra, loving attention to your legs. First apply the Rosewater Body Rub for Elbows and Knees (see page 246), and then follow up with your choice of body butters (see page 247).

Hair

Give your hair an extra boost with the Hair Care Cream (see page 251).

Face-Building Exercises (see page 242).

Nutrition

◎ Breakfast
2 scrambled egg whites
1 piece of fresh fruit

◎ Lunch
Carrot Soup with Madeira

◎ Dinner
Rainbrow Trout with Orange
Steamed vegetables of your choice
Green salad
1/2 cup steamed brown rice

Day 18

Meditation

For today's session, begin with the Progressive Relaxation Exercise II (see page 31), followed by the Awareness Breath (see page 32), and for your meditation technique, choose one of the Nature Meditations (see page 59).

Aromatherapy

To stay invigorated and energized, select an aromatherapy diffuser formula for Surviving Stress and follow the instructions (see page 131).

Exercise

Take a break from aerobic exercise today and perform Yoga Practice Sessions Seven and Eight (see pages 159–160), preceded by Yoga Warm-Ups (see page 154).

Home Spa

Face

Pamper your face today. First, apply the Gentle Oatmeal Cleanser (see page 232); then choose one Facial Sauna formula (see page 233). Next use Fresh 'n' Cool Skin Freshener (see page 234); followed up with the Almond Meal Cleansing Mask (see page 236), or, if you feel your skin needs extra attention, choose either Face Mask for Balancing Oily Skin, Face Mask for Improving Skin Texture, or Face Pack for Normal, Dry, or Sensitive Skin (see page 237).

Nutrition

◎ Breakfast

1/2 cup Bircher Muesli
1 piece of fresh fruit

◎ Lunch

Celery-Leek Chowder

◎ Dinner

Scallops Edam
Steamed vegetable of your choice
Green salad

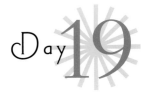

Day 19

Meditation

For today's session, begin with the Tension Release Exercise (see page 30), followed by the Standing Breath (see page 33), and for your meditation technique, choose one of the Four Elements Meditations (see page 61).

Aromatherapy

To keep up the good work, select an aromatherapy mist spray formula for Mood Uplifting, and follow the instructions (see page 129).

Exercise

Go for a 35-minute swim. It's okay to vary your strokes; just make sure that you're constantly moving. After your swim go through Yoga Practice Session Nine (see page 161). Before your yoga, be sure to perform the Yoga Warm-Ups (see page 154).

Stretching

Although swimming causes very little nerve damage, and on its own strengthens and stretches the entire body, be sure to perform these stretches before and after to have a more enjoyable and beneficial swim (see pages 173–183).

1. Open Mouth Stretch
2. Jaw Protrusion Stretch
3. Neck Tilt
4. Neck Turn
5. Neck Tilt with Slight Extension
6. Deltoid Stretch
7. Arm over Head Stretch
8. Rotator Cuff Stretch
9. Shoulder Blade Squeeze
10. Front Press Out
11. Lower Chest Stretch
12. Upper Chest Stretch
13. Wrist Extension Stretch
14. Wrist Flexion Stretch
15. One Leg Stretch
16. Lunge Against Wall
17. Side Lunge
18. Standing Shin Stretch
19. Straight Leg Stretch
20. Outer Ankle Stretch
21. Inner Ankle Stretch
22. Knee to Chest Stretch
23. Supine Groin Stretch

Home Spa

Body

Care for your body with an Aromatherapy Bath (see page 244), or, if you prefer a shower, the Lavishly Smooth Shower Gel (see page 245), followed by Wintergreen Body Rub (see page 247).

Face-Building Exercises (see page 242).

Nutrition

◎ **Breakfast**
2 scrambled egg whites
1 piece of fresh fruit
1 piece of toast

◎ **Lunch**
Fresh Tomato Corn Soup

◎ **Dinner**
Simply Monkfish
Steamed vegetables of your choice
Green salad
Mixed Fruit Compote

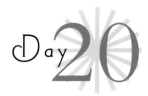

Day 20

Meditation

For today's session, begin with one of the Basic Relaxations (see page 29), followed by the Counting Breath (see page 33), and for your meditation technique, choose one of the Flower meditations (see page 63).

Aromatherapy

Enjoy yourself by selecting an aromatherapy application formula for Relaxing, and follow the instructions (see page 130).

Exercise

Although most of your exercise program today will be devoted to weight training, it's important to get your heart going, so start your workout today with a brisk, 20-minute walk.

Stretching

Be sure to stretch before and after your workout (see pages 173–183).

Walking Stretches

1. Deltoid Stretch
2. Middle Chest Stretch
3. Sitting Twist (on floor)
4. Knee to Opposite Chest Stretch
5. Hamstring Stretch to Bench
6. Ankle Reach
7. One Leg Stretch
8. T Stretch
9. Lunge Against Wall
10. Side Lunge
11. Calf Stretch on a Step
12. Inner Calf Stretch
13. Outer Calf Stretch
14. Standing Shin Stretch
15. Inner Ankle Stretch
16. Outer Ankle Stretch

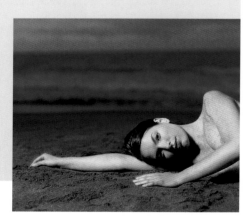

Weight-Lifting Stretches

1. Neck Turn
2. Neck Tilt with Slight Extension
3. Reach Stretch
4. Rotator Cuff Stretch
5. Arm over Head Stretch
6. Middle Chest Stretch
7. Tall Stretch
8. One Leg Stretch
9. T-Stretch
10. Bent Knee Calf Stretch
11. Standing Shin Stretch
12. Straight Leg Stretch
13. Supine Groin Stretch
14. Knee to Chest Stretch
15. Cat Stretch
16. Back Arch

Weight Training: Weekly Workout 4

Legs
One-Leg Squat
Knee Extension/Hip Extension

Chest
Low-Pulley Cable Fly
Pullover

Back
Lat Pull Down, Front, CloseGrip
Wide-Grip Seated Low-Pulley
   Row

Shoulders
Hanging One-Arm Lateral Raise
Front Shoulder Raise with
Olympic Plate

Biceps
Hammer Concentration Curl

Triceps
One-Arm Overhead Extension

Abs
Side Crunch on Roman Chair
Knee-Up

Home Spa

Hands
Pamper your hands with the Sugar Soft Hand Exfoliant (see page 253), followed by the Lemon Protective Hand Cream (see page 254), and finish up with the Nail Cleaner (see page 255).

Face-Building Exercises (see page 242).

Nutrition

◎ Breakfast
1 hard boiled egg
1 piece of fresh fruit
1/2 cup of granola

◎ **Lunch**
Hearty Parsnip–Turnip Soup

◎ **Dinner**
Gorgonzola Cheeseburgers on Crostini
Steamed vegetables of your choice
Green salad
$^1/2$ cup steamed brown rice

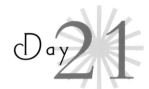

Day 21

◎ *Meditation*

For today's session, begin with the Progressive Relaxation Exercise I (see page 30), followed by the Yogi Complete Breath (see page 34), and for your meditation technique, choose one of the Tree Meditations (see page 65).

◎ *Aromatherapy*

Luxuriate in your invigorated and energized self by selecting an aromatherapy mist spray formula for Appreciation, and follow the instructions (see page 115).

◎ *Exercise*

Strengthen today with the Yoga Warm-Ups (see page 154) and then Yoga Practice Sessions Nine and Ten (see pages 161–162).

◎ *Home Spa*

Feet
Treat your feet with the Refreshing Peppermint Foot Gel (see page 256).

◎ *Nutrition*

◎ **Breakfast**
$^1/2$ cup Bircher Muesli
1 piece of fresh fruit

◎ **Lunch**
Portobello Mushroom Soup

◎ **Dinner**
Curried Beef & Potatoes
Steamed vegetables of your choice
Green salad

WEEK
4
Endure

Continuing to strengthen and tone your body, this week you will also learn the value of both physical and mental endurance by keeping up your meditation, aromatherapy, aerobic exercise, yoga practice sessions, weight-training exercises, spa treatments, and balanced diet.

Meditation

By now, you should be able to hold the more simple postures for longer periods of time, and the more advanced postures for some length of time. Each day, meditate for 15 minutes in a quiet place, but work on creating an outdoor altar to further enhance your experience.

Aromatherapy

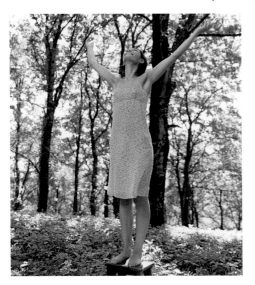

To get through this last week of the *30-Day Revitalization Plan*, you will want to relax using aromatherapy. In addition to helping you prepare your body and mind for the tasks at hand, aromatherapy will help you unwind. Each day the aromatherapy portion of the *30-Day Revitalization Plan* will address a different theme, but you are free to choose the actual formula, depending on what aromas appeal to you.

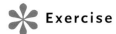 **Exercise**

This week you will continue with four days of aerobic exercise, five yoga practice sessions, and two days of weight-training exercises. Depending on your fitness level, you might want to repeat a practice sesssion from the previous day and build up through the week.

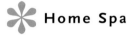 **Home Spa**

This week, indulge your hair with the wonderful Lavender Ylang-Ylang Shampoo (see page 249). Continue to use daily the Strawberry Night Cream (see page 238), the Strawberry Facial Cream (see page 238), the Deodorant (see page 245), and the Liquid Hand Lotion (see page 254).

Nutrition

The daily menu suggestions (see Chapter 8 for specific recipes) offer a wide array of flavors that are healthy and will ensure that you get all of the necessary nutrients for a balanced diet. Supplement each recipe with a steamed vegetable of your choice and a green salad. Dress the salad with olive oil and vinegar or a low-fat bottled dressing.

Remember, as your activity level increases, you need to fuel yourself adequetly. Snack on fresh veggies or a piece of fruit when you are hungry.

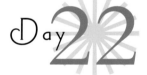

Day 22

Meditation

For today's session, begin with the Progressive Relaxation Exercise II (see page 31), followed by the Awareness Breath (see page 32), and for your meditation technique, choose one of the Rainbow Color meditations (see page 78).

Aromatherapy

To continue to strive for the best, select an aromatherapy application formula for Improvement and follow the instructions (see page 117).

Exercise

Get your heart going and your blood pumping with a 30-minute jog, either outdoors or on a treadmill. Run until you are out of breath, then change to fast-paced walking, then run again, then walk, then run, then walk, and so on. Then switch gears to yoga first with the Yoga Warm-Ups (see page 154) followed by Yoga Practice Session Eleven (see page 162).

Stretching

To avoid injury from your jog, be sure to do the following stretches before and after your workout (see pages 173–183).

1. Deltoid Stretch	9. Lunge Against Wall
2. Middle Chest Stretch	10. Side Lunge
3. Sitting Twist (on floor)	11. Calf Stretch on a Step
4. Knee to Opposite Chest Stretch	12. Inner Calf Stretch
5. Hamstring Stretch to Bench	13. Outer Calf Stretch
6. Ankle Reach	14. Standing Shin Stretch
7. One Leg Stretch	15. Inner Ankle Stretch
8. T-Stretch	16. Outer Ankle Stretch

Home Spa

Hair

Focus on your hair today with the Sandalwood Hot Oil Treatment (see page 250) and Ravishing Rosemary Hair Conditioner (see page 252), followed by the Hair Care Cream (see page 251).

Face-Building Exercises (see page 242).

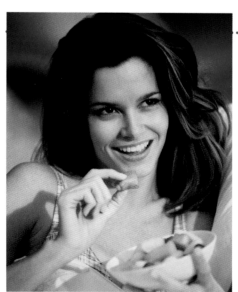

Nutrition

◎ Breakfast
2 egg-white omelet
1 piece of fresh fruit
1 piece of toast

◎ Lunch
Shallot-Watercress Soup

◎ Dinner
Egg Noodles with Chicken & Vegetables
Steamed vegetables of your choice
Green salad
Mocha Bread Pudding

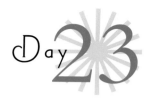

Day 23

Meditation

For today's session, begin with one of the Basic Relaxation Exercises (see page 29), followed by the Standing Breath (see page 33), and for your meditation technique, begin with Day 1 of the Eightfold Path meditation (see page 41).

Aromatherapy

To evaluate your progress, select an aromatherapy diffuser formula for Introspection and follow the instructions (see page 118).

Exercise

Go for a fast, 35-minute bicycle ride, then change the pace with yoga: first Yoga Warm-Ups (see page 154), then Yoga Practice Session Twelve (see page 163).

Stretching

To avoid pain and injury from your bicycle ride, be sure to do the following stretches before and after your workout (see pages 173–183).

1. Neck Turn	13. Figure Four Stretch
2. Neck Tilt with Slight Extension	14. Lying Hamstring Stretch
3. Deltoid Stretch	15. Cat Stretch
4. Rotator Cuff Stretch	16. Back Arch
5. Middle Chest Stretch	17. Lying Back Extension
6. Squatting Chest Stretch	18. Pelvic Tilt
7. External Rotation Stretch	19. One Leg Stretch
8. Internal Rotation Stretch	20. T-Stretch
9. Wrist Extension Stretch	21. Straight Leg Stretch
10. Wrist Flexion Stretch	22. Half-Kneeling Shin Stretch
11. Open Hand Stretch	23. Outer Ankle Stretch
12. Closed Hand Stretch	24. Inner Ankle Stretch

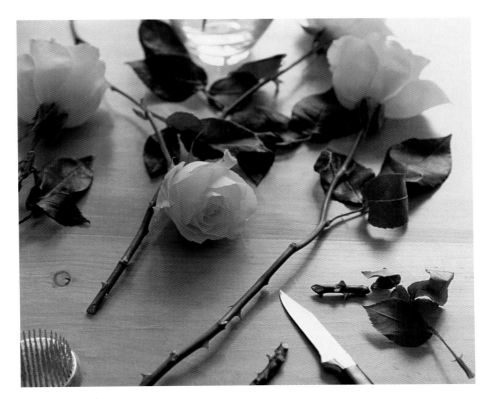

Home Spa

Arms

Today, pay extra, loving attention to your arms. First apply the Rosewater Body Rub for Elbows and Knees (see page 246), and then follow up with your choice of body butters (see page 247).

Face-Building Exercises (see page 242).

Nutrition

◎ **Breakfast**
1 hard-boiled egg
1 piece of fresh fruit
1/2 cup of granola

◎ **Lunch**
Tuna & White Bean Salad

◎ **Dinner**
Thai Pork Chops
Steamed vegetables
Green salad of your choice

Day 24

Meditation

For today's session, begin with the Progressive Relaxation Exercise I (see page 30), followed by the Awareness Breath (see page 32), and for your meditation technique, begin with Day 2 of the Eightfold Path meditation (see page 41).

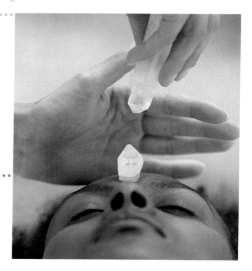

Aromatherapy

To stay invigorated and energized, select an aromatherapy mist spray formula for Loving Yourself, and follow the instructions (see page 120).

Exercise

Although most of your exercise program today will be devoted to weight training, it's important to get your heart going, so start your workout today with a brisk, 20-minute walk.

Stretching

Be sure to stretch before and after your workout (see pages 173–183).

Walking Stretches

1. Deltoid Stretch
2. Middle Chest Stretch
3. Sitting Twist (on floor)
4. Knee to Opposite Chest Stretch
5. Hamstring Stretch to Bench
6. Ankle Reach
7. One Leg Stretch
8. T-Stretch
9. Lunge Against Wall
10. Side Lunge
11. Calf Stretch on a Step
12. Inner Calf Stretch
13. Outer Calf Stretch
14. Standing Shin Stretch
15. Inner Ankle Stretch
16. Outer Ankle Stretch

Weight-Lifting Stretches

1. Neck Turn	9. T-Stretch
2. Neck Tilt with Slight Extension	10. Bent Knee Calf Stretch
3. Reach Stretch	11. Standing Shin Stretch
4. Rotator Cuff Stretch	12. Straight Leg Stretch
5. Arm over Head Stretch	13. Supine Groin Stretch
6. Middle Chest Stretch	14. Knee to Chest Stretch
7. Tall Stretch	15. Cat Stretch
8. One Leg Stretch	16. Back Arch

Weight Training: Weekly Workout 5

Legs
Knee Extension
Leg Curl/Hip Extension
Step-Up
Squat

Biceps
EZ Bar Preacher Curl
High-Pulley Cable Curl
One-Arm Hammer Curl on
    Preacher Bench

Back
Low-Pulley Cable Row
Dead Lift, Straight Leg
Lat Pull-Down
Upright Row

Abs
Center Curl-Up
Crunch
Side Curl-Up
Tailbone Lift

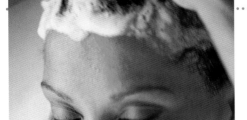

Home Spa

Legs
Today, pay extra, loving attention to your legs. First apply the Rosewater Body Rub for Elbows and Knees (see page 246), and then follow up with your choice of body butters (see page 247).

Hair
Give your hair an extra boost with the Hair Care Cream (see page 251).

Face-Building Exercises (see page 242).

(see page 242).

Nutrition

◎ **Breakfast**
2 scrambled egg whites
1 piece of fresh fruit

◎ **Lunch**
Tomato and Leek Soup

◎ **Dinner**
Greek Chicken Sandwiches
Steamed vegetables of your choice
Green salad
1/2 cup steamed brown rice

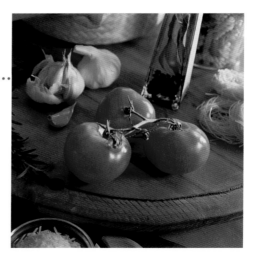

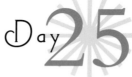

Day 25

Meditation

For today's session, begin with the Tension/Release Exercise (see page 30), followed by the Yogi Complete Breath (see page 34), and for your meditation technique, begin with Day 3 of the Eightfold Path meditation (see page 41).

Aromatherapy

Consider your progress and select an aromatherapy application formula for Meditation and follow the instructions (see page 123).

Exercise

Take a break from aerobic exercise today and perform Yoga Practice Sessions Twelve and Thirteen (see pages 163–164), preceded by Yoga Warm-Ups (see page 154).

Home Spa

Face

Pamper your face today. First, apply Lemon Cleansing Cream (see page 233); then choose one Facial Sauna formula (see page 233). Select the toner you most enjoyed from Week 1, 2, or 3; follow up with the Cucumber Egg Mask (see page 236), or, if you feel your skin needs extra attention, choose either Face Mask for Balancing Oily Skin, Face Mask for Improving Skin Texture, or Face Pack for Normal, Dry, or Sensitive Skin (see page 237).

Nutrition

◎ **Breakfast**
1/2 cup Bircher Muesli
1 piece of fresh fruit

◎ **Lunch**
Juicy Summer Salad
1 small baked potato

◎ **Dinner**
Honey Turkey Fajitas
Steamed vegetables of your choice
Green salad

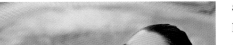

Meditation

For today's session, begin with the Progressive Relaxation Exercise II (see page 31), followed by the Counting Breath (see page 33), and for your meditation technique, begin with Day 4 of the Eightfold Path meditation (see page 41).

Aromatherapy

Think about all that you have accomplished and your reasons for doing so by selecting an aromatherapy diffuser formula for Motives for Our Actions and follow the instructions (see page 125).

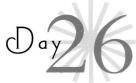

Exercise

Go for a 35-minute swim. It's okay to vary your strokes, just make sure that you're constantly moving. After your swim go through Yoga Practice Session Fourteen (see page 164). Before your yoga, be sure to perform the Yoga Warm-Ups (see page 154).

Stretching

Although swimming causes very little nerve damage, and on its own strengthens and stretches the entire body, be sure to perform these stretches before and after to have a more enjoyable and beneficial swim (see pages 173–183).

1. Open Mouth Stretch
2. Jaw Protrusion Stretch
3. Neck Tilt
4. Neck Turn
5. Neck Tilt with Slight Extension
6. Deltoid Stretch
7. Arm over Head Stretch
8. Rotator Cuff Stretch
9. Shoulder Blade Squeeze
10. Front Press Out
11. Lower Chest Stretch
12. Upper Chest Stretch
13. Wrist Extension Stretch
14. Wrist Flexion Stretch
15. One Leg Stretch
16. Lunge Against Wall
17. Side Lunge
18. Standing Shin Stretch
19. Straight Leg Stretch
20. Outer Ankle Stretch
21. Inner Ankle Stretch
22. Knee to Chest Stretch
23. Supine Groin Stretch

Home Spa

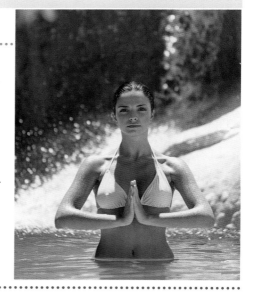

Body

Care for your body with an Aromatherapy Bath (see page 244) or, if you prefer a shower, the Refreshing Sea Salt Scrub (see page 245) or the Lavishly Smooth Shower Gel (see page 245). Moisturize with a body butter of your choice (see page 247).

Face-Building Exercises (see page 242).

Nutrition

◎ Breakfast

2 scrambled egg whites
1 piece of fresh fruit
1 piece of toast

◎ **Lunch**

Spinach and Mandarin Orange Salad

◎ **Dinner**

Grilled Turkey & Tomato Burgers
Steamed vegetables of your choice
Green salad
Warm Fresh Fruit Delight

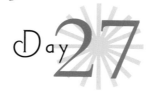

Day 27

Meditation

For today's session, begin with the Tension Release Exercise (see page 30), followed by the Standing Breath (see page 33), and for your meditation technique, begin with Day 5 of the Eightfold Path meditation (see page 41).

Aromatherapy

To stay invigorated and energized, select an aromatherapy mist spray formula for Reflection, and follow the instructions (see page 127).

Exercise

Although most of your exercise program today will be devoted to weight training, it's important to get your heart going, so start your exercise today with a brisk, 20-minute walk.

Stretching

Be sure to stretch before and after your workout (see pages 173–183).

Walking Stretches

1. Deltoid Stretch	9. Lunge Against Wall
2. Middle Chest Stretch	10. Side Lunge
3. Sitting Twist (on floor)	11. Calf Stretch on a Step
4. Knee to Opposite Chest Stretch	12. Inner Calf Stretch
5. Hamstring Stretch to Bench	13. Outer Calf Stretch
6. Ankle Reach	14. Standing Shin Stretch
7. One Leg Stretch	15. Inner Ankle Stretch
8. T-Stretch	16. Outer Ankle Stretch

Weight-Lifting Stretches

1. Neck Turn
2. Neck Tilt with Slight Extension
3. Reach Stretch
4. Rotator Cuff Stretch
5. Arm over Head Stretch
6. Middle Chest Stretch
7. Tall Stretch
8. One Leg Stretch
9. T-Stretch
10. Bent Knee Calf Stretch
11. Standing Shin Stretch
12. Straight Leg Stretch
13. Supine Groin Stretch
14. Knee to Chest Stretch
15. Cat Stretch
16. Back Arch

Weight Training: Weekly Workout 6

Chest
Decline Bench Press
Low-Pulley Cable Fly
Incline Dumbbell Press

Shoulders
Lateral Raise
Bar Press
Rear Delt Raise

Triceps
Black Eye—French Press
Combo Kickback

Forearms
Reverse Curl
Wrist Curl—Flexion and Extension

Abs
Bar Twist
Side Crunch on Roman Chair
Knee-Up
Center Curl-Up

Home Spa

Hands
Pamper your hands with the Lemonade Hand Exfoliant (see page 253), followed by the Hand Cream for Chapped Hands (see page 254), and finish up with Nail Whitener (see page 255).

Face-Building Exercises (see page 242).

Nutrition

◎ **Breakfast**

1 hard boiled egg
1 piece of fresh fruit
1/2 cup of granola

◎ Lunch
Greek Salad
1/2 cup steamed brown rice

◎ Dinner
Skillet Salsa Beef
Steamed vegetables of your choice
Green salad
1 small baked potato

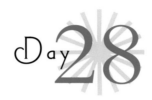

Day 28

Meditation

For today's session, begin with the Basic Relaxation Exercise (see page 29), followed by the Counting Breath (see page 33), and for your meditation technique, begin with Day 6 of the Eightfold Path meditation (see page 41).

Aromatherapy

Enjoy yourself by selecting an aromatherapy application formula for Appreciation and follow the instructions (see page 115).

Exercise

Strengthen today with the Yoga Warm-Ups (see page 154) and then Yoga Practice Sessions Fourteen and Fifteen (see pages 164–165).

Home Spa

Feet
Treat your feet with the Banana Foot Lotion (see page 256).

Nutrition

◎ Breakfast
1/2 cup Bircher Muesli
1 piece of fruit

◎ Lunch
Caribbean Stewed Vegetables
1/2 cup steamed brown rice

◎ **Dinner**
Spicy Orange Beef with Broccoli
Steamed vegetables of your choice
Green salad

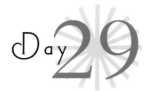

Day 29

Meditation

For today's session, begin with the Progressive Relaxation Exercise I (see page 30), followed by the Yogi Complete Breath (see page 34), and for your meditation technique, begin with Day 7 of the Eightfold Path meditation (see page 41).

Aromatherapy

Continue to strive for the best by selecting an aromatherapy diffuser formula for Improvement and follow the instructions (see page 117).

Exercise

Go for a fast, 35-minute bicycle ride then unwind with yoga: first Yoga Warm-Ups (see page 154), then Yoga Practice Session One (see page 155).

Stretching

To avoid pain and injury from your bicycle ride, be sure to do the following stretches before and after ypour workout (see pages 173–183).

1. Neck Turn	13. Figure Four Stretch
2. Neck Tilt with Slight Extension	14. Lying Hamstring Stretch
3. Deltoid Stretch	15. Cat Stretch
4. Rotator Cuff Stretch	16. Back Arch
5. Middle Chest Stretch	17. Lying Back Extension
6. Squatting Chest Stretch	18. Pelvic Tilt
7. External Rotation Stretch	19. One Leg Stretch
8. Internal Rotation Stretch	20. T-Stretch
9. Wrist Extension Stretch	21. Straight Leg Stretch
10. Wrist Flexion Stretch	22. Half-Kneeling Shin Stretch
11. Open Hand Stretch	23. Outer Ankle Stretch
12. Closed Hand Stretch	24. Inner Ankle Stretch

Home Spa

Shop

Indulge your new body with a shopping trip!

Body

Relax with an aromatherapy bath of your choice.

Face-Building Exercises (see page 242).

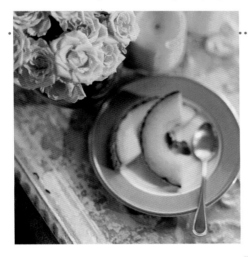

Nutrition

◎ **Breakfast**

2 egg-white omelet
1 piece of fresh fruit
1 piece of toast

◎ **Lunch**

BLT Salad

◎ **Dinner**

Baked Fish & Vegetable Packets
Steamed vegetables of your choice
Green salad
1/2 cup steamed brown rice

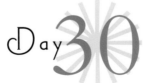

Day 30

Meditation

For today's session, begin with the Progressive Relaxation Exercise II (see page 31), followed by the Awareness Breath (see page 32), and for your meditation technique, begin with Day 8 of the Eightfold Path meditation (see page 41).

Aromatherapy

Bask in your accomplishments and select an aromatherapy mist spray formula for Introspection, and follow the instructions (see page 118).

Exercise

Get your heart going and your blood pumping with a 30-minute jog, either outdoors or on a treadmill. Run until you are out of breath, then change to fast-paced walking, then run again, then walk, then run, then walk, and so on. Then switch gears to yoga first with the Yoga Warm-Ups (see page 154), followed by Yoga Practice Session Two (see page 155).

Stretching

To avoid injury from your jog, be sure to do the following stretches before and after your jog (see pages 173–183).

1. Deltoid Stretch	9. Lunge Against Wall
2. Middle Chest Stretch	10. Side Lunge
3. Sitting Twist (on floor)	11. Calf Stretch on a Step
4. Knee to Opposite Chest Stretch	12. Inner Calf Stretch
5. Hamstring Stretch to Bench	13. Outer Calf Stretch
6. Ankle Reach	14. Standing Shin Stretch
7. One Leg Stretch	15. Inner Ankle Stretch
8. T-Stretch	16. Outer Ankle Stretch

Home Spa

Face

Select the scrub, Facial Sauna formula, and toner you most enjoyed; follow up with the Lemon and Honey Face Mask (see page 237), or, if you feel your skin needs extra attention, choose either Face Mask for Balancing Oily Skin, Face Mask for Improving Skin Texture, or Face Pack for Normal, Dry, or Sensitive Skin (see page 237).

Nutrition

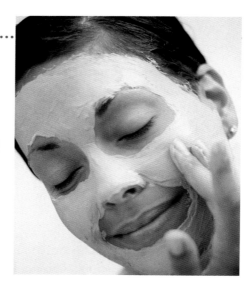

◎ **Breakfast**
1 hard-boiled egg
1 piece of fresh fruit
1/2 cup of granola

◎ **Lunch**
Slivered Cucumber & Chicken Salad

◎ **Dinner**
Stir-Fried Sesame Lamb
Steamed vegetables of your choice
Green salad
Chocolate-Cappuccino
  Dream Creams

Index

A

Activity level, 265-266
Aging, 266-267
Alanine, 15-16
Alaskan Salmon Salad Sandwiches,
    286-287, 342
Almond Meal Cleansing Mask, 236,
    354
Altars, 25, 26-27
Apple-Plum Crisp, 305, 340
Apples, 304, 305, 306
Aromatherapy, 85-132, 312, 333-334,
    347, 359
    baths, 244-245, 355, 368, 373
    body butters, 247-248
    for Appreciation, 115-116, 314,
        340, 358, 371
    for Breathing, 131-132
    for Improvement, 117-118, 317,
        341, 360, 372
    for Introspection, 118-120, 319,
        343, 362, 373
    for Loving Yourself, 120-122, 323,
        345, 364
    for Meditation, 123-124, 325, 348,
        366
    for Mood Uplifting, 129, 335, 354
    for Motives for our Actions,
        125-126, 327, 350, 367
    for Reflection, 127-128, 330, 351,
        369
    for Relaxation, 130, 336, 338, 353,
        356
    for Surrendering Your Stress, 130,
        338, 353
    formulas, 115-132
    hair care creams, 251
    methods of application, 86-87
    safety guidelines, 88-89
    scents, 91-114
    themes, 115-132
Arthritis, 138
Asparagus, 274, 285
Asparagus Soup, 274-275, 346
Avocado Coconut Conditioner, 250,
    336
Avocados, 281

B

Bacon, 281, 282
Baked Cod with Seasoned Tomatoes,
    288, 336
Baked Fish and Vegetable Packets,
    293-294, 373
Banana Foot Lotion, 256, 371
Basil, 299
Basil Oil, 299
Baths and showers, 244-245, 326

wrists, 224–225
Wheatgerm Hot Oil Strengthening
    Fingernail Treatment, 255, 328
Wintergreen Body Rub, 247, 355

Y

Yamas, 82–84
Yoga, 152–166
    poses, 155–166
    practice sessions, 155–166, 335,
        336, 340, 341, 345, 349, 350,
        353, 354, 358, 361, 362, 366,
        367, 371, 372, 374
    tips, 153
    warm-ups, 154, 161, 335, 336,
        340, 341, 345, 349, 350, 353,
        354, 358, 361, 362, 366, 367,
        371, 372, 374
Yoga poses, 155–166
    archer, 156
    arm variations, 166
    backward arm stretch, 158
    boar with strap, 162
    bound angle, 155
    chair corpse, 154, 161, 162, 165
    chair lower back stretch, 154, 158
    chair twist 1, 162
    chair twist 2, 162
    child's, 154, 159
    cobra, 160–161
    dead bug, 155
    desk, 154, 161
    double inner thigh stretch, 156
    downward facing dog, 159
    feet on the floor twist, 161
    5-second pre-headstand, 159–160
    foot on knee twist, 162
    forward arm stretch, 158
    full forward bend, 156
    full locust, 161

head to chair, 156
hero, 165–166
knees to chest, 154, 155
leg lifts, 163
leg-to-chair, table, or wall pose—
    front angle, 157
leg-to-chair, table, or wall pose—
    side angle, 157
locust variation 2, 161
lunge, 164, 165
plank, 159
quadriceps stretch, 163
reclining hamstring stretch, 156
reclining inner thigh stretch, 156
right angle (Geometry 101), 160
rock the baby, 164
seated double hamstring stretch,
    164
seated hamstring stretch, 164
seated wide angle, 155
side angle, 159
staff, 155
standing hamstring stretch, 164
standing forward bend 1, 163
standing forward bend 2, 165
supported chest opener, 157
tree, 157
triangle, 158–159
upward arm stretch, 158
wall hang, 160
warrior I, 165
warrior II, 159, 165
warrior III, 160
wide angle, 155
yoga sit-ups, 163
Yogurt, 298

Z

Zucchini, 274
Zucchini Soup Margherita, 274, 341

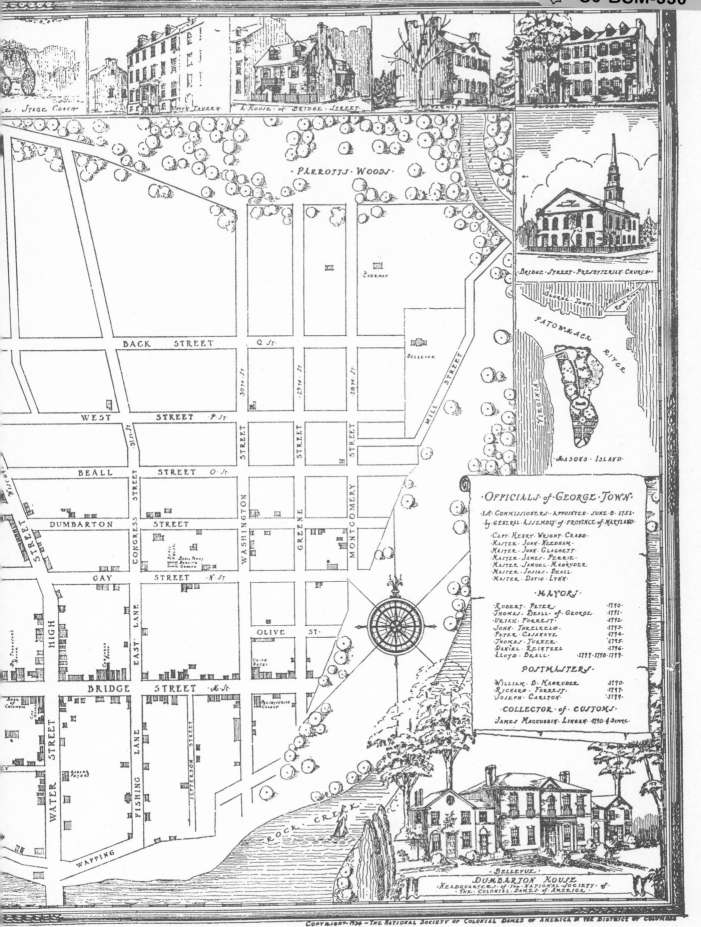

OFFICIALS of GEORGE TOWN

A. COMMISSIONERS APPOINTED JUNE 8. 1751.
by GENERAL ASSEMBLY of PROVINCE of MARYLAND.

CAPT. HENRY WRIGHT CRABB.
MASTER JOHN NEEDHAM.
MASTER JOHN GLAGOLY.
MASTER JAMES PERRIE.
MASTER SAMUEL MAGRUDER.
MASTER JOSIAS BEALL.
MASTER DAVID LYNN.

MAYORS

ROBERT PETER.   1790.
THOMAS BEALL of GEORGE.   1791.
URIAH FORREST.   1792.
JOHN THRELKELD.   1793.
PETER CASANAVE.   1794.
THOMAS TURNER.   1795.
DANIEL REINTZEL.   1796.
LLOYD BEALL.   1797. 1798. 1799.

POSTMASTERS

WILLIAM B. MAGRUDER.   1790.
RICHARD FORREST.   1797.
JOSEPH CARLTON.   1799.

COLLECTOR of CUSTOMS

JAMES MACCUBBIN LINGAN. 1790 & since.

BELLEVUE.
DUMBARTON HOUSE
HEADQUARTERS of the NATIONAL SOCIETY of
THE COLONIAL DAMES of AMERICA.

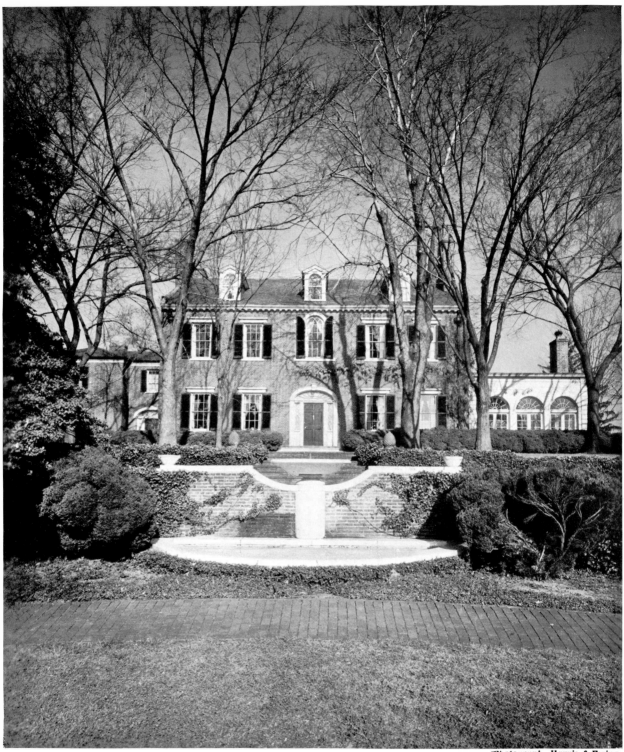

EVERMAY

GEORGETOWN
HOVSES

OF THE
FEDERAL PERIOD

WASHINGTON · D · C ·

1780~1830

★ ★ ★

By · DEERING · DAVIS · A · I · D ·
STEPHEN · P · DORSEY · &
RALPH · COLE · HALL

Foreword by
NANCY · McCLELLAND · A · I · D ·

BONANZA BOOKS · NEW YORK

FOREWORD

INVITED BY THE AUTHORS to sponsor this work on "Georgetown Houses," the American Institute of Decorators accepts the honor with pride and pleasure, believing that the book will prove to be an important contribution to the architectural history of this country.

Illustrated here are twenty-two houses just one mile from the White House and leading hotels of Washington. With travel curtailed, interest in everything American increased by our National crisis, and the Capital crowded with people from every part of the globe, this book should serve a valuable purpose by presenting, in well-documented form, an account of part of our heritage that is too little known.

Although the pages that follow are concerned primarily, indeed, with one exception, exclusively with Georgetown, its personal history, and its architecture after 1780, it does not seem amiss in this foreword to say a few words about the family relation of Georgetown to our National Capital. For Georgetown in a manner was the parent city of Washington.

The little town first came into National prominence in 1783, when Congress, weary of moving about from New York to Philadelphia, to Trenton, to Baltimore, to Lancaster and York, to Princeton and Annapolis, decided to fix on a permanent residence for the Capital. At the outset a location on the Delaware was selected. Two weeks later it was decided that, in addition, there should be a second National Capital, *"at or near the lower falls of the Potomac at Georgetown."*

This idea of the two Capitals was not received with great enthusiasm. Francis Hopkins flicked it with a sly touch of ridicule by proposing that the statue of Washington which was authorized at the same session be put on wheels so that it could follow wherever Congress went!

Seven years later Georgetown learned that the plan of one Federal City had finally been adopted; that it was to be on the Potomac and that the President of the United States himself was coming to view the proposed site with his three commissioners.

In his diary Washington records using Suter's Tavern as his Georgetown headquarters, and makes note of several visits there. He first came from Mount Vernon on October fifteenth, 1790, and set out with his commissioners and the principal citizens of the town to inspect the surrounding country. The following year in March he visited Georgetown again. Major L'Enfant, who was to lay out the new city, had arrived on March twelfth, as noted in the Georgetown Weekly Record. Andrew Ellicott, the official surveyor, was also there.[1] Washington's Diary describes the great occasion:

March 28, 1791. Breakfasted at Georgetown about 8; where having appointed the commissioners under the residence law to meet me, I found Mr Johnson, one of them (and who is Chief Justice of the State) in waiting—and soon after came in David Stuart and Dan'l Carroll, Esqs, the other two. A few miles out of Town, I was met by the principal citizens of the place and escorted in by them; and dined at Suter's tavern, (where I also lodged) at a public dinner given by the Mayor and corporation—previous to which I examined the surveys of Mr Ellicot, who had been sent on to lay out the district of ten miles square for the Federal seat: and also the works of Majr L'Enfant, who had been engaged to examine and make a draught of the grds. in the vicinity of Georgetown and Carrollsburg on the Eastern branch, making arrangements for examining the ground myself tomorrow with the commissioners.

[1] Records of the Columbia Historical Society, Vol. II, 1908.

7

Then came the President's proclamation about the decision on the permanent seat of Government; the "Ten Miles Square" authorized by Congress had finally been selected. The proclamation concludes;

Done at Georgetown aforesaid, the 30th day of March, in the year of our Lord 1791, and in the independence of the United States the fifteenth.

                                         By the President

                Thomas Jefferson   *George Washington*

Work on the Federal City began October 12th, 1792, when the cornerstone of the President's House was laid, without any special ceremony. James Hoban, the architect and builder, advertised for "good carpenters and joiners at two dollars per day at the President's House." When Washington laid the cornerstone of the Capitol in his capacity of a Mason the following September, the Mayor and Corporation of Georgetown were at the head of the procession.

The Capital, however, at this time was a city only in name, and for many years was obliged to rely upon Georgetown for its living accommodations, its supplies and its social life. There is ample evidence of this in the correspondence of the senators and representatives after Congress moved to Washington in 1800. John Cotton Smith in a letter to his wife recounted; "A large proportion of the Southern members took lodgings at Georgetown, which, though of a superior order, were three miles distant from the Capitol, and, of course, rendered the daily employment of hackney coaches indispensable."

Oliver Wolcott, Secretary of the Treasury, soon after arriving in the Federal City wrote; "There are few houses in any one place, and most of them small, miserable huts, which present an awful contrast to the public buildings. . . . You may look in almost any direction, over an extent of ground nearly as large as the City of New York, without seeing a fence or any object except brick kilns and temporary huts for laborers." Again, in a letter to his wife, Wolcott said; "I do not perceive how the members of Congress can possibly secure lodgings unless they will consent to live . . . crowded ten or twenty into one house and utterly secluded from society. The only resource for those who wish to live comfortably will be found in Georgetown, three miles distant, over as bad a road in winter as the claygrounds near Hartford."

Georgetown newspapers and the National Intelligencer of Washington were at this time full of advertisements of lodgings, addressed to the Congressmen. The Georgetown Mansion House even went so far as to print an announcement from its enterprising owner that, "for the accommodation of such members of Congress as may favor him with their patronage he will keep horses and carriages to convey them to and fro Congress Hall *free of expence.* (sic)"

Gouverneur Morris of New York, reaching Washington after days of bumping along bad roads, sent this spicy letter to Princesse de la Tour and Taxis; "We only need here houses, cellars, kitchens, scholarly men, amiable women, and a few other such trifles to possess a perfect city, for we can walk over it as we would the fields and woods. . . . I hasten to assure you that building stone is plentiful, that excellent bricks are baked here, that we are not wanting in sites for magnificent mansions . . . in a word, that this is the best city in the world to live in—*in the future!*" Morris added that, as he was not "one of those good people whom we call *posterity,*" he would meanwhile certainly prefer to live somewhere else.[2]

It would seem that the President from the very beginning desired government workers to establish themselves in Washington proper, rather than in Georgetown. His note sent on May 17th, 1795, to Alexander White, one of the Commissioners, says rather severely: "I shall intimate that a residence in the City, if a house is to be had, will be more promotive of its welfare than your abode in Georgetown."

Such warnings must have been repeated, for a year later the Commissioners informed the

[2] Diary of Gouverneur Morris, Vol. 2, pp. 394-5.

President that they intended to establish themselves in the Federal City "as soon as ever decent houses could be had."

It is not difficult to understand the partiality of Government members and their families for quiet comfortable, beautiful, well-bred old Georgetown. In contrast with the swampy ground of Washington, its dreary wilderness of open fields, its few scattered dwellings and the crowded boarding houses on Capitol Hill, the ordered comfort of the small city across Rock Creek was a blissful refuge. "From the steps of the Capitol," says Claude Bowers, describing the Federal City in his Jefferson and Hamilton, "one could count seven or eight boarding houses (Jefferson lived in one of them) one tailor's shop, one shoemaker's, one printing establishment, the home of a washwoman and a grocer's shop; a stationery store, a drygoods house and an oyster market. And this was all." A vivid picture of Washington in the year 1800!

Georgetown, on the other hand, had been in existence for almost a hundred and fifty years. Its foremost citizens "were not men of wealth in the present acceptation of the word, but they were men of birth, education, high character and influence for good in the community, and their wives and daughters were women of charming personality and greatest refinement. Together with their near neighbors, they constituted a society sought by the most cultivated and distinguished in the public and private life of the Capitol." [3]

* * * * * *

Georgetown is a city of brick. The abundance of good clay on every hand, made it the natural building material to use for homes. There are many indications that claypits were dug on or near the sites where houses were to be built, and brick-yards established there. The same procedure was followed in Williamsburg, you will remember.

The Reverend Francis Makemie, first Presbyterian minister to arrive on the Eastern Shore of Maryland, wrote a book descriptive of the country, which was published in London early in the eighteenth century. "Here we have a clear and serene Air," he said, "a long and hot summer, a short and sharp winter, a free and fertile soil. . . . Here are vast quantities of Timber for Shipping, Trade and Architecture. . . . Here are in most places Bricks to be made at every man's Door for building." [4]

Bricks made in Virginia in the seventeenth century were rated at eight shilling a thousand. In England between 1650 and 1700 they could not be purchased for less than eighteen shillings a thousand. Had they been sent over for use in the Colonies, transportation across the ocean must have been added to this price, as well as import duties.

Mr. George A. Townsend's article on "Houses of Imported Bricks" written for the Records of the Columbia Historical Society sheds light in a very interesting manner on the old discussion about home-made versus imported bricks. He cites the fact that in 1695, "good brick clay having been found in the neighborhood of Annapolis, contracts were made with Casper Hermann, a burgess from Cecil County, for the erection of the Parish Church, Schoolhouse and State House." In Virginia in 1736, a contractor named George Dudley "Doth agree, for satisfaction of four years servitude, to make Isham Randolph one hundred thousand bricks and to set and burn them." [5]

The great abundance of clay on the Eastern coast may be attributed to the country's geological structure, which is that of an old mountain range, steadily eroding toward the ocean. This wash has taken the top soil off the level bench, from the foot-hills to the fall-line, leaving a band of soil better suited to brickmaking than to agriculture. East of the fall-line is the extensive tidewater area, with deep alluvial soil containing no stones but plenty of good clay.

[3] From "Old Homes on Georgetown Heights," by William Gordon.
[4] From "A Plain and Friendly Perswasive to the Inhabitants of Virginia and Maryland for Promoting Towns and Cohabitation, by a Well-Wisher of Both Governments," reprinted in the Virginia Magazine of History and Biography, Vol. IV.
[5] George A. Townsend in Records of the Columbia Historical Society, Vol. 7, pp. 195-210.

In Georgetown many of the old brick sidewalks and brick street-gutters still exist. And among the beauties of the place, in addition to the dwelling-houses, are the high brick walls smothered with ivy, which surround the lovely gardens.

The bricks used in these constructions are larger than those made today and they are set in a special way which is well described by Arthur Holden and Lewis A. Coffin, Jr.,[6] who say, in writing of Annapolis Houses: "The brickwork is most interesting from many points and of great import to an architect. The color of the brick approximates a dull salmon and is distinctly different from the brick-color found anywhere else in the country. It is very agreeable to the eye, giving a refreshing and not too glaring contrast with the white trims and cornice. The jointing employed is also uncommon, being seldon as much as one-quarter of an inch, struck with a fine line. The cement is a clean white in color, being made of white sand and pulverized sea-shells, which supplied oftentimes the lime for the mixture. When the brick was laid, the joint seems to have bulged slightly and then to have been carefully struck, making a clean straight line about one-sixteenth of an inch wide on the face of the bulge. The effect of this fine line on a narrow white joint gives an added crispness and refinement to the brickwork."

The same workmanship is often found in the Georgetown Houses, for example, on the recently restored Patterson house, whose mortar-joints Mr. Waterman calls "hand-tooled." (See photograph on page 107.)

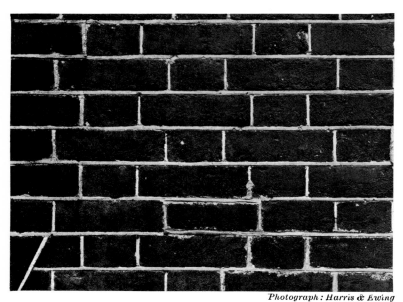

Photograph: Harris & Ewing

The brick work of the Hyde House facade laid up in 1798 is a fine example of "tooled joint" work.

No glazed-end bricks have been used in Georgetown as they were in Williamsburg.

Under a coating of dirt and dust the bricks of these old houses have sometimes turned a chocolate-brown. If cleaned, however, they would undoubtedly reveal the original warm, pinky salmon color that seems to be characteristic of the locality.

In the letters of Gouverneur Morris and of Secretary Wolcott we have already seen references to the use of brick in the new city of Washington. The "History of the National Capital" by W. B. Bryan says; "As it was known that the clay in the vicinity was excellent for brick, by the first of October gangs of men were employed in getting out this material for building in the vicinity of the two public buildings, and later on kilns were erected there, where the brick used in these structures was made."

Daniel Carroll, one of the three Commissioners named by the President, made every exertion to provide accommodations for the First Congress in the Federal City, erecting numerous buildings on Capitol Hill and also furnishing brick for these houses, "as he was one of the largest brick-makers of that day."[7]

Brickyards and rubbish—an ever-present element of ugliness—surrounded the President's House. Dolly Madison complained that this was all she could see from her windows!

It is not generally known that a brick plant had to be moved to make place for the Penta-

[6] See "Brick Architecture of the Colonial Period in Maryland and Virginia."
[7] "Greenleaf and Law in the Federal City" by Allen C. Clark.

gon Building when it was erected. The plant was not abandoned but, re-established on a new site provided by the Government and on the same clay deposit, is still operating today.

* * * * * *

For many years after the establishment of "the permanent Capital," there were grumblings and complaints about it. A bill was even introduced into Congress eight years later, urging reconsideration of the site and presenting valid reasons for removing the seat of Government to Philadelphia!

Fortunately the original plan was not abandoned. Our present magnificent Washington has developed from the genius of Major L'Enfant, and from the far-sightedness of our first President, who insisted that "the public buildings must look far beyond the needs of today."

What a distinguished group of gifted architects and designers was gathered together in one spot at that time! You will find much about them in the following pages—James Hoban, William Thornton, Benjamin Henry Latrobe, Thomas Jefferson, Stephen Hallet and, a little later, Charles Bulfinch of Boston. In one way or another each one of them has left his hall-mark on private dwellings in Washington and Georgetown, as well as on public buildings.

As Washington grew, the parent city of Georgetown declined. In 1800 its population had about equaled that of the Capital; ten years later Washington had doubled in size and Georgetown decreased forty percent. In 1851 the question of annexing Georgetown to Washington was discussed, and the Georgetown Advocate published the following amusing article:

"Is it best to marry Widower Georgetown to Miss Maryland or to Lady Washington?

"Miss Maryland has been accustomed to high living. She has given soirées and parties frequently at her palace at Annapolis, and invited the surrounding country to feast on champagne and oysters, while old Georgetown has been accustomed to live upon Potomac herring and corn bread, and by his economy has laid up a little property; which he is now going to throw away upon his extravagant lady-love Maryland. . . .

"Now, would it be well to marry Widower Georgetown to such an extravagant lady as this? The best we can do is to unite Georgetown to Washington. Lady Washington is little in debt compared to Miss Maryland, and she has an uncle, called Uncle Sam, who is very liberal towards her. He has a large revenue of fifty millions. . . .

"Now, as old Georgetown is rather poor, and hard pushed for money to get along, would it not be well to marry him to Lady Washington, so that he can share in her prosperity and wealth?"

Lady Washington won. Georgetown's charter as a city was revoked in 1871 and the area was incorporated into the District of Columbia, the streets being later joined with letters and numbers that continued those of Washington.[8]

It is still a regret among people who love the historic atmosphere of Georgetown and who wish to keep it intact that the charming old names like "Duck Lane" and "Gay Street," as well as the names of Jefferson, Madison, Monroe, Lafayette and Stoddert Streets, and the names of our Generals Greene, Montgomery and Washington, have all been discarded in favor of the Washington system, which is perhaps practical but certainly not poetic.

Far more serious than the loss of the old names, however, is the fact that many buildings recorded by the Historic American Building Survey have been destroyed. Under present conditions many others may disappear.

From a report to the Secretary of the Interior on the Preservation of Historic Sites and Buildings by J. Thomas Schneider in 1935, we learn that "there is no existing authority by which the National Park Service or any other Federal Agency can take appropriate steps to

---

[8] From "Origin and Government of the District of Columbia" by William Tindall.

prohibit or prevent the threatened destruction of a building not in Federal ownership which possesses historic interest, nor means by which the Federal Government can effectively cooperate with States, Private organizations and individuals toward such an end."

In Boston there is the Society for the Preservation of New England Antiquities, which has saved many beautiful old houses from destruction. In New York there is the Historical Society. The Colonial Dames, the D.A.R. and the Garden Clubs have all exerted their efforts to preserve historic spots in various parts of the country. And there are many other organizations with the same interest in safeguarding our national heritage. Is it not possible to link together the Presidents of all these separate groups, to include with them the heads of the large museums, and so to form a great National Association which could operate like the *National Monuments Commission in England* or the *Commission des Monuments in France?* Surely proper legislation could be obtained by such a group which would give it the power to protect and care for places connected with the history of this country and to preserve them for future generations.

*   *   *   *   *   *

The three men who have created this book on "Georgetown Houses" are now in Washington, in the service of the nation. In the past two years they have been able to devote only their hard-won leisure moments to accomplish this project, which has become an absorbing interest to each one of them.

Deering Davis, a member of this Institute, conceived the idea, persuaded the others to help, did the research, supervised the photography and compilation and arranged for the publication of the book.

Commander Ralph Cole Hall, USNR, contemporary St. Louis architect acted in the capacity of architectural advisor in the project.

Stephen P. Dorsey, descendant of the Dorsey and other distinguished Maryland families, a keen student of architecture and a writer of historical manuscripts, is responsible for the charming and readable text.

In conclusion, the authors wish me, first of all, to thank the owners of the houses shown for the gracious permission to photograph their homes. They also wish to extend their most sincere thanks to Miss Virginia Daiker of the Art Department, and Mrs. Clara E. LeGear of the Map Department, Library of Congress; Miss Mercedes Jordan, Chief of the Washingtonia Room, K Street Public Library; Miss Eva Nelson Gilbert of the Peabody Room, Georgetown Public Library; Dr. Herman Kahn, Chief of the Interior Archives; Mrs. Walter G. Peter, authoress and authority on Georgetown; Lieutenant Commander Charles E. Peterson, U.S.N.R., President of the Thornton Society of Washington; The National Society of Colonial Dames of America in the District of Columbia; Mr. Robert E. Lammond, Jr., of the Columbia and Real Estate Title Insurance Companies; Mr. Rex Curtiss of Harris and Ewing, and the Office of General U. S. Grant III for their many courtesies.

NANCY V. McCLELLAND,
A.I.D.

TABLE OF CONTENTS

LIST OF ILLUSTRATIONS

THE HISTORICAL BACKGROUND

GEORGETOWN—once in Maryland—now part of the District of Columbia—scene of many important historical events—was founded three years after nearby Alexandria. By the latter part of the Eighteenth Century each had become a thriving port, daring to hope that it would eventually compare with New York or Philadelphia.

The locality, originally the site of the Indian village of Tahoga, was visited as early as 1608 by Captain John Smith. About 1703, it caught the fancy of a sturdy Scot, Colonel Ninian Beall, Commander in Chief of the Provincial Forces of Maryland, who in 1699 had been rewarded by an "Act of Gratuity" passed by the Assembly in recognition of his services "Upon all incursions and disturbances of neighboring Indians." Beall Patented 795 acres here and, probably thinking of the great Rock of Dunbarton, above the Firth of Clyde, near Glasgow, he gave that name to his new holding. In 1734 George Gordon became the owner of "Gordon's Rock Creek Plantation" of 300 acres next to Beall and since the majority of those who followed the first settlers were Scots, the area came to be called New Scotland Hundred. Pleasantly situated at the head of navigation, the land was a natural site for an urban center and the development of the surrounding region inevitably resulted in the establishment of the town itself.

On June 8, 1751, the Assembly of the Province of Maryland appointed six Commissioners whose survey was completed in February of the following year. "Knaves Disappointment," owned by George Gordon, as well as "Bealls Levels," and the "Rock of Dumbarton," owned by George Beall, son of the original settler, were the tracts found "most convenient" for the new center which was named for George II, the reigning king. Each owner was offered two town lots plus the price of condemnation. Gordon accepted, and Beall, after refusing to recognize the proceedings, finally agreed, with the declaration, however, that "I do hereby protest and declare that my acceptance of the said lots, which is by force, shall not debar me from future redress from the Commissioners or others, if I can have the rights of a British subject. God save the King." Two hundred and eighty pounds were paid for the sixty acres of townsite extending from the river about to the present N Street and from the site of Georgetown University approximately to 30th Street. The boundary stone marking the town's northeast corner still stands in the garden at 3014 N Street. The new town flourished as a port and tobacco inspection point. Its original eighty lots were supplemented by six further additions, but it was not until 1789 that it was formally incorporated.

The province had been founded at St. Mary's in 1634 by Leonard Calvert for his brother Cecil, second Lord Baltimore, and from that point settlement rapidly spread northward up Chesapeake Bay and the Potomac. Under the manorial system land grants were large, often consisting of thousands of acres, and through the unique feudal system established by the Lord Proprietor, many of the great planters became manorial lords, with rights of court baron and court leet over their tenants.

By the beginning of the Eighteenth Century most of the Potomac tidewater region had been taken up by aristocratic Maryland and Virginia families, but due to the size of the plantations, and the distances between neighbors settlements were sparse and many of the planters spent much time in the saddle. Their hospitality was abundant. Indeed, George Washington wrote that his family had not sat down alone to dinner in twenty years. Horse races, hunt meets and card parties were frequent, and except at "public times" in the provincial capitals when the courts and assembles were held with their attendant races, slave auctions, cock fights and theatricals, it was not until late in the colonial period that life centering about the great manors became gradually directed to the urban centers. Obviously the great planters were not the sole residents of these colonies. Certainly the largest segment of the population was made up of negro slaves upon whose labor the plantation economy was based. There were, too, very considerable numbers of white mechanics, artisans and laborers—the "little people"—most of whom had arrived as indentured servants who had bound themselves to their masters for five years of service in payment for their voyage to the new world. Then there were the small farmers who worked the less fertile tobacco lands themselves, perhaps with the help of a slave or two. It was difficult for this group to consign its product profitably to the English agents and gradually the larger planters became traders, buying the tobacco of their smaller competitors to whom they sold a variety of necessary goods and stores.

Out of this transition grew the need for Georgetown, laid out, as it was, at a natural place for an inspection and shipping point at the end of the "rolling" roads over which the great tobacco casks were rolled from the plantations, and where the western channel of the Potomac beyond Analostan Island offered water deep enough for large sailing ships. Already in 1755 General Braddock was able to write back to England that "never have I attended a more complete banquet, or met better dressed or better mannered people than I met on my arrival in George Town, which is named after his gracious Majesty." Men from the old plantation families and from the mother country saw promise in the place and they were joined by a substantial number of New England merchants. The warehouses grew, and by 1791 Washington himself described the town as "the greatest tobacco market in Maryland if not in the Union."

During the last quarter of the Eighteenth and the first quarter of the Nineteenth centuries, this busy seaport saw its ships carrying tobacco, flour, lumber and fish to its sister colonies, to the West Indies and abroad, and returning with sugar, spices, molasses, textiles, furniture and supplies of all sorts. Here too, by 1800 were a rope walk, a paper factory, a textile mill, numerous counting houses, shops and stores. Guns made at Henry Foxall's foundry during the war of 1812 contributed to Perry's victory on Lake Erie. Newspapers were published and banks were opened. The Great Conestoga wagons that rumbled through the streets carried Georgetown's products overland, and the new Potomac (later Chesapeake and Ohio) Canal was organized to open a water route to the west.

It has been said that "Colonial Williamsburg occupied during colonial times an area of about one mile square; had approximately 300 houses and a resident population of about 3,000 which increased to 7,000 during "public times." Of these colonial buildings sixty-six have been repaired or restored, while 84 have been reproduced on colonial foundations. During the first twenty years of the Nineteenth Century Georgetown also occupied about one square mile but according to census records had a resident population of 5,000 to 7,000. By the same ratio of dwellings to population as at Williamsburg, Georgetown probably consisted at that time of about 700 buildings of which 400 are estimated to have been of brick and 300 of wooden construction. Of these buildings 300 were probably brick dwellings of the type shown in this book, with the balance made up of stores, warehouses, schools, churches, etc. Today 200 structures of this period remain, or over 25%, a remarkable tribute to the builders of the day. The streets on which they stood, since alphabetized and numbered, bore such delightful names as Cherry, Duck, and Fishing Lanes, Gay, High, Water, Back, and Bridge Streets, and simply Wapping, Causeway and Keys. The modern system, although perhaps more practical, is certainly less pleasant, and there are those inhabitants who still resent it.

Early Georgetown was the site of a number of schools, and here in 1789 Georgetown College was founded by Bishop John Carroll. The town was frequently visited by theatrical companies, and it abounded in dancing and drawing masters. Here about 1803 Gilbert Stuart spent two years painting the portraits of the great of the town and of the new capital city adjacent to it. The Anchor, The Sailors, The Sign of the Indian King and other inns were vigorous centers of life. The Fountain Inn, also called Suter's Tavern, was the scene of many of the transactions in connection with the establishment of the Federal City across Rock Creek, and here the disputed presidential election was decided by the House of Representatives in favor of Thomas Jefferson rather than John Adams, his Federalist opponent. The great Union Tavern, later Crawford's Hotel, built in 1796, became famous for its Pompeian ballroom, its gentlemen's arched corridor or colonnade opening on the courtyard, and its stables for fifty horses. A large coach, The Royal George, took legislator guests to the Capitol and back. Here at various times stayed Louis Philippe, Jerome Bonaparte, Talleyrand, John Adams, Washington Irving, Robert Fulton and many other famous personages. Here the night before his duel with Henry Clay, John Randolph of Roanoke played whist and quoted poetry while his will was amended. Jefferson lived here for a time while he was Secretary of State. Here Francis Scott Key lived for twenty years as a lawyer and District Attorney and from his house on Bridge Street left for his rendezvous aboard a British man of war lying below Fort McHenry and the creation of the verses that epitomize love of country for all Americans everywhere. The town was visited at one time or another during the Early Federal Period by practically all of the great and near great who passed through the capital city painfully coming into existence on the other side of the creek. Washington, in his journeys north from Mount Vernon, was a frequent visitor to the town where he had both family connections and business interests. He was one of the founders of the Potomac Company to promote a canal westward to the Ohio and it was in Georgetown that he organized the survey and purchase of the land for the new Federal Capital. On such visits he frequently stopped with the family of Mr. Thomas Peter. He dined at Wise's Tavern enroute to New York to his inauguration as first President of the United States, and The *Pennsylvania Packet* of May 5th, stated:

"George-Town, April 23.—Last Thursday, passed through this town, on his way to New-York, the Most Illustrious the President of the United States of America, with Charles Thomson, Esq.; Secretary to Congress. His Excellency arrived at about 2 o'clock, on the banks of the Potowmack, escorted by a respectable corps of gentlemen from Alexandria, where the George-Town ferry boats, properly equipped, received his Excellency and suite, and safely landed them under the acclamations of a large crowd of their grateful fellow-citizens—who beheld their Fabius in the evening of his days, bid adieu to the peaceful retreat of Mount Vernon, in order to save his country once more, from confusion and anarchy. From this place his Excellency was escorted by a corps of gentlemen, commanded by Col. William Deakins, Jun. to Mr. Spurrier's Tavern, where the escort from Baltimore take charge of him."

During the following eight years which kept him from residence at Mount Vernon, he crossed Maryland on visits to his home on an average of twice a year, making the sixteen trips, by fast coach almost continually enveloped in the clouds of dust kicked up by his mounted escorts.

After seven years of bitter conflict between North and South over the location of the Federal City, the Residence Bill was passed in July 1790 and under it the following October President Washington assumed his role as agent for Congress to choose the site for a permanent seat of government, to acquire the lands and to appoint building commissioners. In January 1791 the Potomac site east of Georgetown was selected, and happily against almost universal opposition the President supported the plan of the French military engineer, Pierre Charles l'Enfant, sufficiently strongly to secure its adoption. Today it is considered America's foremost achievement in municipal planning. Inevitably the human desire to secure the best locations in the new city, actually still only in the planning stage, resulted in a veritable tempest of speculation though it was not until June 1800 that the seat of government was removed from Philadelphia and established in its permanent location in Washington. Building of the new Federal City did not at once affect the commercial development of its neighbor. In fact, for the first decade of the nineteenth century the older sister in many ways overshadowed the sprawling infant, and continued to be the home of many of the foreign envoys who gave it a certain world consciousness and cosmopolitanism in addition to the quieter and more established culture that comes with greater age. In August 1814 all of the public buildings in the new city, with the exception of the Post and Patent Office, were burned by British forces under General Ross and Admiral Cockburn. Although very little private property was destroyed and the public buildings were rebuilt in three years, the shabbiness of Washington was in decided contrast to older Georgetown.

As late as 1835 a British visitor, Harriet Martineau, wrote:

"The city itself is unlike any other that ever was seen, straggling out hither and thither, with a small house or two a quarter of a mile from any other; so that making calls 'in the city' we had to cross ditches and stiles, and walk alternately on grass and pavements, and strike across a field to reach a street—Then there was the society, singularly compounded from the most varied of elements; foreign ambassadors, the American government, members of Congress, from Clay and Webster down to Davy Crockett, Burton from Missouri; and Cuthbert; with the freshest Irish brogue, from Georgia; flippant young belles, 'pious' wives dutifully attending their husbands, and groaning over the frivolities of the place; grave judges, saucy travellers, pert newspaper reporters, melancholy Indian Chiefs and timid New England ladies, trembling on the verge of the vortex."

Although certainly less beautiful, this earlier Washington sounds not unlike descriptions of the wartime city we know today. Nor was it greatly improved physically by 1862 when Mary Clemmer Ames described it:

"Capitol Hill, dreary, desolate and dirty stretched away into an uninhabited desert,—arid hill and sodden plain showed alike the horrid trail of war. Forts bristled above every hill-top.—Shed hospitals covered acres in every suburb.—the rattle of the anguish-laden ambulance, the piercing cries of the sufferers whom it carried, made morning, noon and night too dreadful to be borne." while "The streets were filled with—new regiments,—their banners all untarnished as they marched up Pennsylvania Avenue, playing 'The girl I left behind me.' "

This was the new Washington under siege, the Washington that for four years was an Army headquarters. During the preceding quarter century, Georgetown's importance as a commercial port, industrial center and canal terminus had gradually gone into eclipse with the advent of the railroads. It was natural that, during this period of growing conflict of opinion between North and South, the sympathy of a great many of its people should lie with the South—the land of their origin—and their blue cockades were worn openly in the same streets that were later to be hung with black after Lincoln's assassination and to witness Southern girls crossing to the other side rather than pass under the National colors hanging over the doors of the Union hospitals located in the town.

With the flamboyance and excitement of the reconstruction years that followed the war, however, came a physical regeneration that transformed Washington from the shabby village that it had been to something like the present metropolis. It was natural that Georgetown, many of whose residents had lost their wealth in Washington real estate speculation, should become principally a residential section while the warehouses crumbled along its once busy water front. Indeed its face became considerably altered by new rows of ugly Victorian dwellings, many of which remain. In 1871 it relinquished the separate charter which it had kept even after its inclusion within the District of Columbia, and by Act of Congress became a part of Washington. Georgetown's golden age became a memory, and the principal glory of the community became the lovely relics of its past.

Still the quiet suburb has retained a unique self-entity within the great capital that now entirely surrounds it. The elements of other days remain in a personality that has caused it to be described poetically as a beautiful old dogwood, always in flower, standing beside the oak in its prime which is Washington proper.

FEDERAL ARCHITECTURE OF GEORGETOWN, D. C.

GEORGETOWN, quiet suburb of the Nation's Capital, is in itself a living record of the Republic's architecture since its founding. Federal, Classic Revival, Victorian and Modern homes —all are here, but the architectural significance and the greatest charm of the town lie in those structures built during the first fifty years of the Nation's existence. These homes have seen many wars come and go, and to them the confusion of the Capital in a time of emergency is nothing new. Through Georgetown passed part of Braddock's forces on their fateful way to defeat at Duquesne in 1755. From Georgetown, men, ships, supplies went forth in the cause of the thirteen colonies, and here Washington, victorious, directed the planning of the new Federal Capital to bear his name. From its heights, Georgetown's residents watched the fires in 1814. In the sixties they knew the legion of the wounded and the feel of a beleaguered city, and they opened their doors to the war workers who packed the city of 1917.

Overshadowed by the city she had helped to build, Georgetown fell into neglect late in the last century. In recent years, however, government officials, officers of the services, newspapermen and others have restored many of the smaller houses whose charm was obvious even under their cloak of neglect, and other more enterprising restorations have contributed to the re-establishment of a proper setting for a brilliant social life similar to that for which Georgetown once was famous. Uniquely too, this living "town within a city" retains its individuality, its entity, and its pride in its tradition. Here one feels the qualities of a small, very charming and very old town, and in these qualities is its architectural significance.

Fiske Kimball has said in his "Regional Types in Early American Architecture" that "in the South it is only at Charleston that we find really urban types. Even at Annapolis the houses are semi-rural." However, in Georgetown, developed principally in the half-century from 1775 to 1825 there does exist an urban type of dwelling with a distinct local idiom adapted to the lives of its builders and to local climate and materials.

From a glance at Georgetown houses of the type which flourished during the town's "golden age" it is evident that they are not "Colonial" in the literal sense of the word. Rather they are true examples of the Federal tradition, influenced by Colonial antecedents, but built during the early days of the new Republic—examples of a school which flourished under the patronage of Thomas Jefferson who, as Secretary of State under Washington and as President, had very considerable influence in fostering America's Federal style. Here the Colonial style of Georgian derivation gave way to a transitional one of greater Classic feeling which became our first national architectural expression.

In reflecting, it may be conjectured that the transition from the Colonial of Georgian derivation consciously paralleled the interest of the new republic in its prototypes, the Greek and Roman Republics. Washington himself, as we shall see, was an enthusiastic patron of the Federal style with an interest in architecture more profound than he himself realized— a fact made obscure by the Colonial features of most of Mount Vernon, and the preoccupation with them of the public mind.

The homes of the period possess a delicacy of scale which distinguishes them, and which was the result of a masterful adaptation of elements of Classic precedent, reduced from the scale of stone to that for work in wood. The brickwork is most frequently of Flemish bond, expertly laid up in large-size bricks, sand-moulded by hand, and now turned a beautiful shade between cherry and chocolate color. Corbeled courses frequently form the eave ornament beneath a simple gutter. Almost without exception these houses are of the simple gabled type, with the roof pitch becoming less acute toward the end of the first quarter of the nineteenth century. The larger houses frequently have chimneys in pairs at the roof-ends flush with the walls, and a flat deck between, with sloping roofs to the front and rear. Dormers are gabled, often with a circular-head upper sash with ingenious arrangements of muntins separating small panes. Muntins, mouldings and vertical treatment of the dormers with pilasters or colonettes were beautifully contrived, and a similarity exists which suggests the work of the same draftsmen or millwrights.

The fenestration is thoughtfully arranged, and in the earlier examples consisted of windows in the first storey having six panes in the lower sash and nine panes above, while the second storey windows were, typically, twelve-light openings. While a simplicity exists in the surrounding mouldings, an ingenious variation occurs which is evidence of a scholarly application to detail. Frequent use of delicate wrought iron work in handrails foreshadows the early Victorian popularity of this decorative medium in Georgetown and is, in certain cases, reminiscent of New Orleans, although it is of a simpler type than the fine ornamental examples in the South.

The larger houses carry porticoes of good proportion and moderate size. Examples are to be found in Tudor Place and Dumbarton House (illustrated on pages 89 to 103). Neither of these houses is characteristic of the Georgetown urban type. They are instead manorial in character, each with a large central mass flanked by wings which were added at a different time. However, they constitute excellent examples of the work of Thornton and Latrobe. Occasionally a balustrade was used over the porch, as at Mackall Square, and there was excellent application of recessed panels beneath windows—sometimes ornamented by cast lead swags as in Cox's Row—and of recessed blind arches where the monumental scale permitted. A consistency of restraint and simplicity prevail in these structures which remind one of the general "quality" evident in the life and effort of the new Republic.

Outside trim is of a simple type using classic mouldings and is delicate in scale. Sills and lintels are typically of stone, frequently with a finely moulded key block or with raised, square corner blocks bearing an indented circular ornament. Doorways are found with circular or eliptical heads, and often with sidelights separated from the door opening by finely reeded or moulded mullions. A few examples remain of leaded glass transoms which are rich and beautiful in their design. Shutters and entrance door were invariably painted dark green with all other wood trim white.

Four basic types of Georgetown houses stand as a document of the time: the manorial type flanked by lower wings which occupy generous plots of ground, the larger ell-shaped house having a two storey wing for servants extending back through the near garden, the small urban dwelling of either rectangular or ell-shape which is the principal subject of this book, and lastly, the small New England type of frame house. The typical, small houses are the most often illustrated in the following plates although some examples of others are included. Frequently they are of the English basement type, and entrance to the main living floor is by steps from the sidewalk, sometimes curved, and built of stone or of brick with stone treads having a "bull-nose" moulding around the front and ends. Others are entered directly from the sidewalk and have one step to gain the level of the floor.

The entrance and hall are at the side, the hallway having two or three living rooms opening from it, and at the rear, access to the ell or servants' wing, should the house have one. Such wings were built either at the time of the erection of the main house or as later additions were required by growing families. The kitchens were located in the wings or in the half-basements, with the dining room adjacent to it or on the floor above as may have suited the tastes of the occupant. This type of dwelling was built abutting directly on the street, which at the time was usually unpaved and through which cattle, pigs and turkeys were often driven to market. To the rear one finds lovely secluded gardens, often with fine boxwood or magnolias, and occasionally an original shed or smokehouse. These dependencies were most often of brick and so placed as to be both accessible and artistically pleasant. Overlooking the gardens, frequently one sees pillared galleries opening on each floor from the hallway or from individual rooms,—admirably adapted to the hot summer climate. The owner of this type of house lived at the rear, on the garden side, as we might well do today when automobile traffic crowds the streets.

The photographs which follow have generally been restricted to the original Federal portion of each house, since some have been supplemented by later additions. It may be noted that, in certain instances, the level of the street has been lowered and consequently the consideration of the mass and scale must be from the standpoint of its original location and placement.

The interiors of these Georgetown houses hold even more of interest to the present day architect, interior decorator or house-owner than do their exteriors. Houses of similar medium size maintained very much the same outward appearance for the 150 years from 1680 to 1830, but their interiors, both as to architectural detail and decorative furnishings, had several clearly defined epochs. There are excellent examples of the artistic accomplishments of these early builders in the houses treated in the following photographs. The wood paneling, carving, and heavier wood trim of the preceding eras were completely set aside. Delicately moulded architraves and dadoes were much in evidence and mantels with gesso or cast ornaments in the form of eagles, swags and decorated bands were employed. Arched openings appear frequently in the hall-way and many have reveals cleverly reeded or panelled, and moulded key and impost blocks. Details were generally of classic derivation, used with great restraint, and interiors were singularly free from the more elaborate tendencies of the Brothers Adam.

Plaster from ceiling to base board was the rule. Often no chair rail and sometimes not even a ceiling cornice was employed. Wood trim around doors and windows many times turned back with a moulding from the reveal for less than two inches on the wall. (See page 108.) This moulding was of extreme delicacy and refinement with beautiful clean cut lines. The simple treatment of walls and openings gave an illusion of greater space in these medium size or small rooms, which were a perfect setting for the classic Sheraton, Phyfe, and Regency furniture of the time or acted as a foil for the Queen Anne, Hepplewhite or Chippendale pieces of former eras.

Walls were either painted or papered; stair balusters were straight-sided rectangles. Fabrics for drapery were small patterned chintz, toiles often depicting scenes of American life or history, silks and satins in classic designs. Floors were wide planked hard Georgia Pine oiled and waxed and were covered with rugs from China, Persia, France or England. Hardware, such as doorknobs, was brass; small in scale and very unpretentious. Locks were usually of the large brass or iron box type. Wall colors and trim were often white or cream. Almost as usual was Adam Green or light blue on walls, with white or cream wood trim. However, almost all colors and tones were used according to the owners taste.

The interior photographs which follow demonstrate the suitability of this simple late Georgian type to many styles and kinds of furniture either used together or kept relatively pure as to period. One may have the most costly and rare examples of the cabinet or chair-makers art; simple maple and cherry pieces of less intrinsic value or very inexpensive but appropriate painted pieces such as the Hitchcock chair, which was manufactured in the early 19th Century as the first truly American mass production furniture item. Nor are good Modern examples out of place; in fact, they seem to be enhanced by the superb functionalism of these Georgian interiors.

The scale is, as indicated above, expertly adapted to local building materials, and while the general mass and disposition of motifs shows the influence of the Georgian antecedents of the day, these houses are truly American.

DR. WILLIAM THORNTON, 1761-1828
Architect of the Federal Period

ARCHITECT, inventor, painter and horseracer, William Thornton was a large man of unusually handsome mien, who knew almost everything, who was genuinely interested in letting almost everyone know about it, who might have gained greater fame had he concentrated in one field of endeavor rather than on "architecture, philosophy, politics, finance, astronomy, medicine, botany, poetry, painting, religion, agriculture, in short all subjects by turns."

Born of Quaker parents May 27, 1761 on the tiny island of Jost Van Dyke in the West Indies, he was sent to England as a boy and received his preliminary education while living with indulgent aunts on the family estate, Green Air, in Lancaster. He entered the College of Edinburgh and took his doctor's degree in medicine in 1784. He then went to Paris to continue his studies and attached himself to the Countess de Beauhearnais, an aunt of the Empress Josephine's first husband. While in Paris, the young man who was already such an excellent penman that as a boy he had been able to fool his uncle with a £5 note of his own manufacture, studied drawing and painting with such talent that he created an excellent miniature of his new patroness.

In 1787 he landed in New York, then went to Wilmington and finally to Philadelphia, where his plans for the Library Company of Philadelphia won the competition for its proposed new building.* Thornton stated in a letter that this was his first architectural attempt and that he had never actually studied the subject until later, when he determined to submit a design for the National Capitol and studied "for a number of months night and day" while working on the drawings. However, from the tone of his letter it seems not unlikely that he was playing down his talents. It is more probable that he had been interested in architecture along with his other artistic researches in England and France, for he had been named a member of the Society of Antiquaries before he left Edinburgh.

In Philadelphia he became a member of the fashionable set, a friend of Dr. Franklin's, and at twenty-nine the husband of fifteen-year old Anna Maria Brodeau, talented and lovely daughter of a prominent Quaker family, who was later to study under Gilbert Stuart and acting as her husband's draughtsman, to make detailed drawings of his rough design sketches. After a two years' honeymoon in the West Indies, the newlyweds returned to Philadelphia in 1792, where Mrs. Brodeau had a pleasant house ready on Chestnut Street with some $2,200 worth of furnishings. Thornton had already begun his plans for the National Capitol while in the West Indies and received notice that his plan had won the competition in April, 1793. On September 18 of the same year the cornerstone was laid by President Washington, who, on the occasion, wore a Masonic apron embroidered by Madame Lafayette. Thornton at first declined to superintend erection of the building but came to Georgetown, living at 3221 M Street. However, several superintendents of construction were dismissed for attempting to alter his plan, and eventually its creator was placed in charge. He was appointed one of the District Commissioners and worked in close collaboration with the President and Major l'Enfant on the planning of the capital city. He sold his M Street house in 1797 and moved across Rock Creek to Washington where he maintained a city residence at 1331 F Street until his death in 1828.

Without doubt Thornton became the leader of the triumvirate of great architects of this area during that period. Of this group, James Hoban (1762-1831), who collaborated with

* Since razed. However, good photographs still exist.

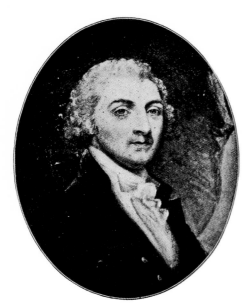

Thornton during the early construction of the Capitol, is best known as architect of the White House or "President's Palace" as it was first known, which he designed in 1792. Unfortunately the present greatly enlarged building has lost much of the charm of the original simpler design and it can hardly be classed as domestic architecture. He planned the original State and Navy buildings which have since been destroyed (though the original drawings remain), as well as several hotels, but there are no known records of his planning domestic structures.

Thornton's principal rival, and the third member of the group, Benjamin H. Latrobe (1764-1820), who succeeded the doctor as Director of Works for the Capitol in 1803, is famous for his quarrels with Thornton over its design. He deserves lasting notice for his creation there of an American order of architecture through the use of cotton blossoms, tobacco leaves, and Indian corn in the columns and capitals of the great structure where they may still be seen. He was the architect of St. John's Church on Lafayette Square, and notable examples of his domestic designs remain in nearby Decatur House and in Dumbarton House in Georgetown, restored according to his plans of about 1809. While other local architects of the period are known, no definite examples of their work exist with the exception of the central portion of the building which houses the United States District Court of the District of Columbia—completed in 1820 as the City Hall from the plans of George Hadfield (1764-1826), an Englishman who had won many architectural prizes in London before coming to Washington to help in the erection of the Capitol.

In any case, it is in the field of domestic architecture that Thornton was by far the most influential local architect of the period. Substantiated documentary and physical evidence proves his designing a double house for Washington on Capitol Hill and one house each for Daniel Carroll, the great landowner, and his brother in the same area. Under the circumstances it is probable that he was also the architect for Carroll's Row, which once stood on the site of the present Library of Congress. Kimball attributes exquisite Homewood in Baltimore—one of Charles Carroll of Carrollton's great houses—to Thornton and we know from Mrs. Thornton's diary that he designed the residence of Thomas Law, wealthy and aristocratic English resident of Washington who married Eliza Parke Custis, granddaughter of Martha Washington. Law built several houses on Capitol Hill as well as some twenty in the Greenleaf Point area where he lost a fortune in an attempt to make it the fashionable residential section of the new city. Surely Thornton, who planned Law's personal residence, greatly influenced these other houses, if he did not actually design them.

There is little wonder that Fiske Kimball, in his foreword to the second volume of Great Georgian Houses, says that his influence in Maryland was so great that even today Baltimore architects feel that they must work sympathetically, or that Glenn Brown terms him the greatest architect of his time.

There is absolute proof that he planned Tudor Place in Georgetown for Thomas Peter and his wife, Martha Parke Custis, another of the three beautiful Custis girls, granddaughter of Mrs. Washington and sister of both Mrs. Thomas Law and Mrs. Lawrence Lewis.

The third Custis granddaughter, Washington's favorite, married his nephew, Lawrence Lewis, who built Woodlawn a portion of which still stands on that part of the original Mount Vernon tract, given the couple by the first President. There is every proof that here too Thornton was the designing architect of this exceptionally lovely structure.

22

Thornton was also the architect of St. Johns Church, Georgetown, as well as of Octagon House, the unusual and beautiful mansion near the White House, completed in 1800 for John Tayloe of Mount Airy, one of the most powerful and wealthy planters of Virginia. Tayloe was persuaded by his close friend General Washington to build his town house in the new city rather than in Philadelphia, as he had first intended. The house, supposed to be haunted by the ghost of the original owner's beautiful daughter who threw herself down the great stairwell as a result of her father's refusal to allow her to marry a young Englishman, was originally connected by secret underground passages with the White House and with the Potomac River. It has served as the executive mansion and it was here that President Madison signed the ratification of the Treaty of Ghent. Its selection in 1902 as the permanent home of the American Institute of Architects is full testimony to its perfection.

Thomas Jefferson, foremost exponent of the New Classic style of architecture, thought highly of William

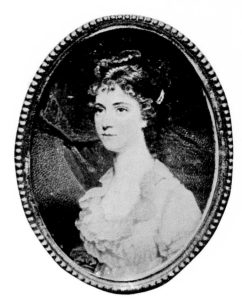

Mrs. William Thornton
By permission of the Columbia Historical Society. Library of Congress photograph
Portrait by Dr. Thornton

Thornton and asked his friend for preliminary sketches for the University of Virginia, which were used in part. President Madison wrote, too, that Thornton was the architect for the main portion of his estate, Montpelier. With such powerful and fashionable patrons as Washington, Jefferson and Madison, it is hardly strange that seemingly half the houses in Georgetown are attributed to him, and that he exercised so great an influence on the architectural style of the whole District of Columbia. Without doubt, more than any other individual, he was the creator of the Federal type of house characteristic of the Georgetown section of the District, if not the "virtual creator of the Federal Style" as he has been called. Certainly he is the father of the type of urban house illustrated in the following pages as the best of its period, singularly suited to city living today.

A sketch of this amazing figure, however, would be incomplete if his other varied activities were not at least mentioned. He painted beautifully, still lifes and miniatures, and his excellent portraits of Washington, Jefferson, Dolly Madison, Mrs. Thornton as well as a self-portrait are still in existence. The first Patent Commissioner, he was an inventor in his own right, an extensive patent holder, and a close collaborator of both John Fitch and Robert Fulton in the development of the steam boat. He was a magistrate and, though a Quaker, a fearless and active captain of cavalry militia.

A member of the Medical Society of Edinburgh, he organized a fire insurance company and drew up a prospectus for a North Carolina Gold Mine Company and for a public market. He first proposed a Washington monument and advocated a Panama canal. A sheep breeder and horse lover, he built a race track in Washington. A poet, a novelist, a philosopher, he advocated eventual union of North and South America, the abolition of slavery, and establishment of a republic of freedmen in Africa, such as Liberia. Continuous candidate for a diplomatic mission to Latin America, he was an early advocate of the good neighbor policy.

Considered a dreamer by many in high places, this intimate of Washington, Jefferson, Adams, Madison and Monroe was nevertheless a factor in government because of his acquaintance with the powerful at home, his accord with the ministers from abroad and his correspondence with scientists the world over. How prophetic were the members of Congress who told him that he had lived a hundred years too soon, and the wife who wrote after his death "His views were too extended, his plans too vast to be embraced by men generally." Such a man was this old world son of the new Republic, who gave so much beauty to his country.

THE WALKER HOUSE
C. 1805
2806 N Street, N. W.

The history of this house—probably built about 1805—is as incomplete as its interior detail is lovely. Thomas Beall sold the property in 1804 to John M. Gannt. The title records for the intermediate period are lost, but it was purchased from Elisha Williams by Thomas Robertson in 1810, and resold to Thomas Clarke in 1811. It then became the property of Thomas Corcoran, originally of Limerick, who had come to Georgetown in 1788 after five years in Baltimore. However, the prosperous leather merchant, mayor, magistrate and postmaster, who died in 1830, lived for many years in the house which he had built at 3119 M Street in 1791.

The house has been beautifully and intelligently restored by its present owners, Mr. and Mrs. John Walker, 3rd.

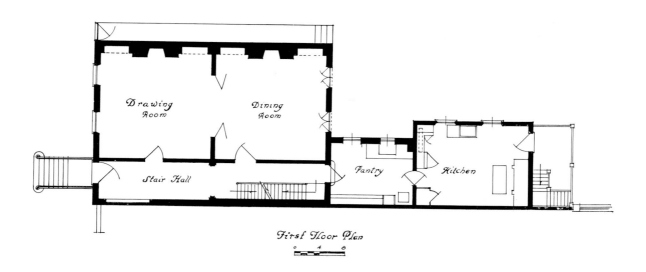

First Floor Plan

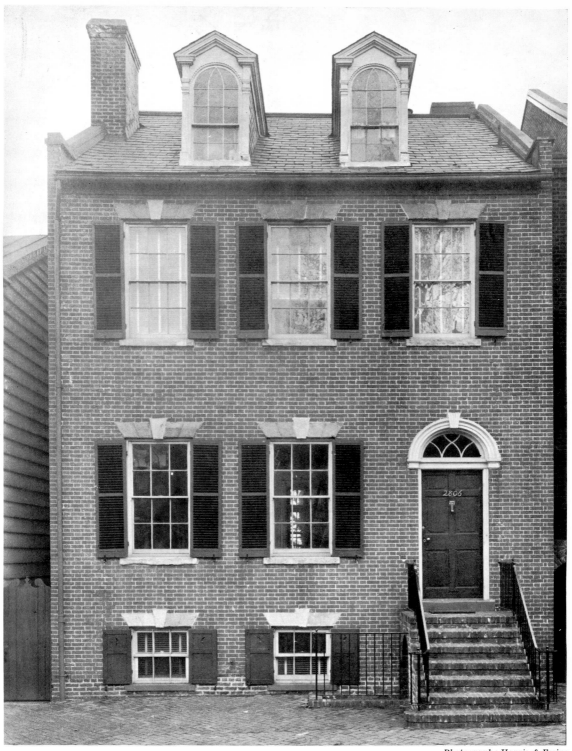

Photograph : Harris & Ewing

The new appearance of the facade was caused by the necessity of sand blasting to remove many coats of paint. Note the multiplicity of detail on the dormers.

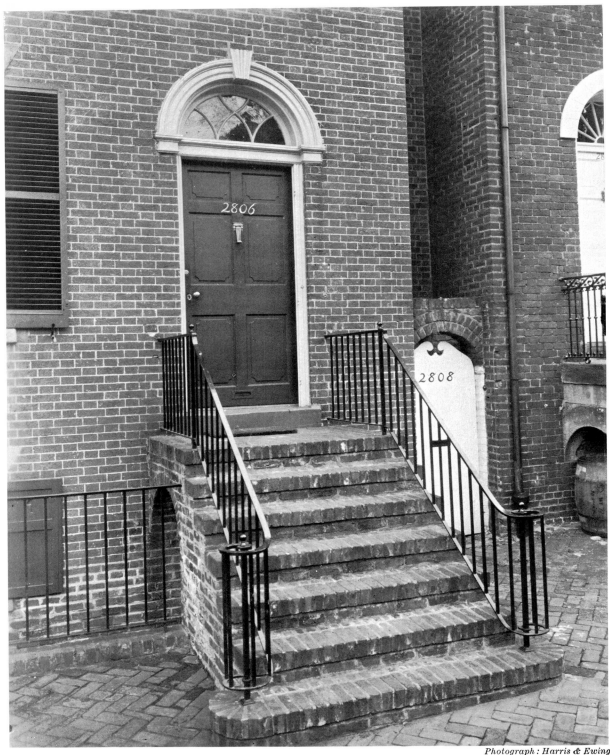

Photograph : Harris & Ewing

Simplicity of scale can be most effective as shown by these mouldings and the stone overdoor

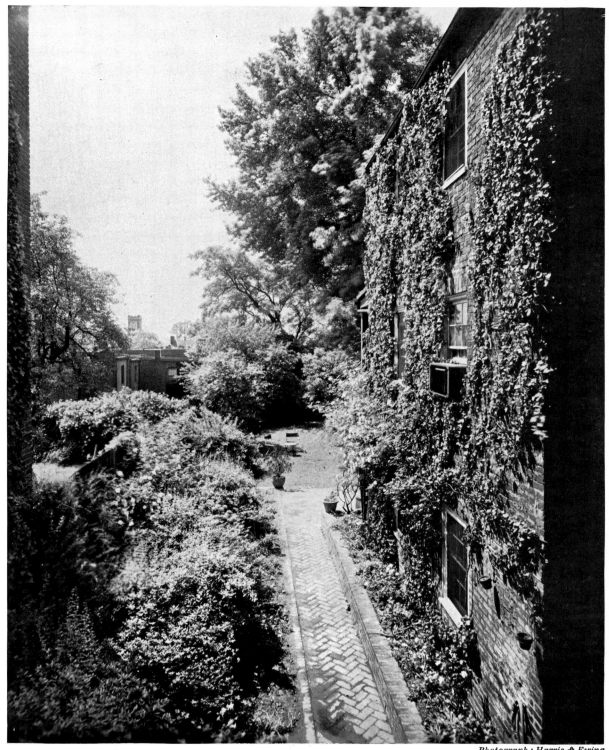

Photograph: Harris & Ewing

The garden is typical and very lovely

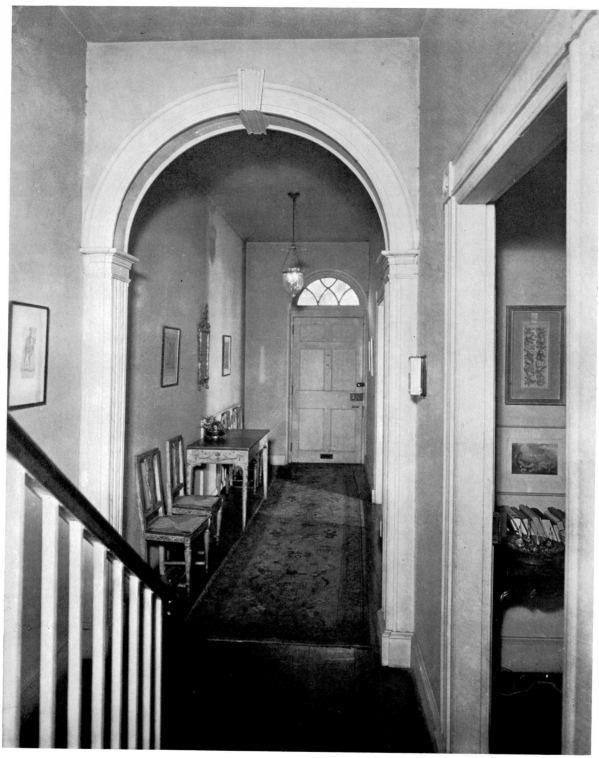

The entrance hall. An interior arch of equisite design complements the front overdoor

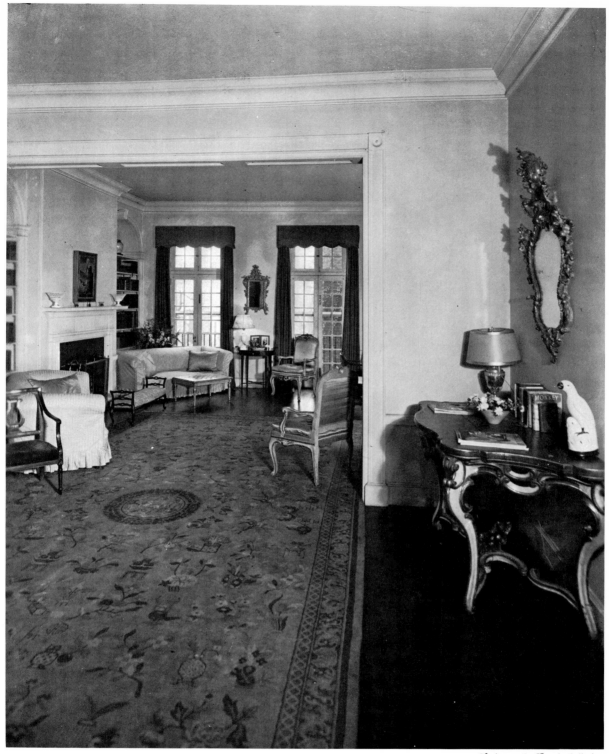

Photograph : Harris & Ewing

Vista of the living room. The original opening between "parlors" has been greatly enlarged to make them one room. A corresponding fireplace and bookcases are not shown.

THE JOHN STODDERT HAW HOUSE
C. 1812
2808 N Street, N. W.

Little is known of this fine example of the Federal town house except that it was built by John Stoddert Haw, nephew of Benjamin Stoddert, one of the founders of Christ Church, Georgetown, probably in the first decade of the Nineteenth Century. It was purchased by the late Admiral and Mrs. Spencer Wood who were among the first to begin the restoration of this section of the town. The garden is lovely and the interior of the house is unusual in its freedom from the Victorian alterations that have marred many other superb buildings of the period.

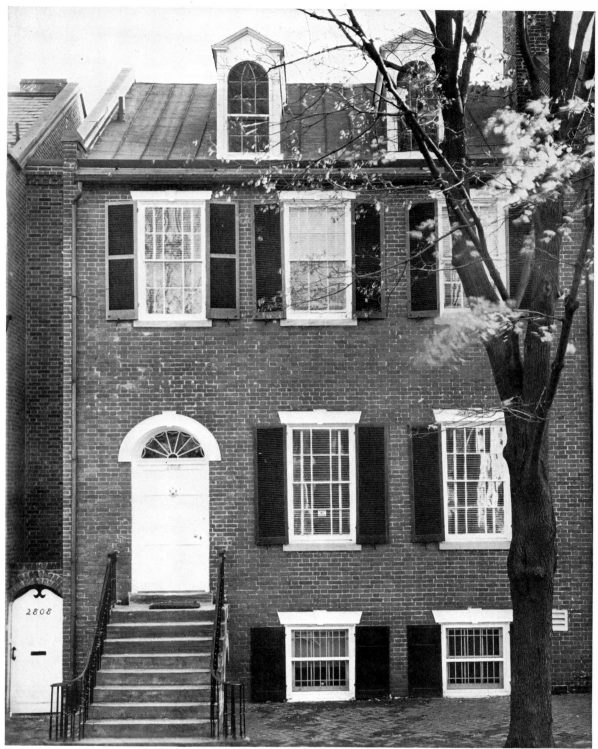

An example of simple dignity achieved in a house of moderate size

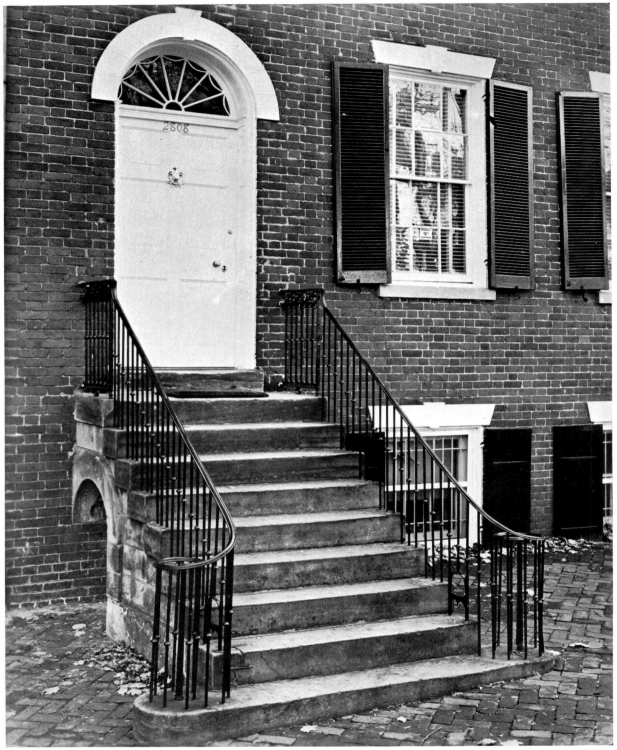

Photograph: Harris & Ewing

A true interpretation of the Federal feeling. Lintels and sills are of painted wood—a common practice in 1800—giving an attractive, fresh, yet soft appearance. The worn stone shows that even the stair treads are original.

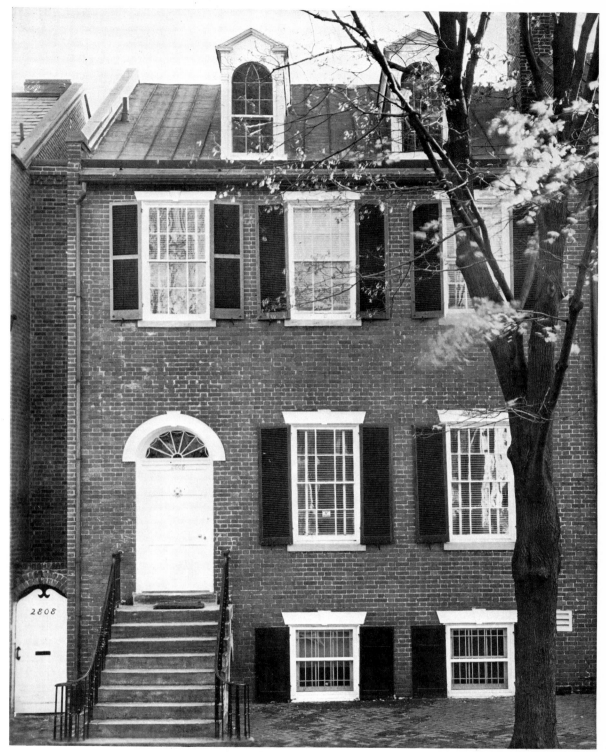

Photograph: Harris & Ewing

An example of simple dignity achieved in a house of moderate size

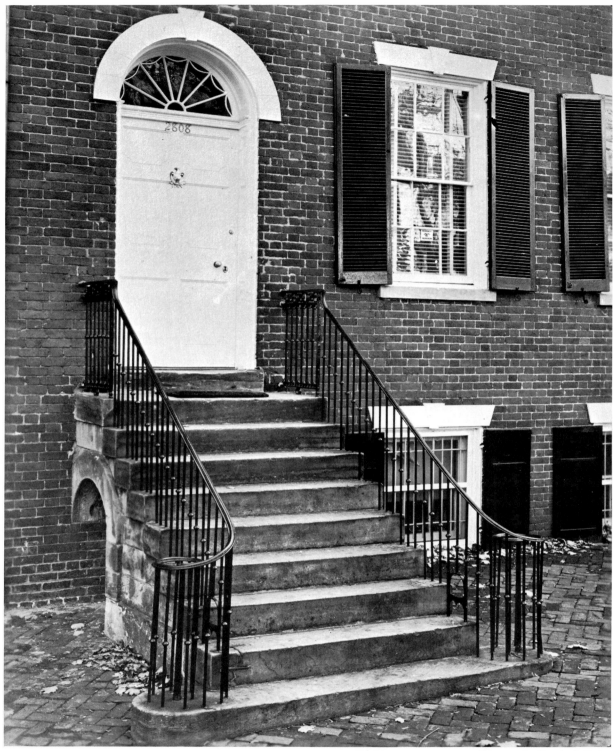

A true interpretation of the Federal feeling. Lintels and sills are of painted wood—a common practice in 1800—giving an attractive, fresh, yet soft appearance. The worn stone shows that even the stair treads are original.

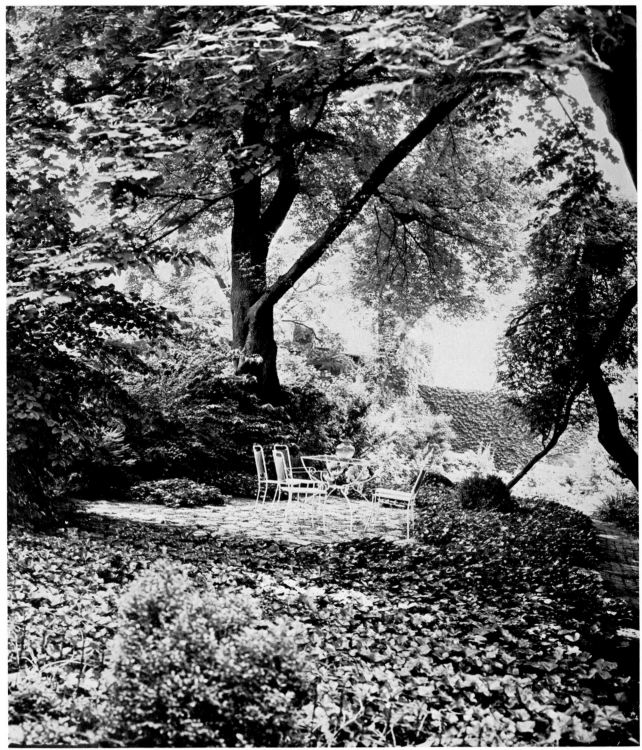

Photograph: Stewart Bros.

The branches of fine old trees protect this sylvan garden at the rear—a perfect setting for *al fresco* dining.

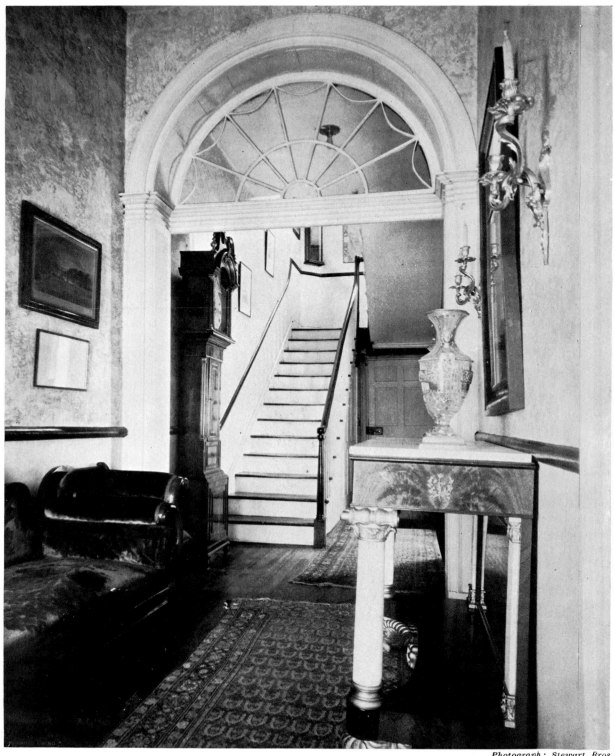

A particularly fine interior arch and fan light occupy the entrance hall

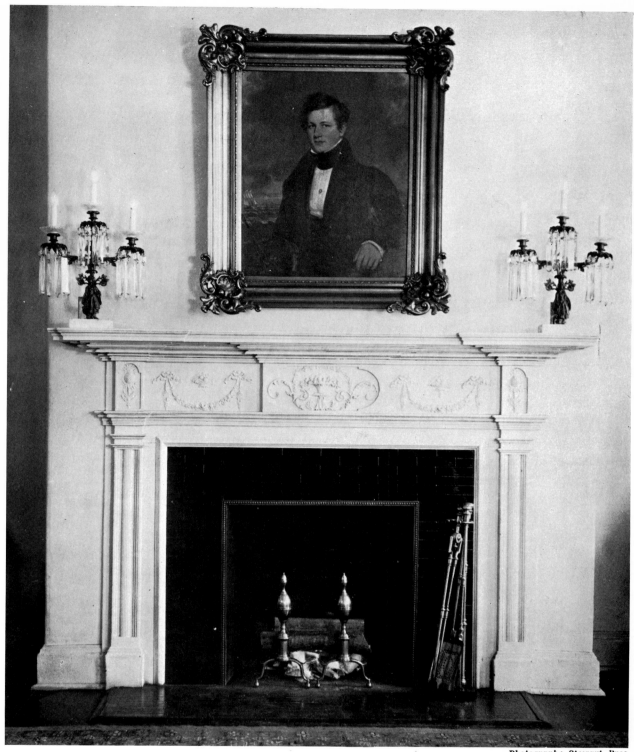

An exquisite classic mantel

THE DECATUR HOUSE
C. 1779
2812 N Street, N. W.

This house has persistently been associated with the name of Decatur although no authentic sources for the legend are known. It is said to have been erected in 1779 and is known to have been the home of Judge Morsell at one time. According to tradition, Mrs. Susan Wheeler Decatur came here to live after the death of the Commodore in his duel with Captain James Barron at Bladensburgh March 22, 1820. Decatur House on Lafayette Square, built by Decatur for his bride according to Latrobe's plans in 1819, shortly after the tragedy was leased to the Russian Minister by the young widow. She then came to Georgetown where she lived until her death in 1860.

Seven years after her husband's death, Mrs. Decatur, still dwelling upon her personal tragedy, refused to enter Washington proper lest she meet his opponent, or his second, whom she considered much to blame. As a result, in the words of an English visitor of that time, "She sees a great deal of company at home." Certainly the walls of her home sheltered many of the great of other days; Mr. W. W. Corcoran, later the philanthropist; General Van Rensselaer, the New York patroon; Mexican Prince Iturbide and his American wife, and many other distinguished persons were her frequent guests.

Later, Mrs. Decatur, who had become a devout Catholic, probably through her close friendship with the Carroll family, moved to a frame house near Georgetown College. Her grave is in the cemetery there, and several mementoes of the Commodore may be seen today at the University. This house, well known for its fine doorway, is the property of Mr. and Mrs. Franklin Mott Gunther and has been leased by the Countess de Martino.

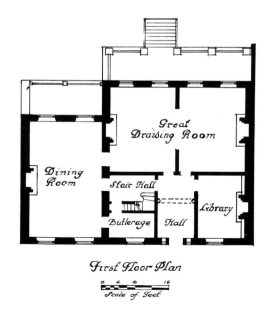

First Floor Plan

Scale of Feet

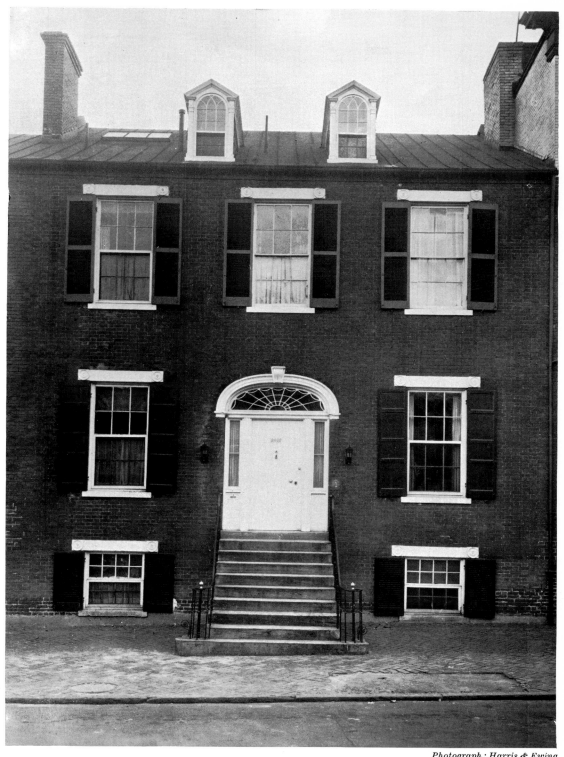

A superb example of function and form

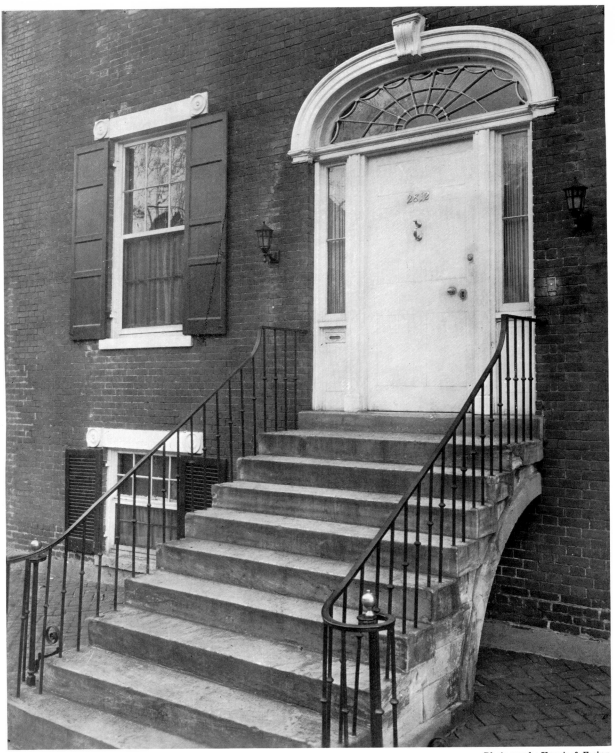

Its hospitable entrance shows carefully worked-out detail. Note graceful stone arch and original iron work. The fan light and stone overdoor are very fine.

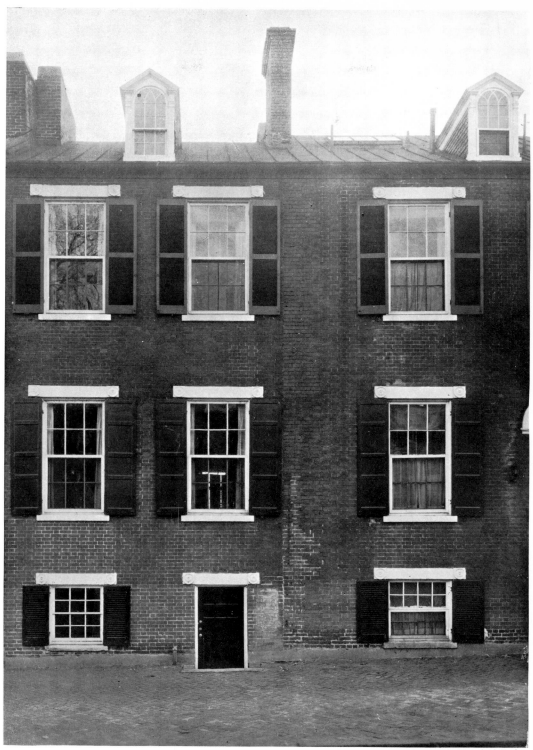

Photograph : Harris & Ewing

Formerly one room in width, this narrow house was joined to its larger neighbor by the simple expedient of knocking out a wall.

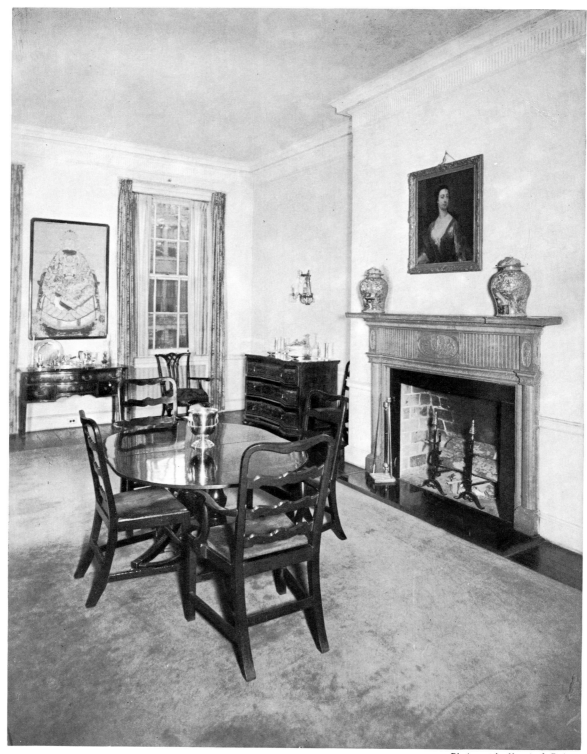

Photograph : Harris & Ewing

This charming room occupies the whole first floor of the little house shown on the preceding page. A fine old pine mantel is used and the carved cornice and chair rail are closely related.

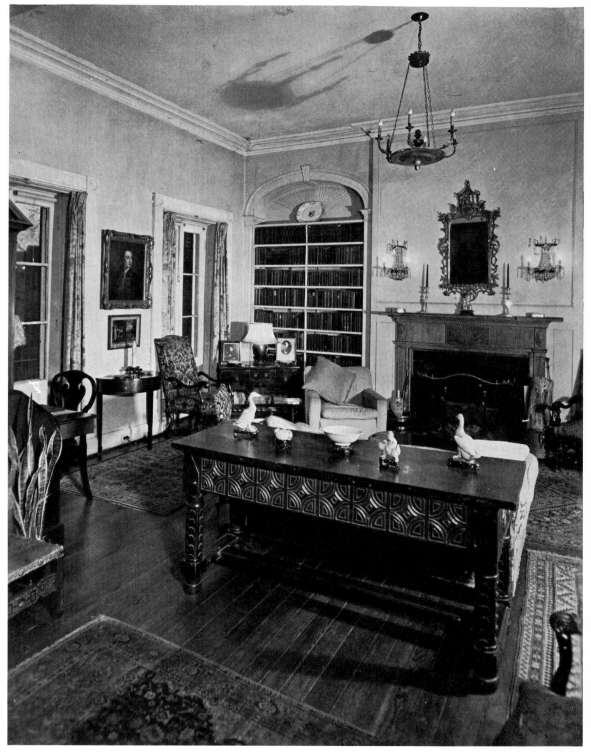

Photograph : Harris & Ewing

Here one large and handsome living room has been made from two. A similar old mantel is at the opposite end; the bookcases are attractive recent additions. The floor plan is unusual as the living room runs across the house. Note fine example of window moulding indicative of the period.

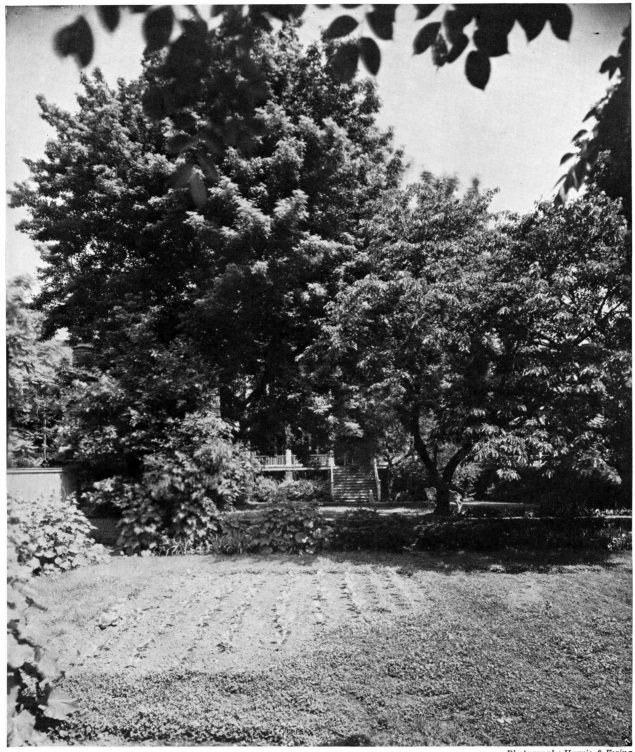

Photograph: Harris & Ewing

The south gallery, almost hidden by the trees—a characteristic feature of Georgetown houses. From it one has a view of the garden, and beyond the housetops a magnificent sweep of the Potomac.

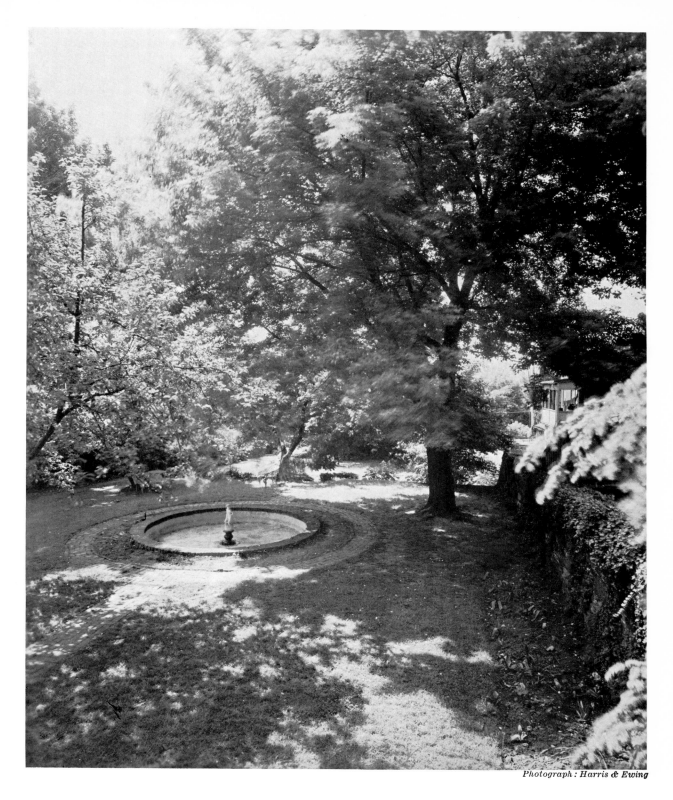

Photograph : Harris & Ewing

The garden as seen from the gallery

THE FOXALL HOUSE
C. 1790
2908 N Street, N. W.

The detail and proportion of this simple little house are intimate and charming. Built in the Eighteenth Century it was once owned as an investment by Henry Foxall, at whose foundry guns were made for the American Forces in 1812. Mr. Foxall, Mayor of the town in 1819, and a convert to Methodism, was known for his strict enforcement of the old "blue laws" against profaning the sabbath and for his practice of buying slaves whom he set free after they had learned a trade.

When the British entered the Capital in 1814 the Foxall foundry was one of the military objectives marked for destruction. Henry Foxall vowed that he would build a church if God would spare his property. The expeditionary force was turned back by a furious hurricane, and Foundry Methodist Church in Washington, the fulfillment of his vow, is the church at which Prime Minister Churchill worshipped with President Roosevelt on the occasion of their meeting in Washington in 1943!

The little house formerly was covered with white plaster. It has now been enclosed within a tall brick wall and is used by Mr. and Mrs. Robert J. Randolph, the owners, as one house in conjunction with the fine replica of a Federal house next door.

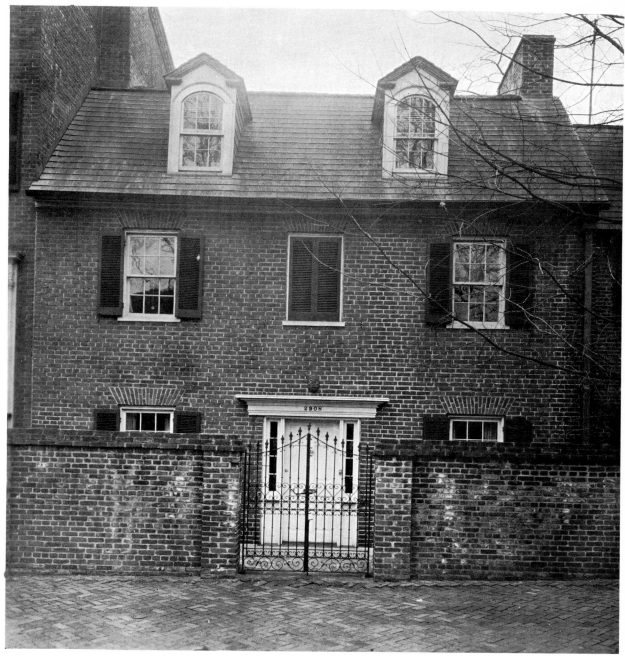

A high wall plays an imposing role in the restoration of this modest house

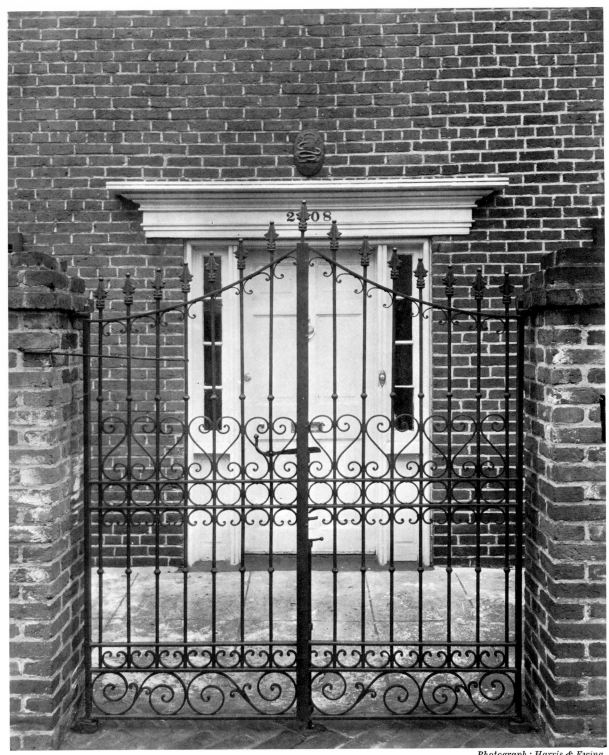

Wrought iron entrance gate—a happy choice

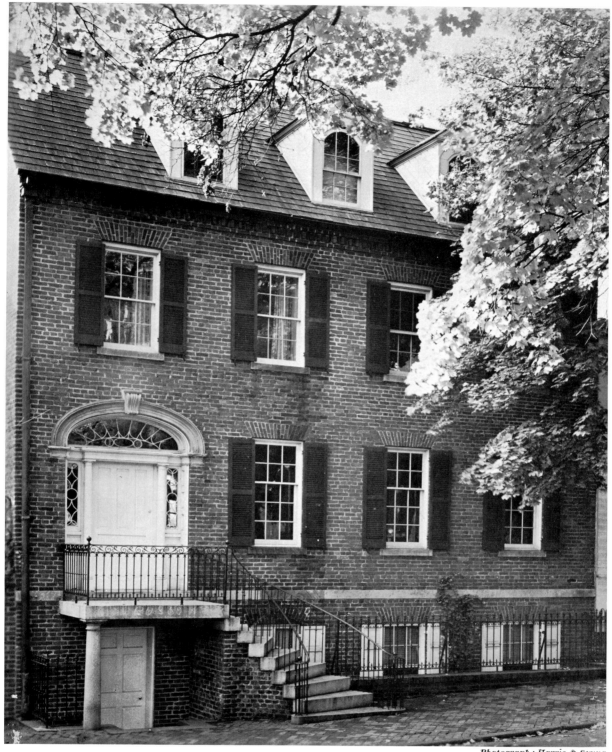

The small house grew by this new addition at the side.   The stone lintel, rail and steps are old.

THE LAIRD-DUNLOP HOUSE
C. 1799
3014 N Street, N. W.

The central portion of this imposing brick mansion was built about 1799 by John Laird, the prosperous owner of one of early Georgetown's great tobacco warehouses. During its construction, he rented Thomas Beall's large house across the street. It is not unlikely that this house was designed by Thornton because of its unusual arched first story windows, which are identical to those of Thomas Law's house on Greenleaf Point, Washington, attributed with reasonable certainty to the great architect.

The house was inherited by John Laird's daughter Margaret in 1833. She lived there with her aunt, Elizabeth Dick, another spinster, for many years devoting much of her time to the Presbyterian Church and the Orphan Asylum. On her death the house passed to her sister, Barbara, (Mrs. James Dunlop) and became known thereafter as the Dunlop house.

Judge Dunlop was at various times Secretary of the Corporation of Georgetown, a law partner of Francis Scott Key, and Chief Justice of the Supreme Court of the District of Columbia until he was removed from the latter office as a southern sympathizer by President Lincoln. His son, William Laird Dunlop, who lived here for a number of years, always kept his own cow and killed his own hogs each fall. The old smoke house remains just east of the house and one of the original town boundary markers still stands in the large garden.

In 1915 the mansion was purchased from William Laird Dunlop's heirs by Robert Todd Lincoln, eldest son of the President, one time Secretary of War and Ambassador to England. His widow lived there until the house was sold to Mrs. Arthur Woods, a granddaughter of J. Pierpont Morgan I, and a direct descendant of Alexander Hamilton. Extensive wings have been added to the original house which today serves as a fitting setting for her beautiful furniture, portraits and tapestries.

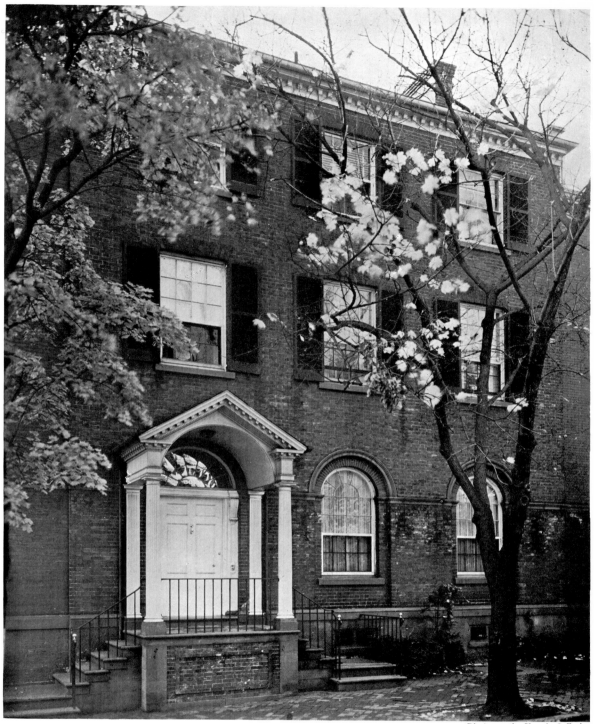

Photograph : Harris & Ewing

There are numerous later additions but this shows the original facade with its imposing entrance. To the left a glimpse of later additions. The fan light carries out the exact semicircle of the heads of the first story windows.

THE RIGGS-RILEY HOUSE
C. 1805
3038 N Street, N. W.

The fine town house of typical smaller "Georgetown" type known to Georgetown citizens for so many years as "old Doctor Riley's" was probably built about 1805. In any case, it was sold on March 24, 1812 by James S. Marshall to William S. Nicholls and Romulus Riggs. The latter, who was born in Brookeville, Montgomery County, Maryland, and who had married a Miss Dorsey in 1810, sometime before 1835 moved to Philadelphia where he became known as an influential and well-to-do merchant. An authority on Georgetown history believes that he lived in this house for some years before he sold it to Dr. Joshua Riley.

A number of medical students received their basic medical training in Dr. Riley's small one story brick office to the east of the house, much as young men once "read law" in the office of an established attorney. Among them were Dr. Armistead Peter, later of Tudor Place, and Waldemer and Boris Bodisco, nephews of the famed Russian Minister. Mrs. Riley's niece, Juliet Murray, was married to John Marbury, Jr., in this house in 1851, and the daughter of the house, Miss Marianna Riley, lived here with her sister-in-law for years after the Doctor's death.

Upon Miss Riley's death the house was sold and resold a number of times, until it became the property of Colonel (U.S. Marine Corps) and Mrs. Henry Leonard. The old office was razed to make way for a large service wing, but the garden and the house itself have been restored to the quaint beauty of their earliest days.

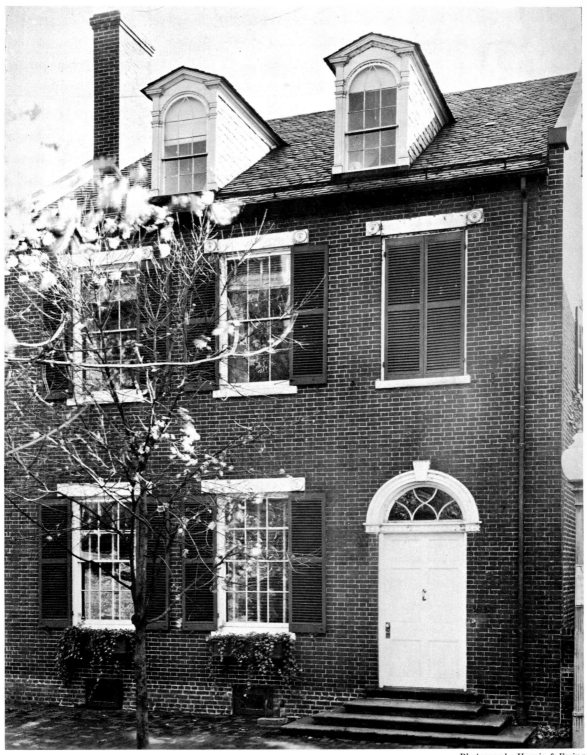

Photograph: Harris & Ewing

One of its beauties is its almost perfect scale—shown clearly in this view of the street facade

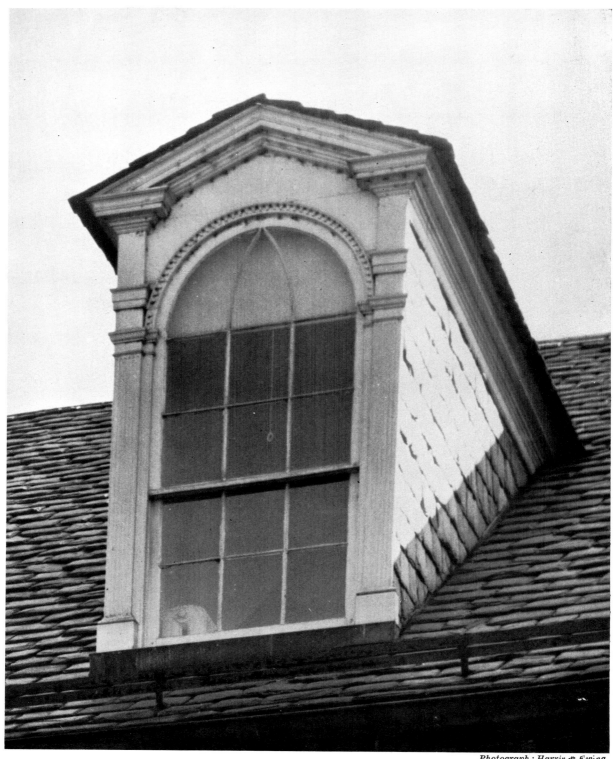

The detail and thoughtful scale of these dormers force great respect for their designers. In some as many as seventeen hand-carved mouldings are used.

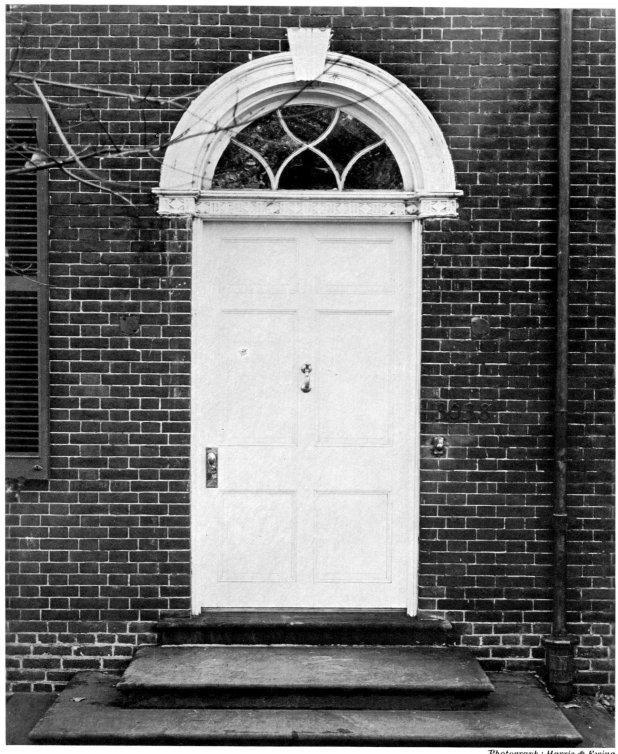

Entrance—Note delicate detail in overdoor

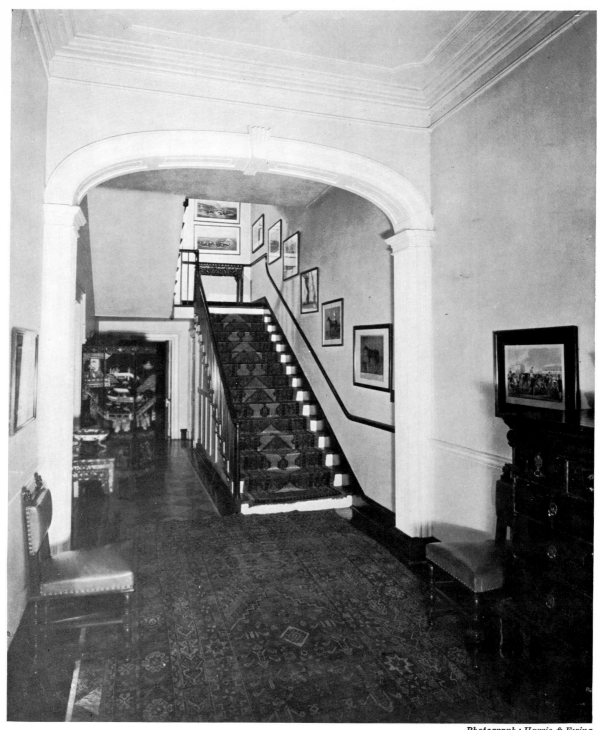

An original interior arch and stair for which no words of praise are necessary

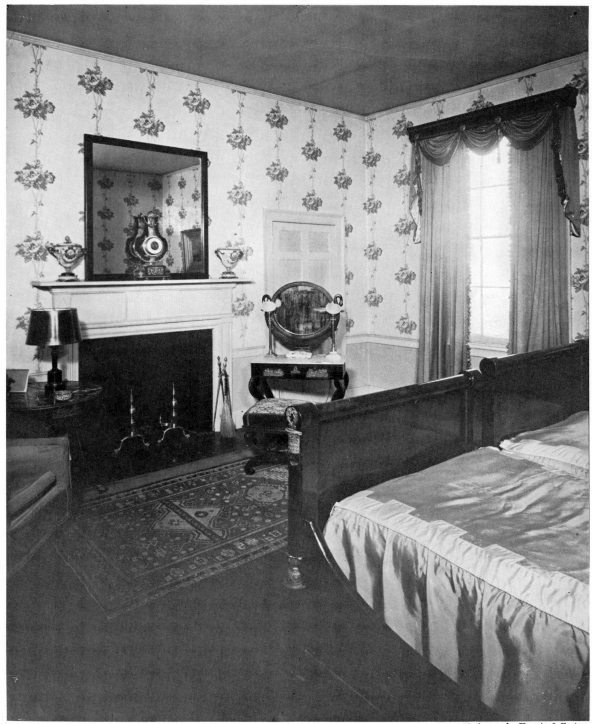

Photograph: Harris & Ewing

A beautiful bedroom with mantel and furniture original

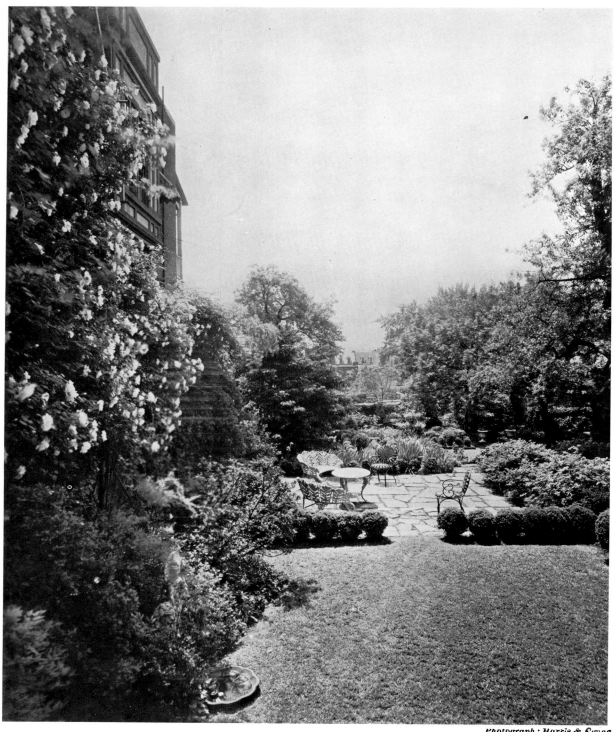

Judging from the exterior facade, it would be difficult to realize that so important and beautiful a garden joined the rear gallery.

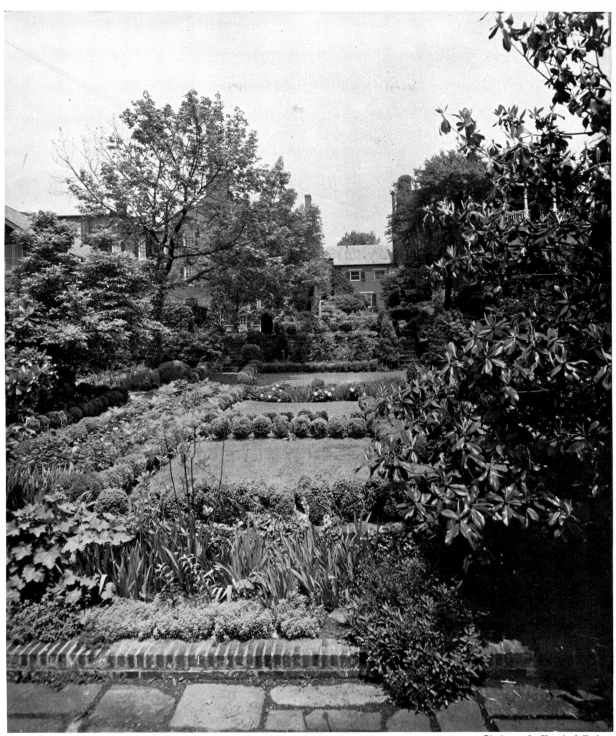

Photograph: Harris & Ewing

The superb planning and great size are even more evident here

THE COLONEL JOHN COX HOUSE
C. 1805
3339 N Street, N. W.

Probably the finest examples of the Federal "row" house standing in Georgetown are those built by Colonel John Cox, about 1805, at the corner of N and 34th Streets. They are large, of ell shape, and are distinguished by their exquisitely fine dormers and leaden swags in the recessed panels which relieve the severity of the facade. They are unique in standing back some distance from the street, which affords them sizable door yards at the sacrifice of the gardens at the rear.

Cox, born in 1775, was a prosperous merchant and real estate owner who served as Mayor of the town for twenty-two years from 1823 to 1845. Well known as a dandy, he served as a Colonel during the War of 1812 and was thrice married; first to Matilda Smith, sister of the first president of the Farmers and Mechanics Bank. They had three children and this corner house is thought to have been the Cox residence during this period. His second wife was the daughter of John Threlkeld of Burleith, Mayor of Georgetown in 1793, and friend of Jefferson. Colonel and Mrs. Cox built a new house, "The Cedars," on part of the Threlkeld estate and were living here when Cox, as Mayor, entertained Lafayette in 1824.

As the arrival of one of the seven children born of this marriage was imminent, Colonel Cox had number 3337, next door to his former home and vacant at the time, completely furnished for the occasion. Even the edges of the floors were decorated by floral garlands drawn in colored chalk. His eldest daughter acted as hostess and a great supper was served which is supposed to have included 600 reed birds.

Number 3339 was at one time the home of Commodore Morris, a hero of the War of 1812, when he served as executive officer of the "Constitution" under Captain Isaac Hull. It was purchased in 1842 by James Keith for his daughter Mrs. Forrest. The old house, almost entirely unaltered, remained in the same family for over 100 years, until its recent purchase and fine restoration by John deBlois Wack.

Among the distinguished residents of the other five houses which make up the row have been William A. Gordon, once Chief of the Quartermaster Corps; Judge Robert Ould; Mayor Henry Addison; William Hunter, Assistant Secretary of State; William Laird, Jr., and many others.

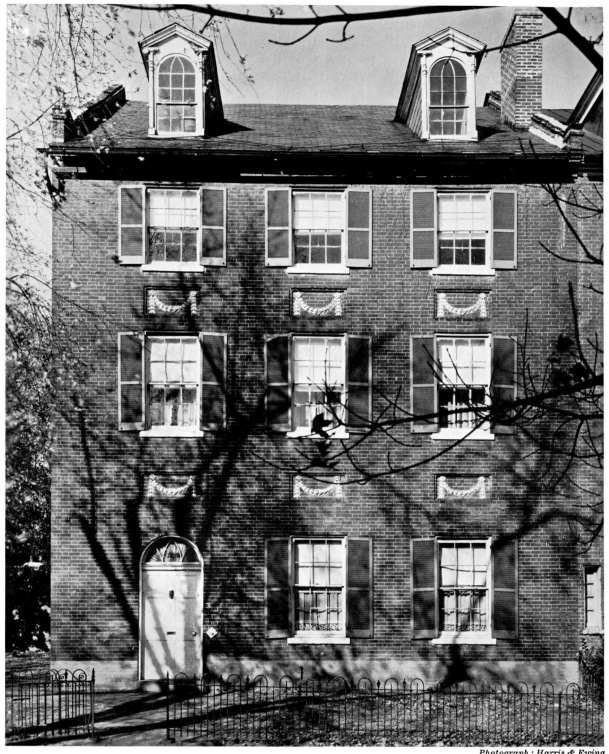

Photograph: Harris & Ewing

One of the finest of its period

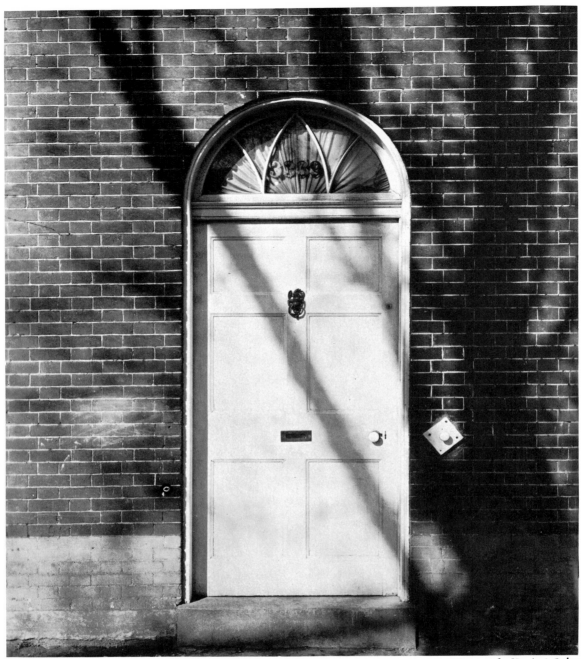

Photograph: Harris & Ewing

Tree shadows form a fascinating pattern on warm brick walls

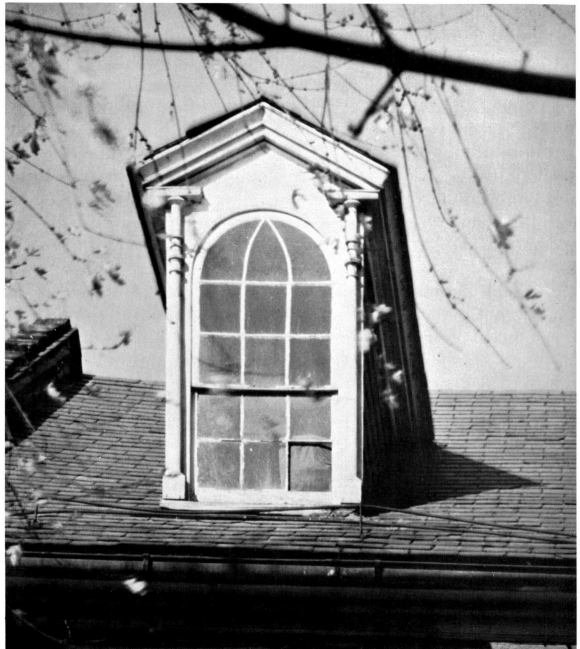

Photograph: Harris & Ewing

Dormer. The grace and delicacy of its colonettes are in perfect harmony with the entrance door on the preceding page.

THE McKENNEY HOUSE
C. 1800
3123 Dumbarton Avenue

Unoccupied in recent years, this notable Federal house was built by Henry Foxall for his only daughter, Mary Ann, on her marriage to Samuel McKenney in 1800. It remained in the McKenney family until the death of Mary Ann Foxall McKenney's granddaughter, Mrs. McCartney,—then a grandmother—a few years ago. Enclosed by a low stone wall and white picket fence, it has fine dormers and a pillared porch with arched ceiling and gabled pediment. The interior trim is very fine.

One of the interesting inhabitants of the house in days gone by, was a spinster from Philadelphia who came for dinner, and being prevailed upon by the children to prolong her stay, remained for forty years until her death. She was somewhat eccentric and insisted that the candles be extinguished by ten o'clock—a peculiarity which her hosts allowed her. After her death, those who slept in the old lady's room found—strangely enough—that their candles went out precisely at ten o'clock; even when no drafts were present.

The old house, surrounded by its garden, is one of the few in Georgetown practically in its original condition. The recent years of desertion and neglect have not been kind to it, but it needs only a new owner with interest and sufficient funds to restore it to happier days again.

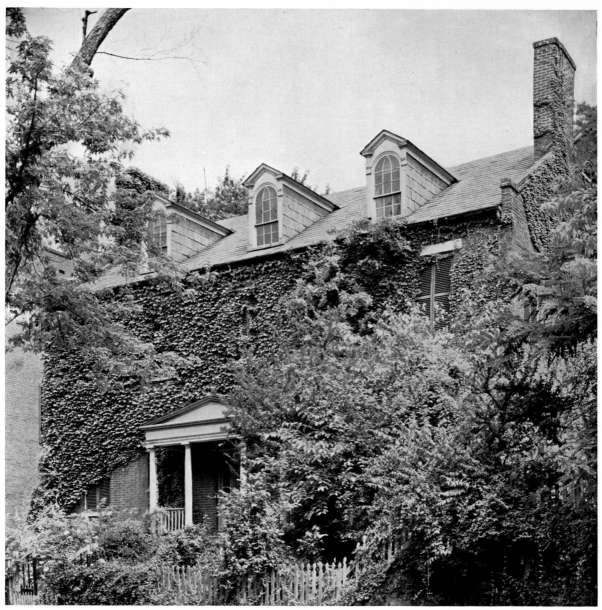

Even the luxuriant growth of ivy cannot completely mask the beauty of this house

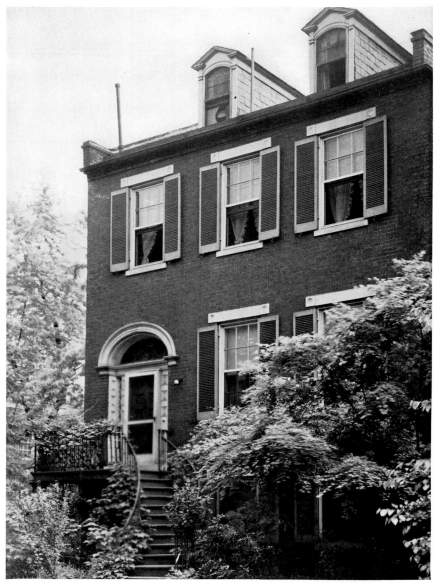

THE BERRY HOUSE
3100 Dumbarton Avenue, N. W.

This house, erected in 1810, was the home of Philip Taylor Berry in 1820. It survived a bad fire about 1900 and now, with the fine rear gallery cut off, and an addition to the west, is divided into apartments. Unfortunately the structure is now much higher above sidewalk level than it was originally, as a result of the cutting down of the street at this point. However, the garden is charming and the front doorway, with sidelights complementing the door panels, is very fine.

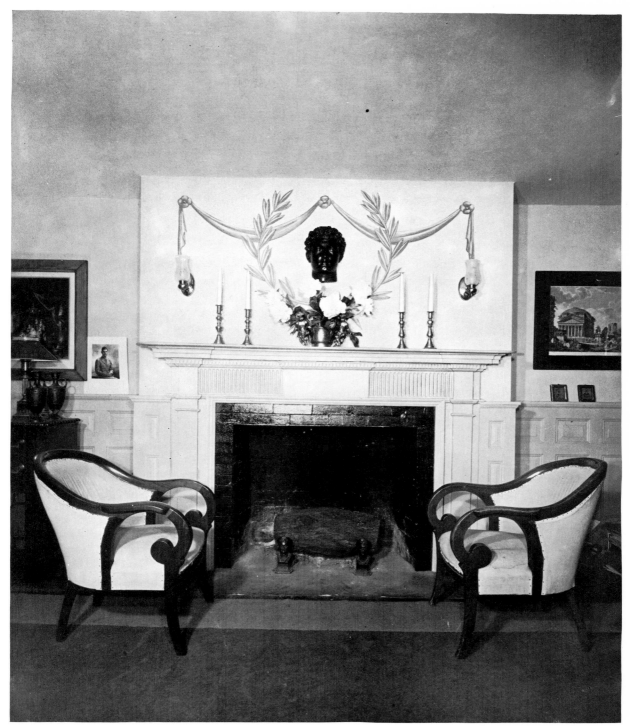

Photograph : Harris & Ewing

The original mantel with the design above it arranged by David Leavitt, well-known mural painter, to nullify the effect of the modern wall lights. The furniture displays similar classic feeling.

THE TENNEY HOUSE
C. 1805
3010 O Street, N. W.

Although part of it is much earlier, the portion of this charming frame house facing the street is thought to have been built in the first years of the Nineteenth Century by a Mr. Tenney who came to Georgetown from Newburyport, Massachusetts, about 1800. The white clapboards and the two end chimneys, in place of the great center type characteristic of its builder's native countryside, are an interesting adaptation of New England architecture to the warmer Maryland climate.

The house with its garden which originally extended to the corner was later the home of the builder's daughters, the three Misses Tenney and their sister Mrs. Brown, who conducted a school for small children. It was purchased in recent years by Major General Louis Mc-Carty Little, USMC. Mrs. Little, the internationally known decorator, Elsie Cobb Wilson, has restored it as a superb background for her fine collection of antique furniture and objects d'art.

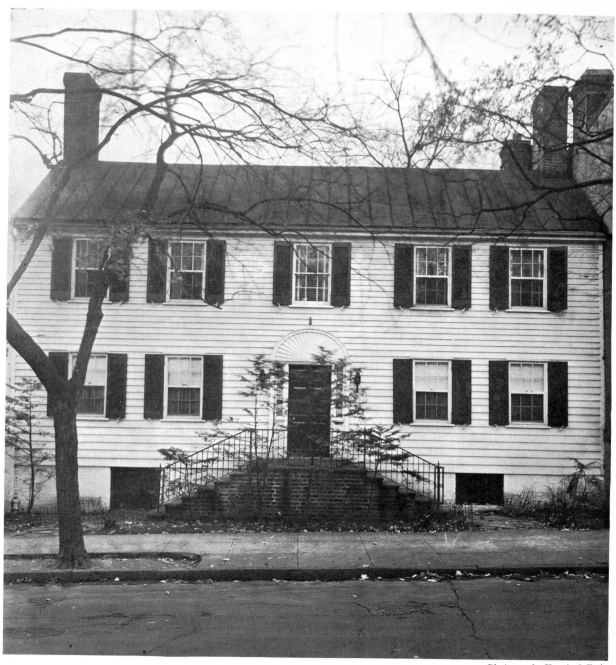

Photograph: Harris & Ewing

Residence of Major General and Mrs. Louis McCarty Little

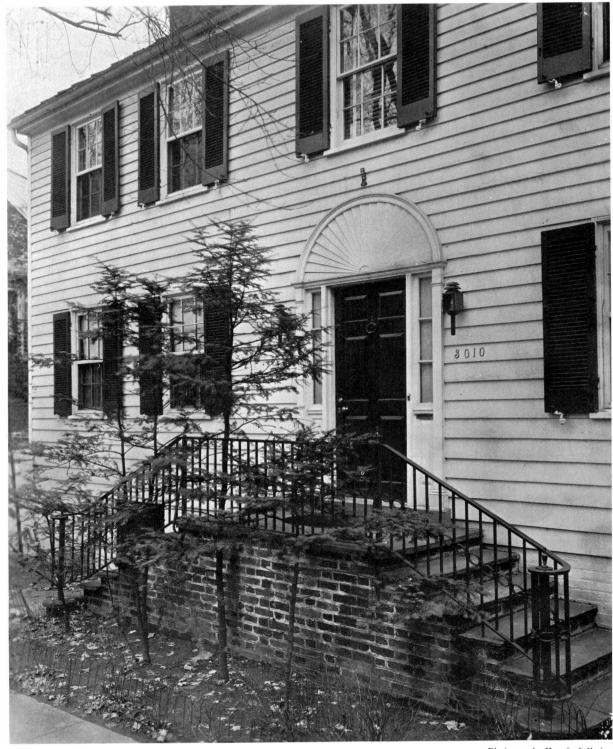

This charming doorway has been restored to its old form

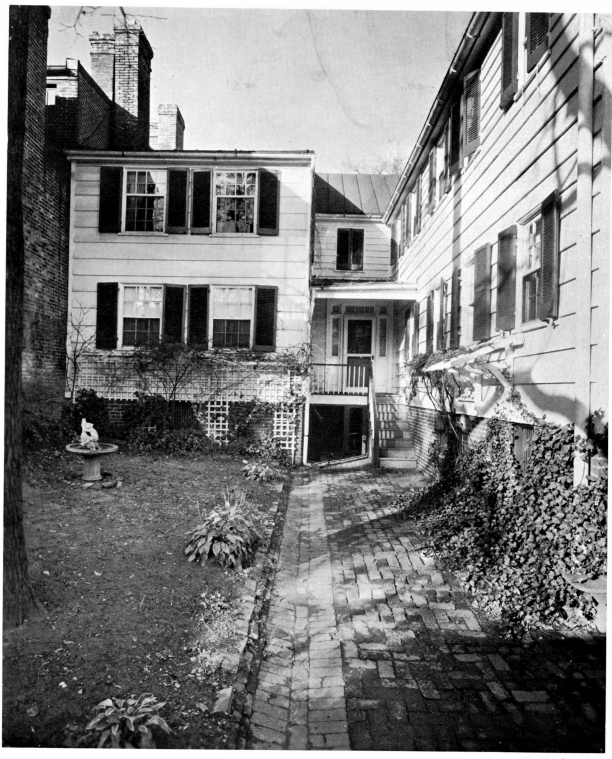

From the garden—the house has grown through several additions

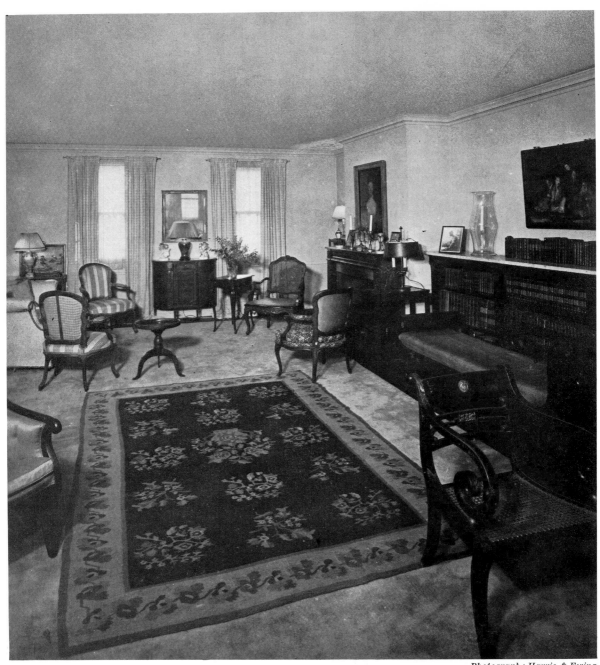

Another conversion from two rooms—hence two fireplaces

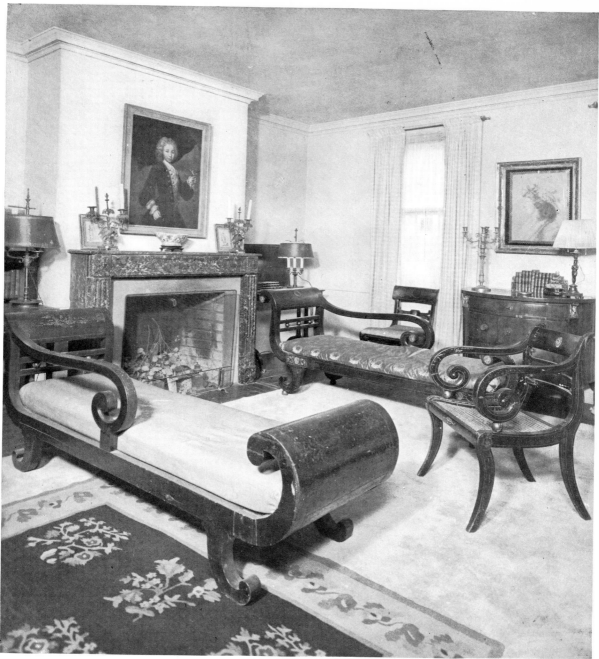

The other end of the Living Room. An unusually fine grouping of furniture of the period

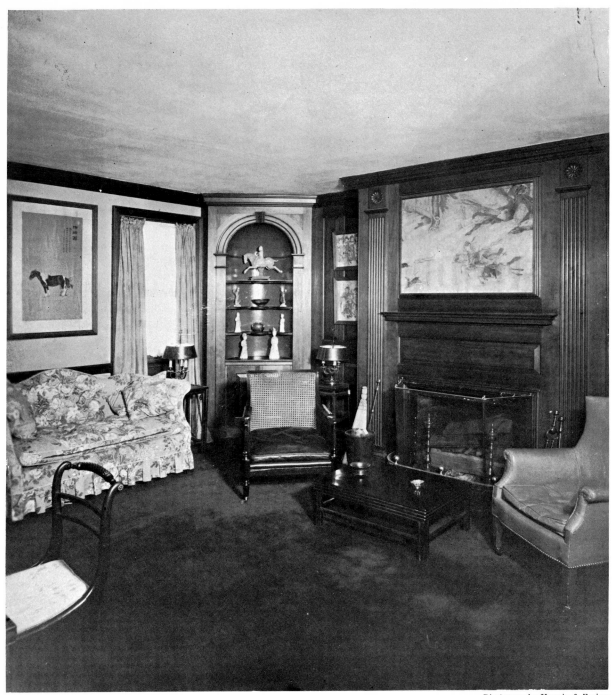

These photographs show three walls of a beautiful small, partially panelled room, a restoration of an earlier period.

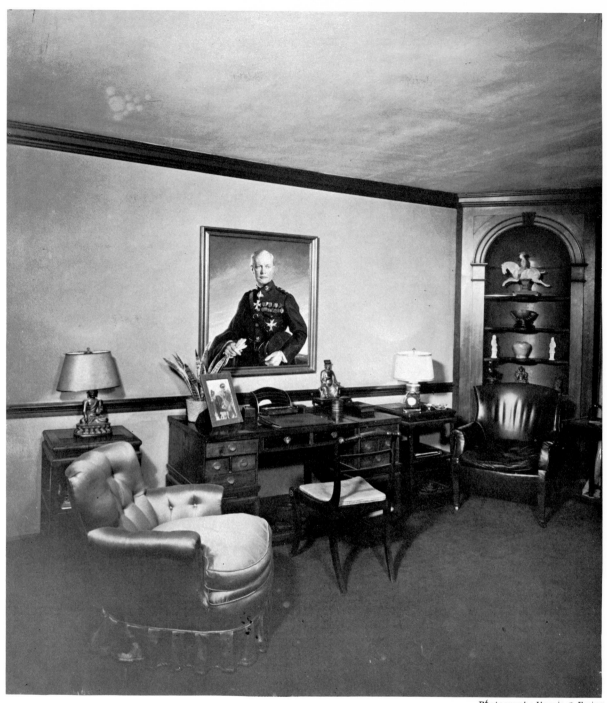

Photograph : Harris & Ewing

A portrait of General Little. The chinoiserie is some of the finest in the world

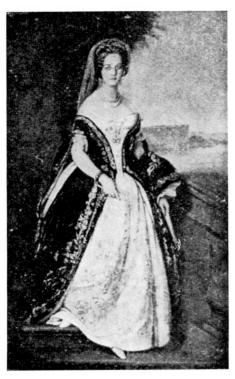

Madame Bodisco

THE BODISCO HOUSE
C. 1820
3322 O Street, N. W.

The old Russian Legation is perhaps better known for its romantic history than for its severe and distinguished beauty. Here, at a fabulous Christmas party which he gave for his nephews, Waldemer and Boris, then students at Georgetown College, Baron Alexander de Bodisco, Imperial Russian Minister to the United States for the seventeen years before his death in 1854, met his future wife, the beautiful Harriet Brooke Williams. He immediately became infatuated with the blonde loveliness of the school girl of sixteen, and his sixty-two years seem in no way to have dampened the ardor and impetuosity of his courtship.

In spite of the opposition of the Williams family they were married in June 1849 at the home of the bride's mother. The bride was given away by Henry Clay and the groomsmen included Senator (later President) James Buchanan; Henry Fox, the British Minister; Mr. Martineau, the Netherlands Minister; Baron Saruyse, the Austrian Minister; Mr. Van Buren, son of the President; Mr. Forsythe, son of the Secretary of State; and Mr. Paulding, son of the Secretary of the Navy. A brilliant reception followed at the embassy where the bride in white and the groom in splendid court dress received a throng of distinguished guests including President Van Buren and Daniel Webster. However brief, the marriage was a very happy one. The great wealth of the Baron allowed him to shower his beautiful young wife with gorgeous jewels and gowns, and the house became famous for the gayety and magnificence of its entertaining.

The house is noteworthy for the severity of its lines, complemented by the great door, the fine pedimented portico, and the extremely graceful double stairway at the entrance. Extending to the side and rear is its spacious garden which, on the occasion of the Baron's lavish wedding reception, was specially decorated with lemon trees hanging full of golden fruit. It is thought that before its long period as a Legation, the house was occupied for a short time by the mother of General Robert E. Lee during his years at West Point. Later it was the home of Abraham Herr, and finally was used as an apartment until its purchase and sympathetic restoration by Francis C. de Wolf, the present owner.

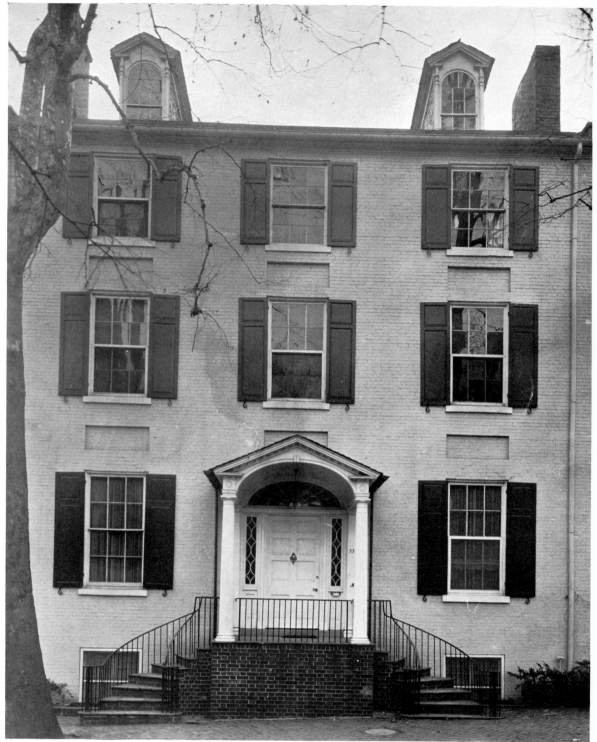

Photograph : Harris & Ewing

A great eight-panelled door, delicate detail of portico, and recessed panels figure prominently in the superb design of this tall mansion; but its dignity is relieved by the wide sweep of its stairs—truly "opening arms."

THE HARMON HOUSE
C. 1810
3025 P Street, N. W.

The quaint little house which is now the home of Mr. and Mrs. Frank P. Harmon, was probably built about 1810. It is noteworthy for the fine stark simplicity of its exterior and for its sympathetically scaled interior trim.

Its later history is lacking, but the property was sold to Thomas and John Wirt in 1805. Between that date and 1816 deeds attest to its ownership at various times by Benjamin and John Pickrell, James and Henry Lunkins, R. Gaines, William Calder and Elisha Lanham.

It is likely that Mr. Calder built the house which was successively bought for investment purposes by Washington Bowie, the shipowner, in 1819 and by Francis Dodge in 1821. The latter had come to Georgetown from Salem as a youth in 1798. In the fifty-three years of his life in the town he became one of the greatest merchants and established one of its largest and most honored families in the huge old house which for many years dominated the block on which this little house still stands.

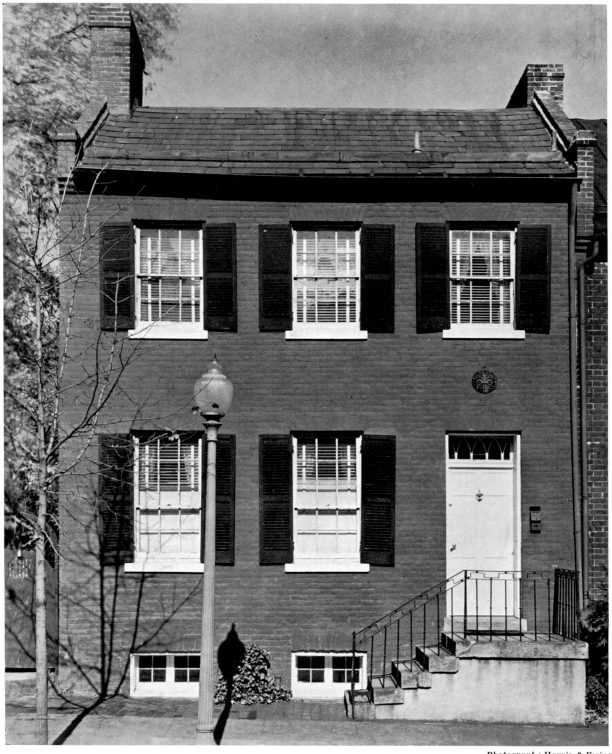

Photograph: Harris & Ewing

This close-up shows the house as a simple, straightforward expression of its purpose

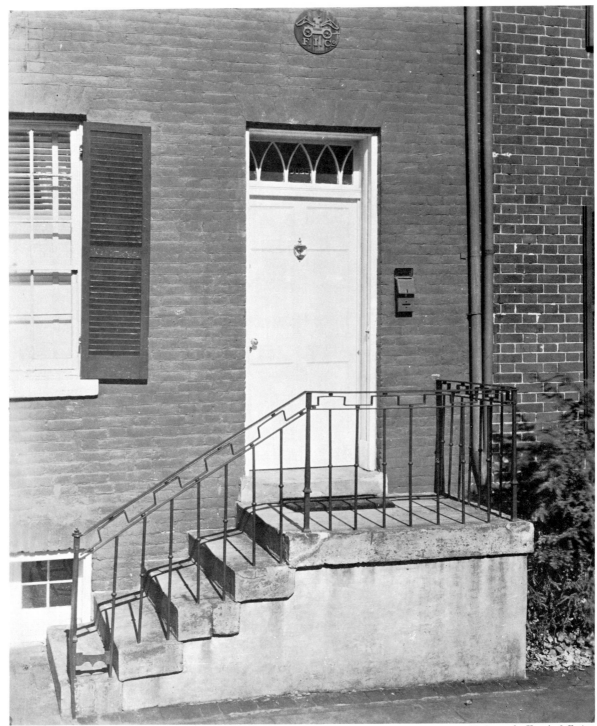

Photograph: Harris & Ewing

Exquisite simplicity. Note the unusual square doorway and complementing details of the handrail.

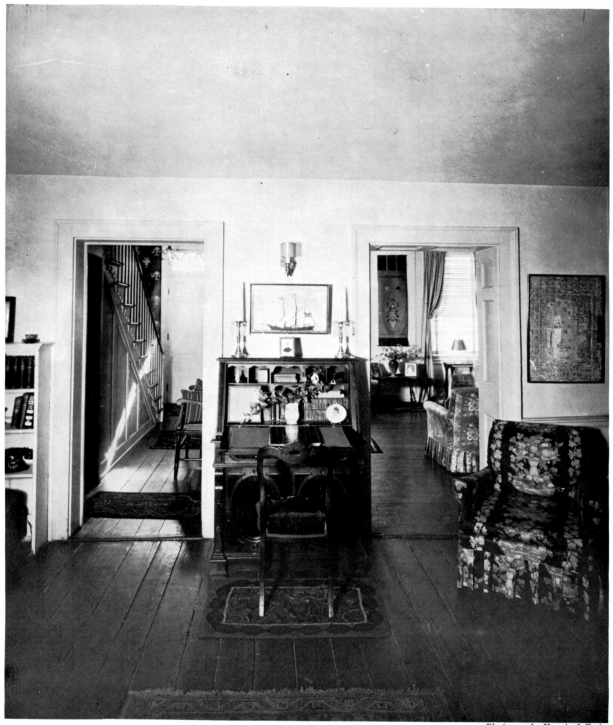

Furniture in proper scale and the lovely soft colors make a perfect complement to this fine small house.

THE LINTHICUM HOUSE
1826
3019 P Street, N. W.

The brick house standing at 3019 P Street was built in 1826 by one of Georgetown's three great philanthropists, Edward M. Linthicum, who lived here until 1846, when he purchased the large house built on Georgetown Heights by William H. Dorsey in 1801, now known as Dumbarton Oaks, but called "Monterey" by Linthicum in commemoration of the great battle of the Mexican War.

While Mr. Linthicum's later mansion became one of the famous estates of the District, this, his earlier home, is possibly a more perfect example of the taste and love of beauty for which this prosperous merchant and civic leader was well known. It is a superb example of the late Federal town house with a particularly fine doorway having both fan and side lights and an exquisite iron railing at the entrance steps. Directly on the street as are its neighbors, behind the house one finds a lovely garden which forms, with the others in the block, a great hollow square of lovely lawns, flowers and trees.

Mr. Linthicum, a merchant, member of the Town Council and trustee of the Methodist Church, left a legacy of $50,000 for the founding of a free school in Georgetown; being convinced, as he wrote, that knowledge and piety constitute the only assurance of happiness and healthful progress for the human race.

The fine house built by this good citizen became the home of Thomas Corcoran, Junior, an older brother of the financier and philanthropist W. W. Corcoran, who sold it to John R. Cochrane in 1856. The latter's sister, Mrs. James A. Magruder, and members of her family, lived here until its purchase by Victor Sutro who has restored it with unusual understanding.

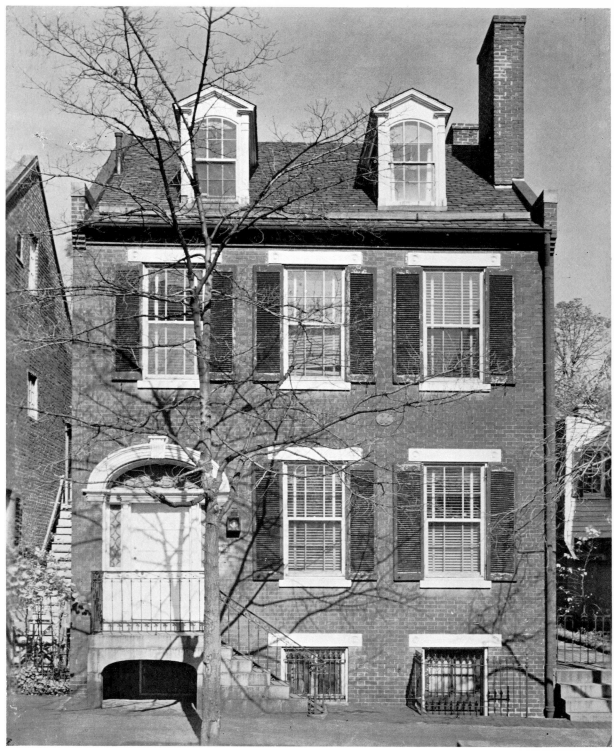

Photograph : Harris & Ewing

The intriguing combination of white stone ornament and red brick wall is an interesting solution of the smaller house problem.

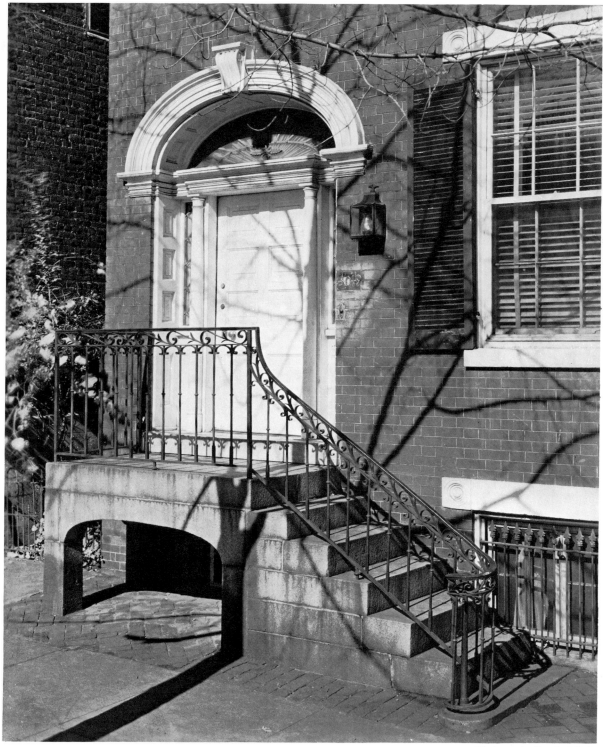

Photograph: Harris & Ewing

The filigree of shadows across this doorway is almost a match for the iron tracery of the handrail.

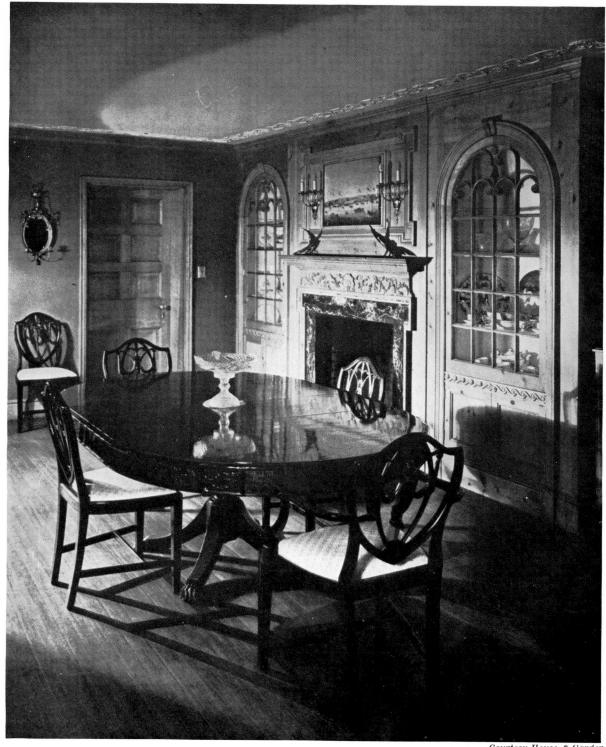

The Dining Room.   Peacock walls plus fine pine panelling of an earlier period

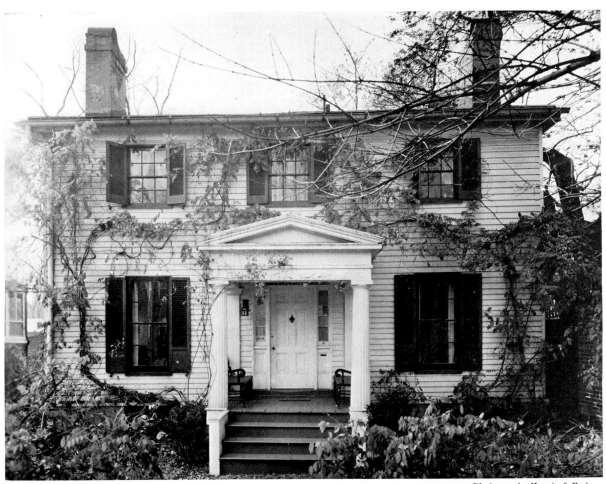

Photograph : Harris & Ewing

THE MILLER HOUSE
1524 28th Street, N. W.

This small frame house was built about 1830 and was at one time the residence of Benjamin Miller of New York, designer and builder of the old Aqueduct Bridge across the Potomac. It is illustrated here as an interesting example of the general Georgetown type employing wood rather than the usual brick. It is distinctly reminiscent of houses of the era built in upper New York State and New England, yet it has the four end chimneys used in Georgetown and the surrounding locality. Its interior trim is noteworthy and its white clapboard walls and doric pillared porch are an interesting deviation from the typical Georgetown house of Federal type. It is today the home of Mr. and Mrs. R. F. Whitehead.

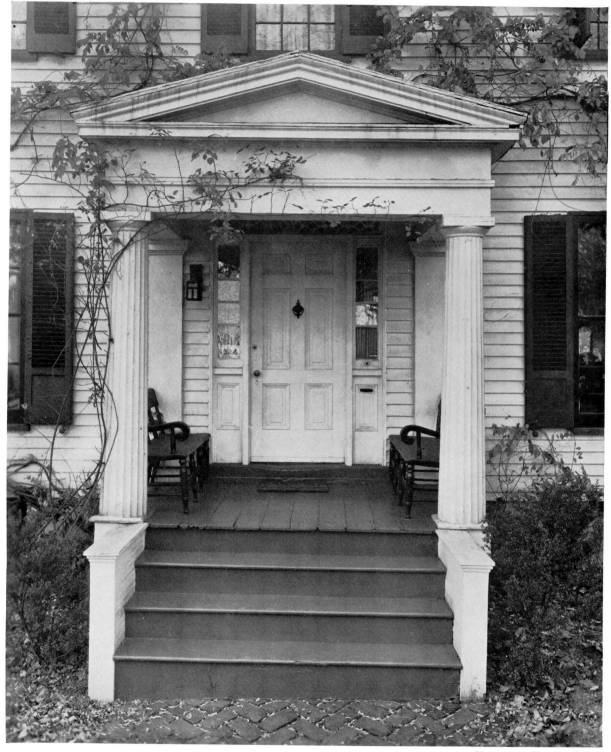

Photograph : Harris & Ewing

The charm of wood, well designed and well executed

SEVIER PLACE
1800
3124 Q Street, N. W.

The south front of the dignified old mansion, built in 1800 by Washington Bowie, may be seen through a maze of boxwood and great trees from the old iron gates of the carriage entrance a block to the south. While the other facade, now high above Q Street is the finer in detail, this secluded garden seems to preserve the very atmosphere of the early Nineteenth Century. The house itself is characterized by very tall ceilings with fine plaster friezes, by finely carved mantels, and great mahogany doors. It has been extended and remodelled during the past fifty years, although the central mass retains the same appearance as when the estate covered the entire block on which it stands. Its builder, who was one of Georgetown's great shipowners, enjoyed the distinction of being a godson of General Washington, whose name is so closely linked with Tudor Place across Q Street. He was a member of the same family as Colonels James and Resin P. Bowie, respectively hero of the Alamo and inventor of the Bowie knife. In 1805 Mr. Bowie sold the property to William Nicholls of Maryland. His two daughters married W. F. Hanewinkel of Richmond and Colonel Hollingsworth, later Curator of Mount Vernon, whose names have since always been closely associated with it.

The old house was sold at auction in 1890 to Mr. and Mrs. John Sevier who happened to be visiting Georgetown at the time. He was the descendant and namesake of John Sevier, hero of Kings Mountain and first Governor of Tennessee. While they had spent a large part of their time abroad, they made this their permanent home, adding one wing to the house and extending the other. It has remained in the same hands ever since, and Mrs. Sevier plans for it to become a museum, similar to Dumbarton House, after her death.

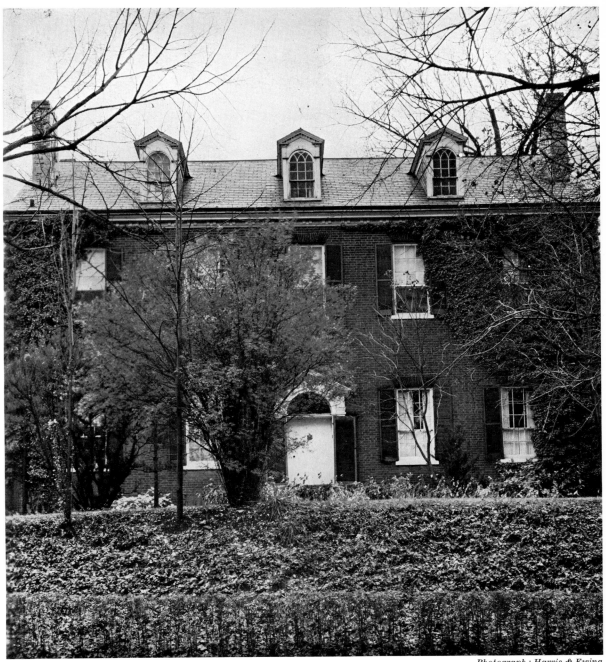

There are wings of much later date but only the original house is shown here

TUDOR PLACE

C. 1815

1644 31st Street, N. W.

Tudor Place, aloof on its shaded lawns, is an unusual example of the Federal house of semi-rural type—unique in its distinguished history, its unbroken chain of family ownership, and its authenticity as one of the few Georgetown examples of the work of the distinguished architect-doctor, William Thornton. An exquisite example of the mansion type with extended wings, it is built of stuccoed brick of buff tone, accented by the white portico and trim, and is practically unchanged from its early appearance.

The property was originally purchased in 1794 from Thomas Beall by Francis Loundes who built the two story wings before he sold it in 1805 to Thomas Peter, Mayor of Georgetown from 1789 to 1798. Here, shortly after their marriage, the latter brought his bride, Martha Parke Custis, one of the three beautiful granddaughters of Martha Washington.

It is thought that the Peter's first used the west wing as their home and the east wing as a stable. In any case, Mrs. Peter decided to use the inheritance left her by the first President to build a mansion here, and the house was completed about 1816 according to Thornton's design. Here Lafayette was entertained when he visited Georgetown in 1824 and the house for many years became the background for a brilliant social scene stemming from the family's associations. Today it contains a notable collection of Washington family relics.

The south facade of the house is characterized by a masterful treatment of both mass and detail and is remarkable for the great main windows surmounted by arches, as well as for Thornton's two story "temple" or domed circular portico, half of which is a niche recessed into the center hall. The northern front, in contrast, is severely treated, and overlooks a circular "turn-around" and a great garden with fine old box. The north, or carriage entrance, opens into an unusual transverse hall backing three large rooms. Those at the sides contain handsome crystal chandeliers, delicate marble mantels, plaster friezes, and unusual doors of highly polished curly maple with great brass locks. The dining room, conservatory and kitchen are in the wings.

Mr. and Mrs. Peter, who built the mansion, had eight children. To Britannia the youngest child, and widow of Commodore Beverley Kennon, USN, who was killed in the tragic explosion aboard the U.S.S. Princeton in 1844, Mrs. Thomas Peter bequeathed Tudor Place. Mrs. Kennon, left a widow before she was thirty, lived to be ninety-six and died at Tudor Place in 1911. Her only child, Martha Custis Kennon, married her cousin, Dr. Armistead Peter, and thus the Peter name returned to this house which has never been out of the family. Today, it is the residence of their son, Armistead Peter, Jr.

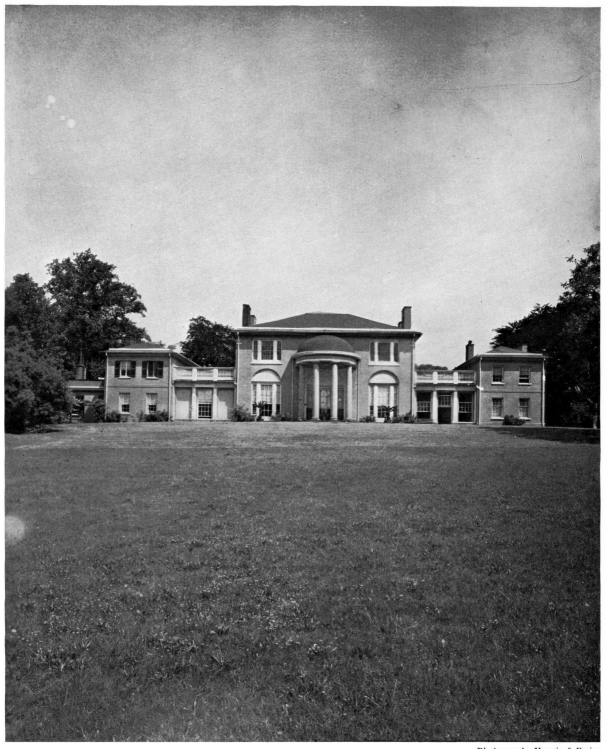

Photograph : Harris & Ewing

The distinguished South front

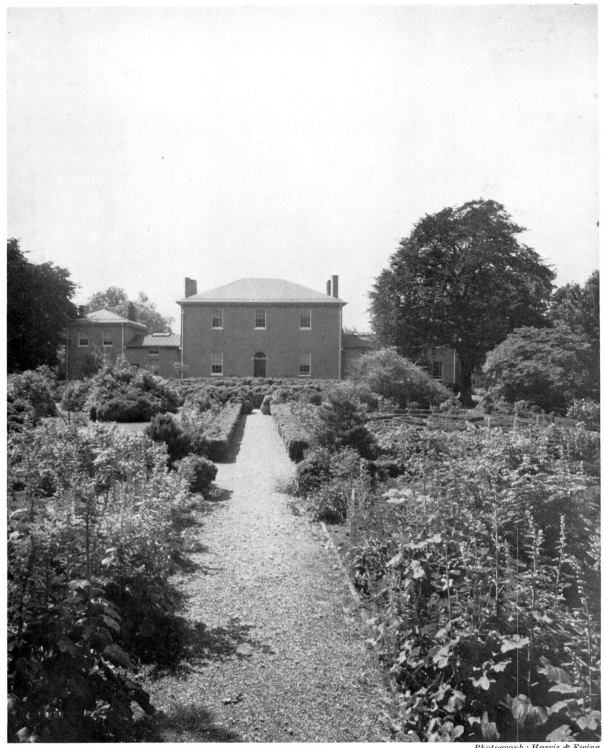

The extreme simplicity of the North facade. Interesting contrast of formal box planting in the background and old-fashioned flower garden in the foreground.

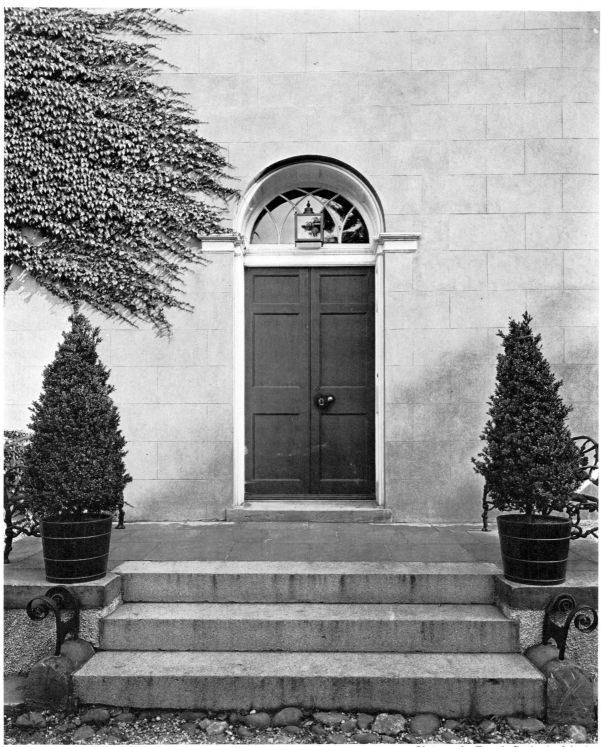

Exquisite precision in a doorway

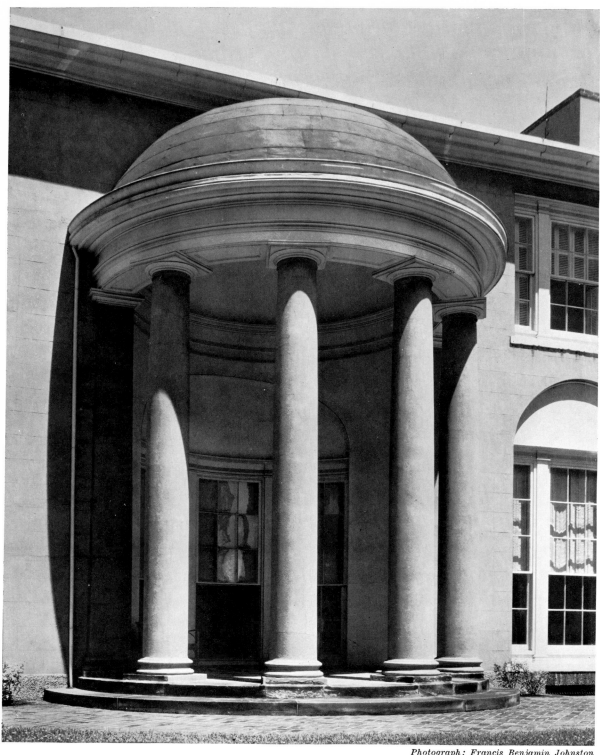

Photograph: Francis Benjamin Johnston

The Temple

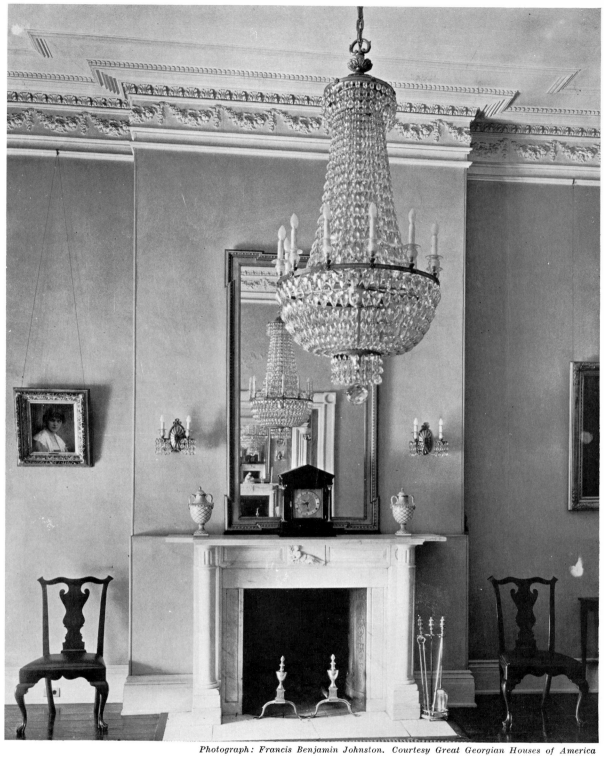

This marble mantel and plaster frieze reflect Thornton's classic mood

EVERMAY
1792
1623 28th Street, N. W.

One of the most beautiful sites in Georgetown is occupied by Evermay, built in 1792 by Samuel Davidson and now the residence of Mr. and Mrs. F. Lammot Belin.

Davidson, a bachelor, well known for his peculiarities, was a successful speculator in real estate, one of the proprietors of the District of Columbia, and with David Burns, owner of the land now occupied by the White House and Lafayette Park. He bequeathed his estate to his nephew Lewis Grant providing that he assumed the name of Davidson. The latter's daughter, Eliza Grant Davidson, who inherited the house, married Charles Dodge in a quadruple wedding June 12, 1847, and Evermay became another Dodge residence. On this occasion four of the Dodges were married at four o'clock in the morning in order that the bridal couples could take the five o'clock stage for Baltimore.

In the later Nineteenth Century the house was owned by the McPherson family and for many years was leased to William B. Orme. The present owners are responsible for its brilliant restoration and improvement. A coat of yellow stucco was removed from the house which was enlarged; the grounds were complemented with a brick wall and gatehouse, and a magnificent formal garden was created which is, in itself, a noteworthy collection of box, magnolia and azalea.

Its eccentric builder's desire to preserve the serenity of Evermay lives in his noteworthy advertisement of June 2, 1810, which forewarned "at their peril, all persons, of whatever age, color, or standing in society, from trespassing on the premises, in any manner, by day or by night; particularly all thieving knaves and idle vagabonds; all rambling parties; all assignation parties; all amorous bucks with their dorfies, and all sporting bucks with their dogs and guns"—and proclaimed, "For the information of those persons who may have real business on the premises, there is a good and convenient gate. But Mark! I do not admit mere curiosity as an errand of business. Therefore, I beg and pray of all my neighbors to avoid Evermay as they would a den of devils, or rattlesnakes, and thereby save themselves and me much vexation and trouble. Samuel Davidson."

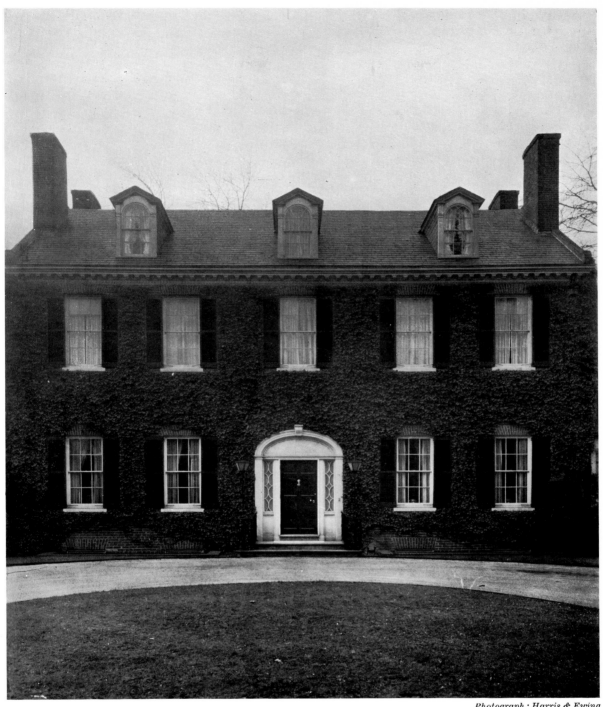

There are wings of later date. However, this photograph shows only the original entrance facade.

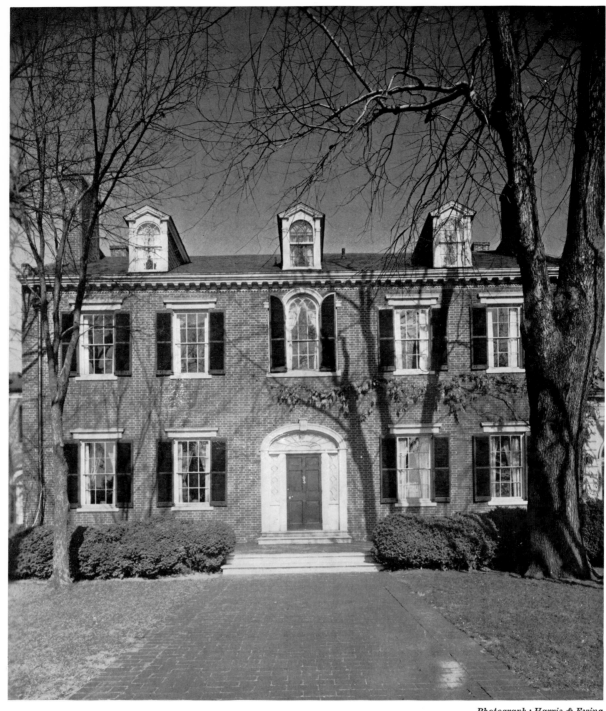

The garden facade. A formal brick house with superb detail

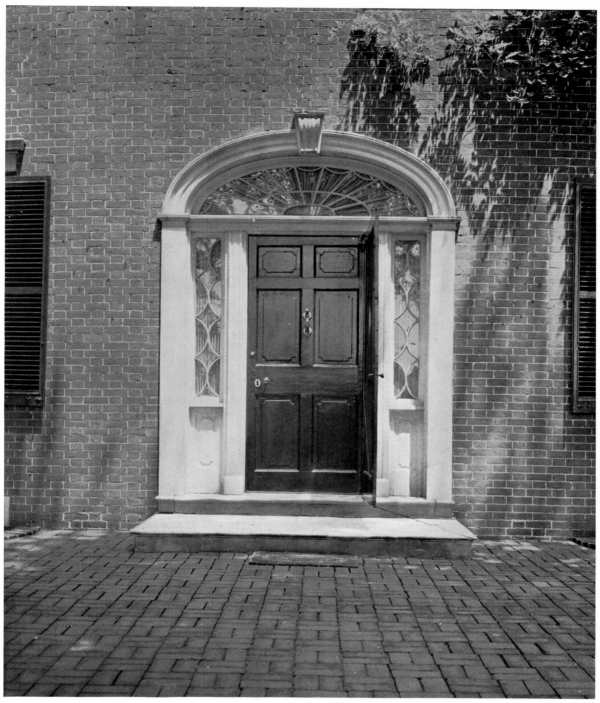

The garden doorway

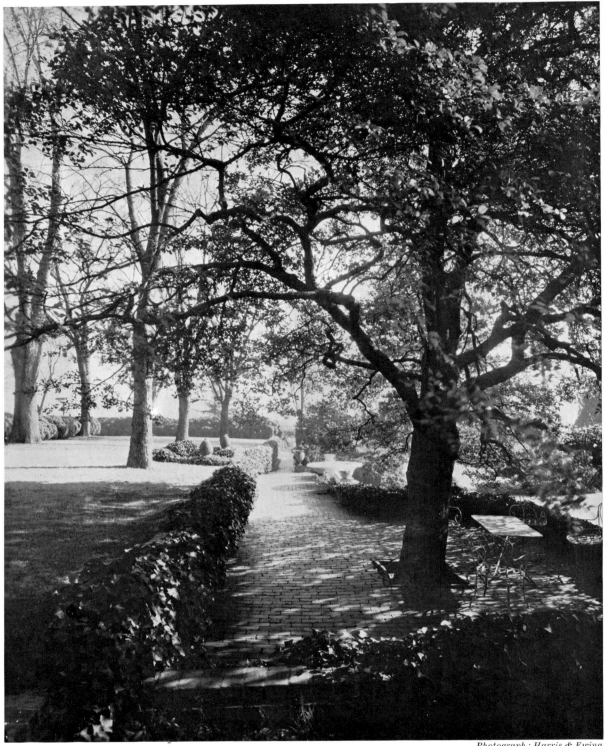

Photograph : Harris & Ewing

A garden walk—Washington in the distance

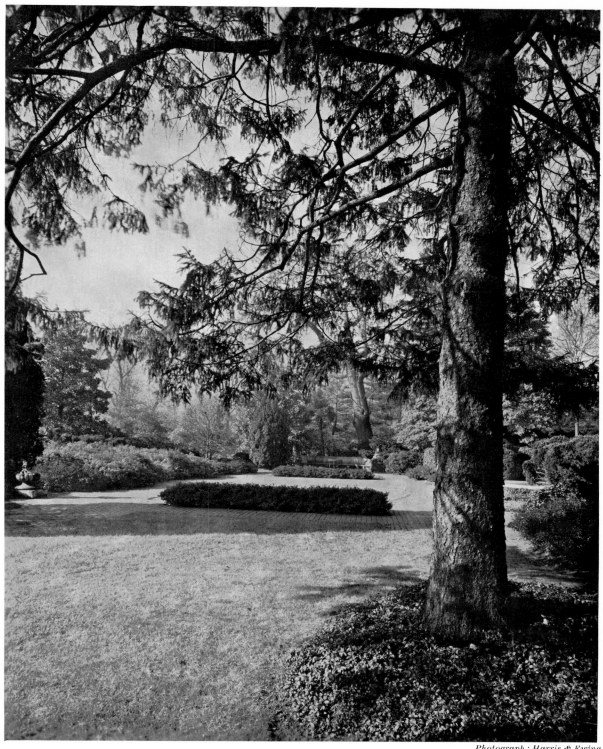

Photograph : Harris & Ewing

Restoration planting at its best

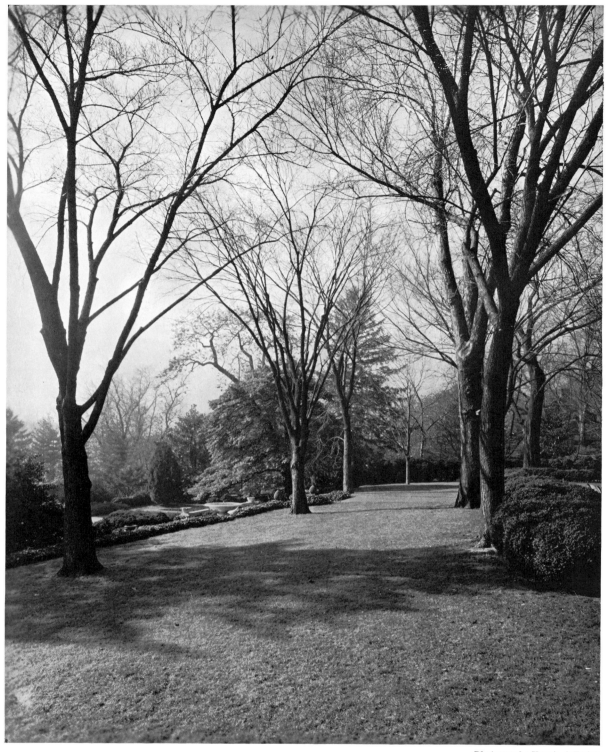

Sky Tracery—Autumn

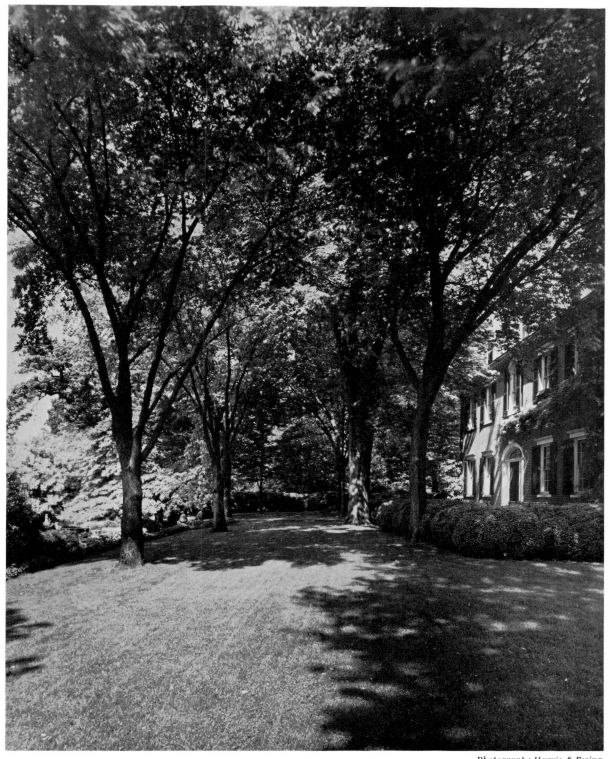

Photograph : Harris & Ewing

Spring Contrast

DUMBARTON HOUSE
C. 1805
2715 Q Street, N. W.

Dumbarton House, or Bellevue as it was called for a hundred-odd years before its purchase by the Colonial Dames in 1928, is possibly the earliest, and certainly one of the loveliest, of the "great houses" of Georgetown. It is a two-story mansion with extended wings, characteristic of the superior pattern of Georgian house popular in Eighteenth Century Maryland and Virginia for country living. It has the usual wide central hall with four large rooms opening into it. The mantels are fine and uniquely those rooms at the rear are oval at their outside ends. The wings are much simpler in treatment than the central mass with its longer windows and delicate fretwork beneath the cornice.

It was thought for a long time that the house was built about 1796 until investigations of old deeds and wills were made at the time of its purchase in 1928 by the Colonial Dames. Those in charge of the project deduced that a house as handsome as Bellevue would not have been built in its original location after the laying out of Georgetown. Addition of four more streets to the North and East of the town would have placed Bellevue at the convergence of two of them, and until the house was moved to its present site by the District Government in 1915 it stood directly in the middle of present-day Q Street.

It is now believed that part of the house was built by George Beall, the son of Ninian Beall, original proprietor of the "Rock of Dumbarton," about 1750. George Beall vigorously protested the founding of Georgetown, complaining that his property might be "totally demolished." He may well have had this house in mind, although no streets were laid out in close proximity until 1783 when his son Thomas, who had inherited this portion of his father's estate, made his first Addition to Georgetown. Moreover, the roof of Bellevue was in danger of falling in when it was leased by Samuel Whitall in 1820 and houses built as this was do not usually disintegrate to that extent in a mere forty or fifty years. In any case, the house in its present form bears close resemblance to handsome Tulip Hill built by the Galloways on West River near Annapolis about 1755 and to His Lordships Kindness near Rosaryville, built by the fourteenth Earl of Shrewsbury as a gift to his niece and ward, Ann Talbot, on her marriage to Henry Darnell.

The property changed hands several times in the feverish land speculation following the selection of the District of Columbia as site of the capital. In 1794 Thomas Beall sold Bellevue to Peter Casanave, who kept it for two months and resold it to Col. Forrest at twenty per cent profit. After a year the Colonel conveyed it to Isaac Pollack for five times its purchase price, but Pollack sold it the following year to Samuel Jackson at less than half its cost. Bellevue was then mortgaged, remortgaged, foreclosed, and finally sold in 1804 to Gabriel Duval, Comptroller of the Currency and later a Justice of the Supreme Court of the United States. In 1805 it passed to Joseph Nourse, Registrar of the Treasury, who remodeled it according to Latrobe's design and who lived there until 1813 when he sold it to Charles Carroll, who had purchased a paper mill on Rock Creek below the house with his brother Daniel of Duddington, and who thereafter styled himself "of Bellevue." According to legend, Mrs. Madison met the President here and agreed on the route of their retreat when the British burned the White House in 1814. Bellevue was leased to Samuel Whitall of Philadelphia in 1820 and was sold to his son by Carroll's executors in 1841. It subsequently was owned by the Rittenhouse family and the Hinkleys until its purchase by John L. Newbold in 1912. Shortly afterward it was moved to its present location and finally purchased and restored by the present owners.

Now handsomely furnished as of the period of 1790 to 1810, and complemented by beautiful gardens, this representative Georgian house has been open to the public until its recent temporary assignment to the Red Cross for war work.

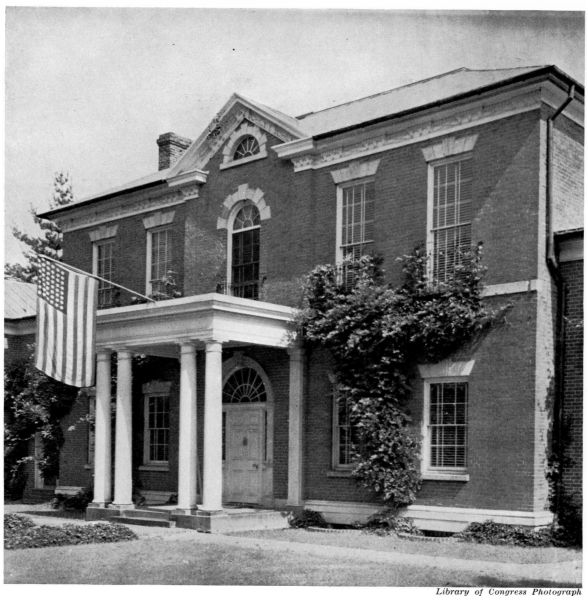

The Central South facade as restored by the National Society of Colonial Dames

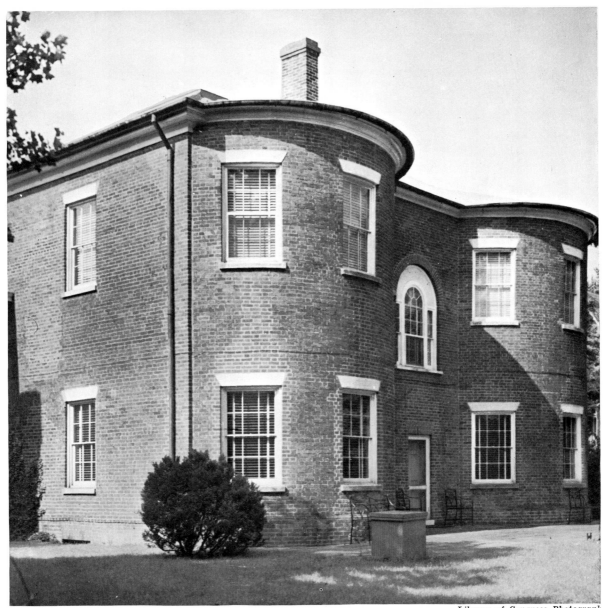

The semi-circular bays are emphasized in this view from the garden

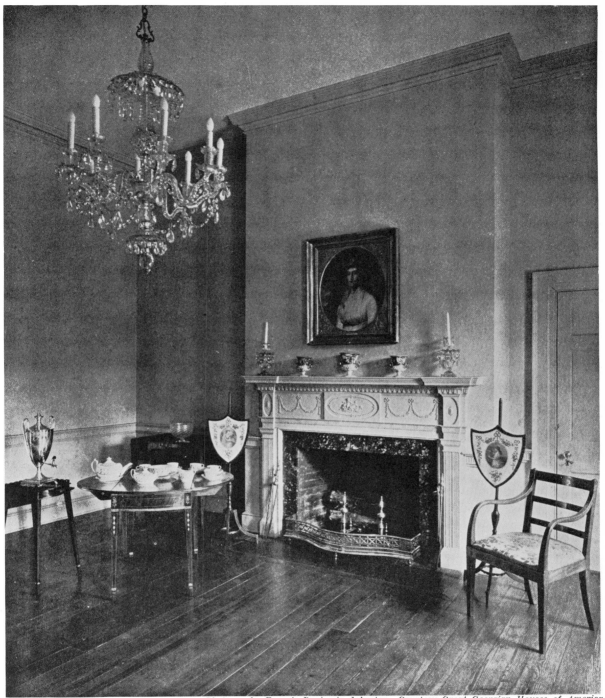

Photograph: Francis Benjamin Johnston. Courtesy Great Georgian Houses of America

Furniture, mantel and bric-a-brac in perfect scale and harmony

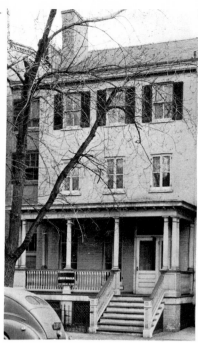

Photograph taken in 1943 showing 150 years accumulation of paint and architectural changes.

THE HYDE HOUSE
C. 1798
1319 30th Street, N. W.

This house was built about 1798 by Charles Beatty who had purchased the lot on which it stands from Thomas Beall the year before. Colonel Beatty owned the ferry which plied the Potomac between the foot of Frederick (34th) Street and the Virginia shore, and in 1806 sold the house to Nicholas Hedges. It passed to James Belt in 1822 and to Joshua Stuart in 1832. The latter is thought to have added the present full third story, as well as a wing to the rear.

The house was later purchased by Thomas Hyde, an early merchant of the town, and was later the residence of his son, Anthony, for many years secretary to the distinguished philanthropist W. W. Corcoran. Recently when Deering Davis restored the house for Morehead Patterson he found a quaint old sign bearing the following bit of doggerel and dating back to the elder Hyde:

> *"Hyde's my name, and Hides I buy*
> *3¢ for wet and 5¢ for dry."*

The small photograph above shows the house as it was in 1943 before restoration began. On page 107 one sees the structure as it now appears and almost as it was in 1797. However the roof was originally of steeper pitch and extended to just above the second story windows. The third floor plan was as it is today but the windows were dormers. About 1830 the roof line was changed and the facade extended to include them. More than 20 coats of paint were removed by steam and chemicals to recover the original fine salmon colored brick. Now the house looks almost too new and passersby remark on the difficulties that must have been encountered in painting all the joint lines white, little realizing that the lime mortar is almost 150 years old.

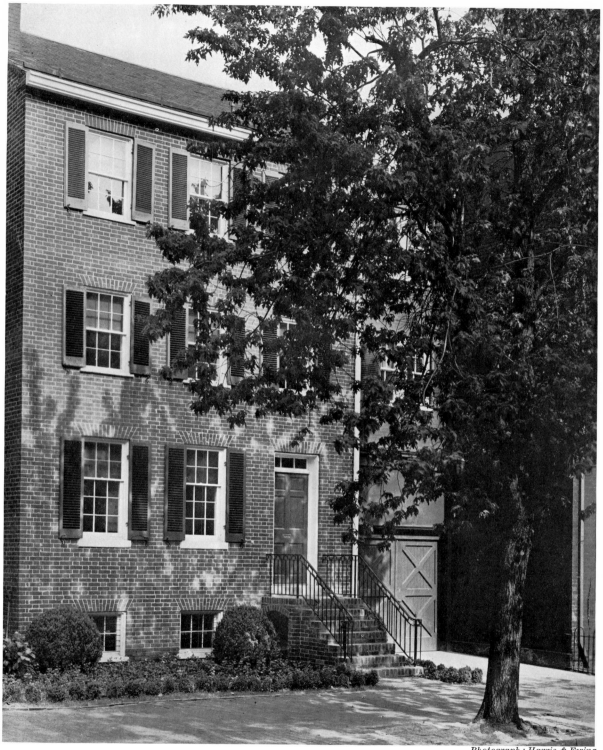

Photograph taken in 1944 illustrates perfectly a restoration to its original state of 1798

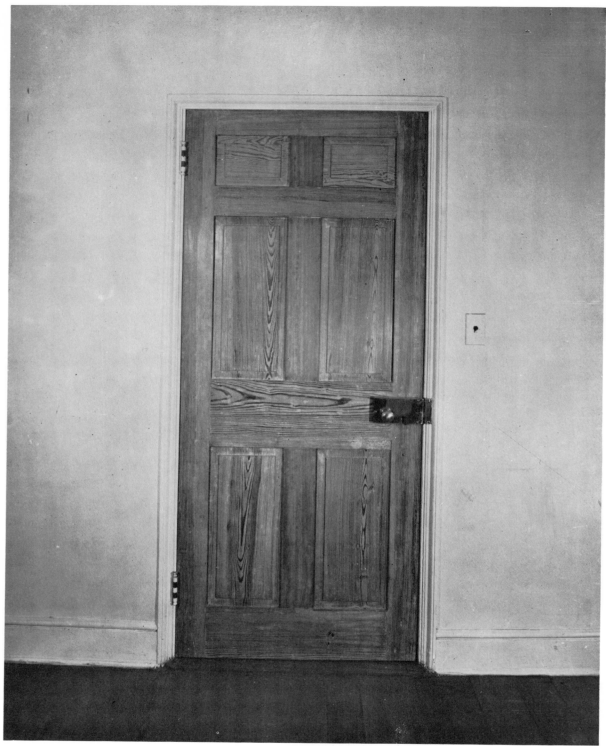

Photograph : Harris & Ewing

The house has original panelled doors of perfect scale with old locks of almost jewel-like re-finement. For years they were covered and caked with numerous coats of paint.

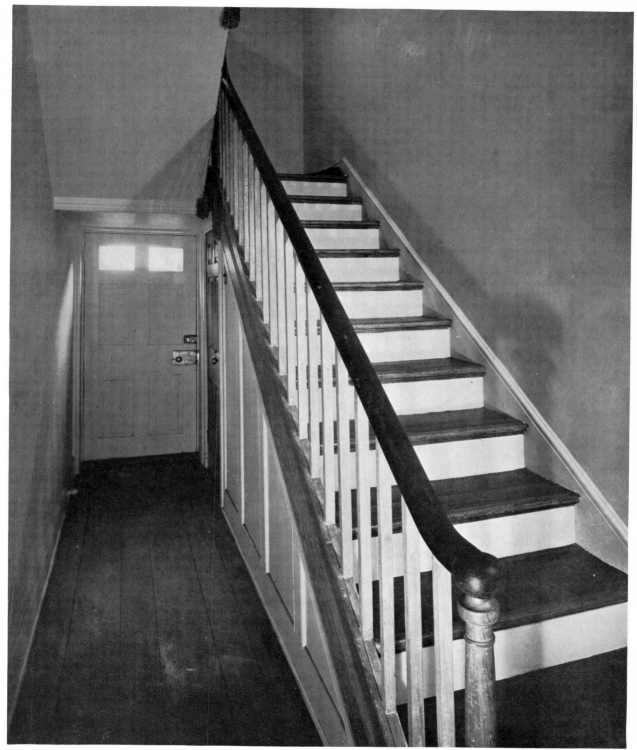

Photograph : Harris & Ewing

An unusual reeded stair panel of waxed red pine running to the third floor. The plain painted panels underneath are typical of the Post-Revolutionary Period in contrast to the raised and beveled type of earlier date. Note original wide pine flooring.

GEORGE WASHINGTON'S HOUSES ON CAPITOL HILL

In the Eighteenth Century an interest in architecture and a taste for decoration seem to have been almost universal characteristics of the gentry. Jefferson's abilities in these directions are well known. Old letters, architectural libraries, estates and houses of the period testify to similar interests on the part of his contemporaries. While Washington inferred in several letters to Dr. Thornton that he was ignorant of architectural principles and claimed that he had "no other guide but his eye," in the same letters he discusses features of two houses which he wished to have built in the new national capital with deep perception and judgment that belie his claims. Other writings as well as the details of the classic state dining room and west parlor which he added to his inheritance, Mount Vernon, are adequate indications of his taste and interest.

The outstanding architects of the day were employed by the leaders of the young Republic to build both public and domestic buildings. In this connection the fact that President Washington engaged Dr. William Thornton to design two private houses for him on Capitol Hill becomes of particular interest. The same architects, of course, designed the outstanding buildings in both Georgetown and Washington itself, but documentary evidence of the work is almost entirely confined to public structures or large houses of mansion or manor type, such as Octagon House and Tudor Place. With few exceptions, the smaller type of town dwelling found in Georgetown, the subject of most of the preceding illustrations, cannot be connected authentically with any prominent architect, even though legend attributes many of them to Dr. Thornton.

These houses were so simple in mass and such a direct adaptation of a well established English prototype that any competent carpenter-contractor could and did build them. However, the design of both exterior and interior trim and detail was copied exactly and directly from the best examples of the known works of Thornton, Hoban and Latrobe.

Therefore, newly discovered details of the building and design of two such town houses actually planned for the first President by William Thornton, the most influential of these architectural leaders, who first planned the new Capitol and whose work there General Washington actively supported, becomes particularly significant.

Several writers have claimed that Dr. Thornton built a double house on Capitol Hill for the President in 1792 or 1793 where he lived for part of three years, stopping on his return from Philadelphia at the close of Congressional sessions to examine the progress of the erection of the Capitol building. These seem to be perfectly reasonable statements, but further research has uncovered several letters written in December 1798 and August and September 1799 giving definite details of the two houses for which Thornton was actually architect and supervisor of construction during the last two years of the President's life. Another letter of Washington's to Alexander White speaks of these houses, indicating that they were being built as an investment as well as for the convenience of Members of Congress, for whom adequate lodging was so difficult to obtain, and stating that at a later date the President would perhaps build a town house for his personal use. Although he had purchased some lots in that section of Washington in 1792 and 1793 the combination of letters mentioned above dispels any thesis that Washington had a residence in the District and that his letters to Thornton referred to two additional houses he wished to build. Washington wrote as follows:

To William Thornton.

(See complete original letter page 114)

Mount Vernon
Dec. 20th, 1798

Dear Sir,

I saw a building in Philadelphia of about the same dimensions in front and elevation that are to be given to my two houses,—which pleased me.—It consisted also of two houses, united Doors in the center, a Pediment in the Roof and dormer windows on each side of it in front, skylight in the rear.—

If this is not incongruous with rules of Architecture, I should be glad to have my two houses executed in this style.

* * * * * *

To William Thornton

Mount Vernon,
30th Dec. 1798

Dear Sir,

Your favor of the 25th. instant, enclosing Messrs. Blagden & Leuthals estimate of the cost of adding a Pediment, and Parapet to the roof of my buildings in the Federal City, has been duly received, but the plan, to which it refers, did not accompany it.—

This plan, on other accounts, I ought to be possessed of, and Mr. Blagden is under promise to take a copy thereof for his own use, to work by, and to send me the original draught.—I pray you to remind him of this promise.—

Presuming that it is not necessary for Mr. Blagden's convenience that I should, at this moment, decide upon the above estimate; nor whether I shall adopt the measure at all; I shall, if no disadvantage will attend the delay, suspend my determination until I can visit the City, & receive some further explanations respecting the consequent alterations which will be occasioned by this Pediment—not at present well understood by me; owing to my entire ignorance of the technical terms in which they are expressed.—At which time also, I will make arrangements for giving him further pecuniary aid.

Rules of Architecture are calculated, I presume, to give symmetry, and just proportion to all the Orders, & parts of buildings, in order to please the eye.—Small departures from strict rules are discoverable only by skilful architects, or by the eye of criticism; while ninety-nine in a hundred—deficient of their knowledge—might be pleased with things not quite orthodox.—This, more than probable, would be the case relative to a Pediment in the Roof over the doors of my houses in the City.—

That a Parapet in addition (for the reasons you have assigned) would have a pleasing & useful effect, cannot be doubted.—When the roof of a building is to be seen—and when it is designed for Chambers it must be seen—something to relieve the view of a plain and dead Surface, is indispensable:—for this reason it was, I thought, and still do think that Dormars are to be preferred to Sky lights in the front;—on the other hand, if the roof is so flat as not to be seen at all, or so low as, in a manner to be hid by a Parapet, I should give a decided preference to Sky lights.—

These ideas, as you will readily perceive, proceed from a person who avows his ignorance of Architectural principles,—and who has no other guide but his eye, to direct his choice:—I never, for a moment, contemplated two Pediments, one over the door of each house, my great object was to give them the appearance of one.—But as I have observed in the former part of this letter, I will suspend coming to any decision until the consequences of the proposed alterations are better understood by me.—

The freedom with which you have expressed your sentiments on this occasion, is highly pleasing to me.—Sorry indeed should I have been on this, as I shall be on any future occurrence, when your opinion may be asked, if they are not rendered with the utmost frankness and candour.—

The compliments of the season are presented to Mrs. Thornton, yourself & Co. by all parts of this family,—and with great esteem and regard I remain, &c.

* * * * * *

To John Francis.

Mount Vernon,
Aug. 25, 1799.

Cost of two Lots in the Federal City, extending from North Capitol Street to New Jersey Avenue in Square 634, together with the expense of the Buildings now erecting thereon, according to

Contract; and an estimate of work not included in the said Contract, occasioned by alterations agreed on since.

viz

	Dollars
For lot No. 16, bought from the Commissioners	535.71
" " " 7, " " Mr. Daniel Carroll**	428.40

On the price of these lots considerable abatement was made, on condition of my building *two* brick houses *three* stories high each.

To Mr. Blagden, Undertaker of the Buildings, according to written Contract. Estimate of Glazing, Painting and Ironmougry* } 11,250.00

Conceiving these charges were high, in the estimate, *I took them, upon myself. But whether I shall lose by so doing, remains to be decided. Mr. Blagden assured me he could not obtain them on better terms than was specified ** of Duddington.

Glazing and Painting, agreeably to this estimate handed in by Mr. Blagden, but not agreed to, nor included in Contract	840.00
Ironmongry Ditto—Do—Do	397.20

A well of fine water at the back doors of both houses; 30 odd feet deep, walled, and a pump therein; the cost of which has not been exhibited, as it was procured to be done by Mr. Blagden, and paid for by him, out of the monies advanced him for general purposes. ....

A Pediment and Parapet, in addition to the original cost of the Buildings. No specific sum agreed on for erecting them ....

	Carried over	$13,451.31
Cost of two lots brought over		13,451.31

...For the original design of.....to add to the appearance of the House: also undefined in the cost ....

Papering all the Rooms, except Cellars and garrets,....being, by Contract to have to... of Plaster than is merely sufficient for that purpose. ....

*The press copy was poorly made. Words indicated by leaders are illegible.

Writings of Washington Col. 37, Nov. 1798-Dec. 1799.

* * * * * *

To Wm. Thornton

Mt. Vernon
Oct. 1, 1799

Painters finding all materials, will do the windows, and cornice, and doors, in short all the exterior of the Buildings, the roof excepted (which must remain for future decision) upon the Terms, etc.

* * * * * *

To John Avery

(In part)

Mt. Vernon,
Sept. 25, 1799.

Although my house, or houses (for they may be one or two as occasion requires) are, I believe upon a larger scale than any in the vicinity of the Capitol, yet they fall far short of your wishes. The largest room, and that occasionally made so, is not more than 40 (sic) feet in length. The houses are three flush stories of Brick, besides Garret rooms; and in the judgment of those better acquainted in these matters than I am capable of accommodating between twenty and thirty boarders. The buildings are not costly, but elegantly plain and the whole cost, at pretty near guess, may be between 15 and 16 thousand dollars.

* * * * * *

Further search has brought to light the photograph of this famous double house with many changes, shown on page 117. It had obviously been converted into a five story hotel

112

with a Mansard roof. When great granite blocks were being hauled for the construction of the Senate wing of the Capitol, the road was much cut down to ease the grade and facilitate the task. This bank was then cut into, and two stories were added underneath the house while the roof was changed to the Mansard type. A better picture was finally discovered which appears on page 116, and shows a third house nearest the camera. This house can be seen at the extreme left with its original entrance undoubtedly similar to the others. Interestingly enough Thornton used similar Ionic columns in the entrance of Octagon House.

The illustration on page 115 shows an interpretation of the front elevation of the two houses as ordered by George Washington who died a few months before their completion in 1799. The day following the Battle of Bladensburg in 1814 they were burned, but the walls remained, and in 1818 these houses were rebuilt. Only four years had passed so that the memory of their appearance must have been very clear and as Dr. Thornton was still active they were undoubtedly restored to their original exterior condition except for the omission of pediment and parapet, the changing of the window lintels and the addition of a string course. The pediment and parapet were not restored in all probability, both to save expense and because the houses were to be used for boarders and the dormers gave additional space and light to the garret rooms. In the rendered drawing the design of the window lintels has been changed from those in the photographs, since the key type of lintel rather than the end block form, was used in all buildings authentically attributed to Thornton. The plaques were also typical of his work.

These buildings were razed in 1913 and we are indebted to the historical interest of two Massachusetts officers for the picture of the houses as they appeared at the time of the Civil War. It was at their request that Brady, the great photographer, took the plate in 1863, and preserved a pictorial record of the only two authentically documented Thornton town houses of the smaller type so popular in Georgetown.

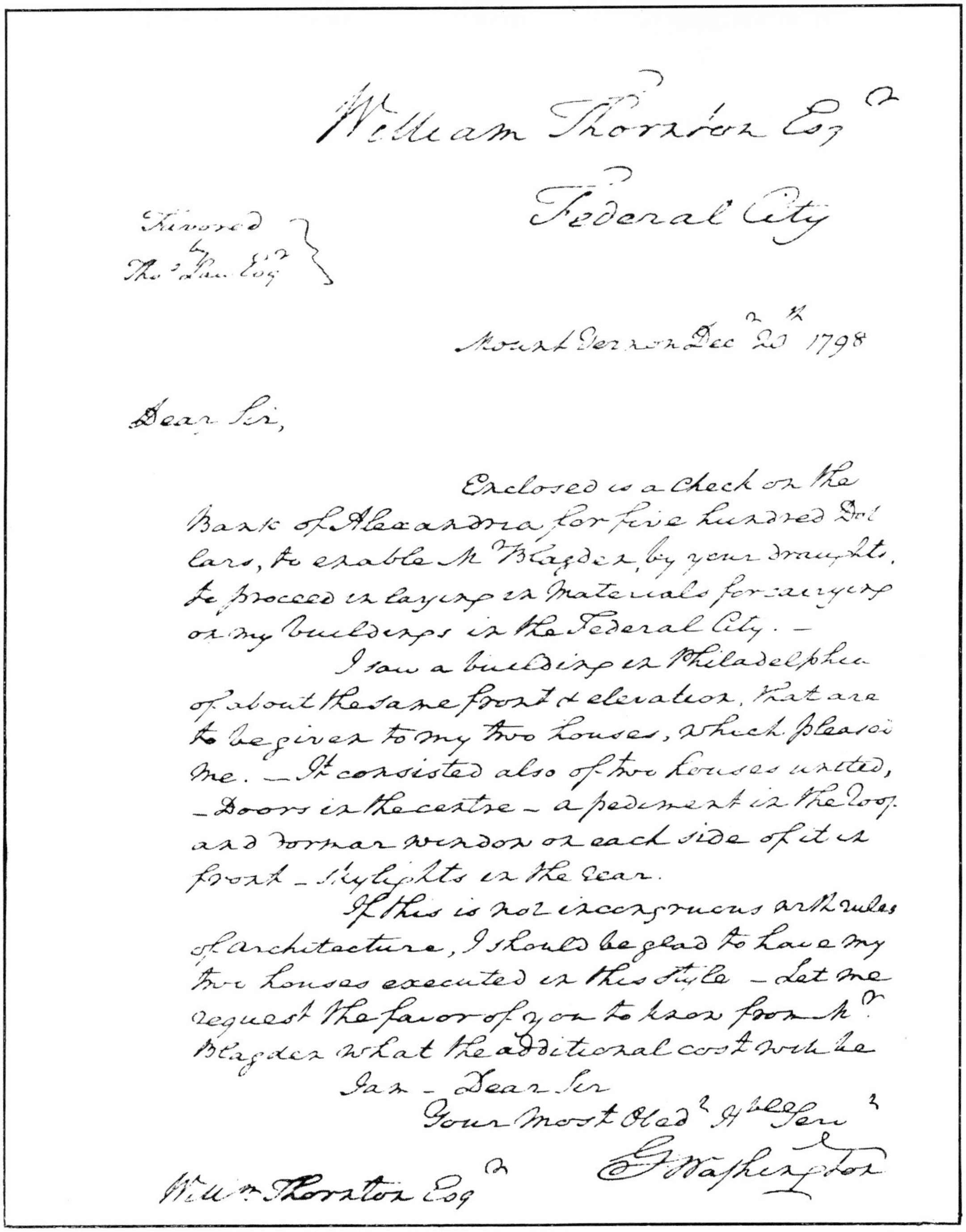

William Thornton Esq^a

Federal City

Favored
_by_
The ^e Law Esq^a

Mount Vernon Dec^o 20th 1798

Dear Sir,

Enclosed is a check on the Bank of Alexandria, for five hundred Dollars, to enable Mr Blagden, by your draughts, to proceed in laying in materials for carrying on my buildings in the Federal City. —

I saw a building in Philadelphia of about the same front & elevation, that are to be given to my two houses, which pleased me. — It consisted also of two houses united, — Doors in the centre — a pediment in the roof, and dormar window on each side of it in front — Skylights in the rear.

If this is not incongruous with rules of architecture, I should be glad to have my two houses executed in this style — Let me request the favor of you to know from Mr Blagden what the additional cost will be

I am — Dear Sir
    Your most Obed^t H^ble Servt
                G Washington

Wm. Thornton Esq^a

By permission of the Columbia Historical Society. Library of Congress Photograph

Photograph of letter. The signature of this letter is unassailable documentary evidence verifying the facts of this chapter.

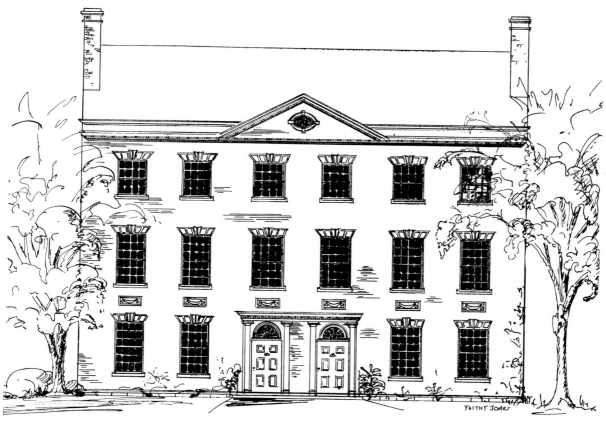

Drawing by Faith Jones

Illustrations on pages 116-117, plus the letters on pages 111-112 clearly demonstrate that **this** drawing shows the original appearance of the distinguished double house ordered by George Washington.

Cut this house in half, remove Pediment, substitute Dormers for Parapet and the prototype of a typical Georgetown house clearly emerges.

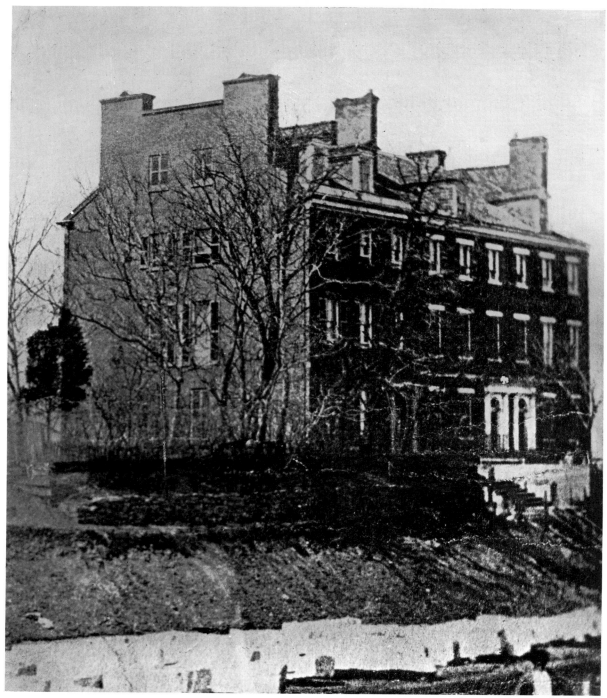

This photograph was taken in 1861 and shows George Washington's double house as it was rebuilt in 1818, after burning in 1814. There is a third house at the end nearest the camera.

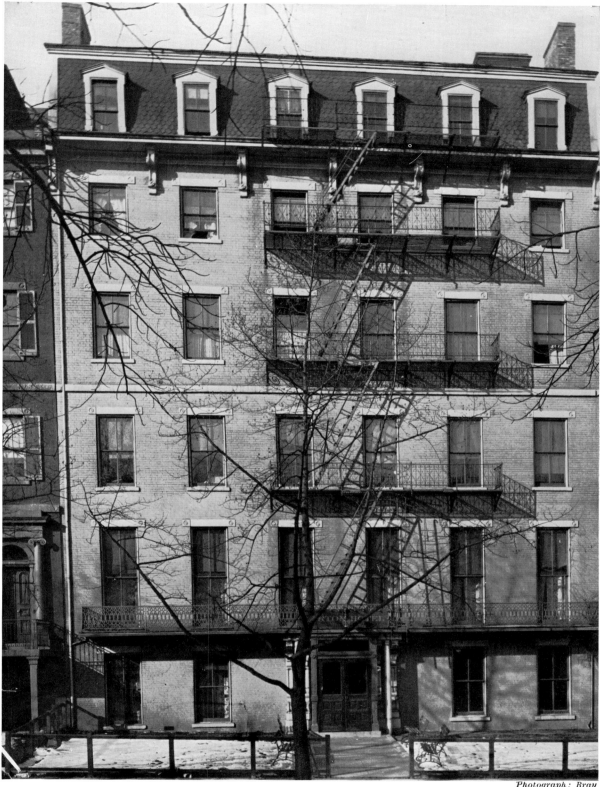

The street much cut down to haul the granite blocks, so plainly visible, is shown on preceding page. The face of the hill was cut away and two stories added underneath to create this five story hotel with added Mansard roof, more dormers, fire escapes, etc.

THE PRE-REVOLUTIONARY DWELLINGS

Georgetown's days of glory were encompassed within the limits of the last quarter of the Eighteenth and the first quarter of the Nineteenth Centuries. It was during this period that the characteristic Federal Houses, for which she is noted, developed; yet any comprehensive account of this town's great architectural idiom, would be incomplete if it did not cover briefly the local antecedents from which its features were derived.

The ordinary conception of Georgetown houses as "Colonial" is, as already indicated, quite erroneous, as few pre-revolutionary structures remain standing. There were perhaps fifty good brick houses in the town in 1775. Of these and their frame counterparts, with the exception of minor portions of later structures, only six authentic examples remain—all, in bad residential areas. Before these few are lost entirely, it is regrettable that several are not moved to good locations and intelligently restored. Already two have been so completely gutted that nothing but the original walls remain. While there are a number of other dwellings—or more correctly parts thereof,—bearing the legend of a building date before 1775, they have been so altered in every exterior and interior feature, that one can only say that their present appearance is that of a considerably later period. Certainly this excludes them from the company of houses which clearly demonstrate the distinct style of the local Colonial or earlier Georgian period.

To the discerning eye there are distinct differences in the exterior appearance of houses built before and after the Revolution. The characteristic local idiom of the post-revolutionary period has already been discussed. In structures of the preceding era bricks are less regular and more obviously of hand moulded origin. The roof angle is generally more pronounced, window openings may have flat arches, and there is usually a water table beneath the principal story capped by an extended course of hand shaped bricks. Dormer details, window size and trim and entrance door details are quite different. Siding in frame structures, is generally of great width. In fact, it is the wood trim both within and without which shows such marked variance that a modicum of serious training is necessary to enable one to distinguish between products of the two epochs with reasonable ease.

The famous stone house on M Street shown on page 120 has been the subject of countless legends and disputes over its identity as Washington's Engineering headquarters and as the renowned Suter's Tavern. In any case, we do know that it was built about 1765 by Christopher Lehman, that it was frequently rented, and that it once served as an ordinary of which Cassandra Chew was at one time proprietess. Its interior paneling and trim is good but rather obviously transplanted to this house from an earlier location. It is of ell shape and the stone terminates at the eave line—the gable ends being of brick. A similar variation in the bonds used may be seen in the treatment of some of the very early Virginia country houses of simple brick type. The large twenty-light window on the ground floor is somewhat reminiscent of those in Alexandria's Ramsey House built in 1755. It is interesting that Washington's small Alexandria town house—recently demolished, shocking as the fact is —was strikingly similar to the Lehman house.

One of the other dwellings is of frame construction. The tiny cottage on 28th Street, now so gaily painted dark blue and yellow, was built prior to 1775 and has remained almost unchanged in a wonderful state of preservation—a tribute to the craftsmen who built it, and the honest timbers used. The extreme width of the hand hewn boards (shown on the ex-

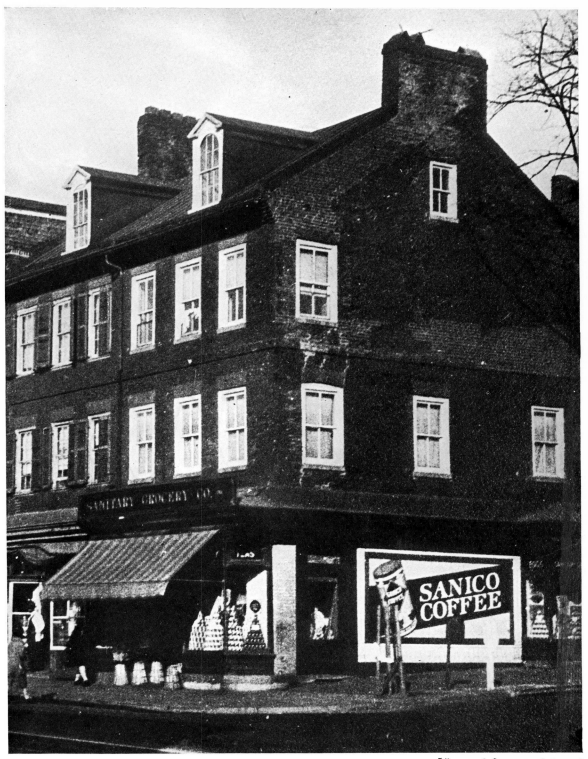

3001 and 3003 M Street

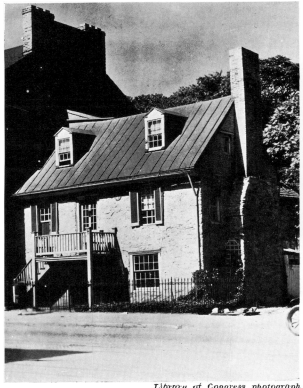 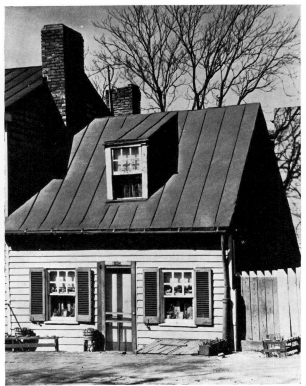

3049 M Street   1222 28th Street

posed end) of the house on page 120 is impressive in an age when great forest timbers are no longer a characteristic of the country.

Of the remaining five, the two brick houses at the corner of 30th and M Streets, shown on page 119 are the finest examples of late pre-revolutionary buildings in the town. The interior trim still extant on the second floor is excellent, and the houses carry the characteristic water table mentioned above, oddly enough, between the first and second stories. Uniquely one of the window openings to be seen in the illustration is topped by a flat arch.

Exhaustive research indicates that these two houses were originally one, a very fine 2½ story mansion house of the Maryland type. The street level has been cut down so that the former basement is now the street level shops as shown in plate. The unusual placement of the water table mentioned above is thus accounted for.

The great significance of these houses lies in their early contribution to the American Architectual tradition. Such structures are becoming more scarce with each passing year. Surely more active measures should be taken to preserve the remaining earlier homes of our forefathers that are still spared.

STRUCTURES NOW STANDING IN GEORGETOWN
ERECTED BEFORE 1825

An accurate list of all structures still standing in the town, erected during the Georgian and early Federal period is extremely difficult to compile. It is expected that omissions in the following—particularly of smaller frame structures—will be found and that some readers will disagree with certain dates in connection with individual buildings.

The site, originally situated in part of Prince George's County, Maryland (organized from part of Charles County in 1695), became part of Montgomery County when it was created in 1776. The town, although organized in 1751, was not incorporated until 1789, and did not give up its charter of separate government, which it had kept even after inclusion in the District of Columbia, until 1871. Records are therefore scanty and scattered, and many have been lost.

Consequently dates with any documentary semblance of accuracy are unobtainable in a great many cases. Thus no dates are given where tradition or research have not afforded reasonable ones in conformity with the original architectural detail of the structure in question. Buildings no longer standing, unrecognizably altered, or containing a very slight portion of the original, as in the case of the Key Mansion, have not been included.

M STREET AND WISCONSIN AVENUE
(Formerly Bridge and High Streets)

These streets, which are primarily commercial today, contain a number of structures which are evidently of this approximate period. Except where otherwise noted they are of brick construction (usually only the fronts are of Flemish bond), of two or three stories and attic, the majority with two or four end chimneys. In every case they are today business or commercial buildings, frequently dilapidated, often almost unrecognizably altered. Most of them are characterized by one or two dormers of widely varying architectural worth and states of repair, and occasional remnants of good architectural detail. Regrettably, those with the most interesting historical associations have been completely razed.

M Street—Numbers 2803, 2919, 3001, 3003, 3005, 3009, 3026, 3041, 3049 (Christopher Lehman House, built by him in 1764 of field stone with brick gables. This small story and a half house of ell shape, with steep pitched roof and dormers is reminiscent of Williamsburg. Its ceilings are low and the rooms are small. Traditionally Washington's engineering headquarters when he planned the Federal city with L'Enfant, the authenticity of this legend has been disputed for many years.) 3053, 3064, 3066, 3068, 3112, 3116, 3204, 3209, 3211, 3232 (clapboard), 3249, 3264, 3350 (built in 1791 by Col. Uriah Forrest, then Mayor. In 1830 it became the home of William Marbury, and is now greatly changed).

Wisconsin Avenue—Numbers 1211, 1218, 1220, 1221, 1255 (John Lutz House—now a home for aged women); N. W. corner of Wisconsin and M Streets (interesting corner store built in 1817 for W. W. Corcoran & Co.);

1322 and 1324 (originally one clapboard house with heavy center chimney), 1503 (clapboard), 1507, 1515, 1517, 1522, 1524, 1525, 1529, 1611.

BELOW M STREET

This area, where most of the business activity of the town took place before 1800, is to-day a region of warehouses, industrial buildings, and dilapidated early structures. Bordering the old Chesapeake and Ohio Canal as it does, it has a unique charm of its own, and there are encouraging signs in the recent renovation of some of its neglected houses, which are generally of much smaller scale than those on or above M Street. Because of its homogeneous character this section of the town has been treated here as if it were one street. Interesting structures of the period are to be found at the following addresses:

3037 K Street (formerly Wapping). A warehouse.

K Street—Second warehouse from the corner of Wisconsin Avenue.

K Street (old West Lane Keys) between Cecil Alley and Potomac Street. A three-story warehouse. The Eastern section has a water table characteristic of pre-Revolutionary houses and was probably erected ca 1760. The roof line has been changed.

K Street (formerly Water Street) between 33rd and 34th Streets. A large four story warehouse, ca 1790.

1068 and 1070 30th Street (formerly Washington Street). Two interesting one story brick cottages, each with two dormers.

1058 Jefferson Street, Potomac Masonic Lodge No. 5. This small building with dilapidated classic facade, stands next to the Canal and was built in 1810. The Lodge participated in the laying of the cornerstone of the Capitol, September 18, 1793.

1041 Jefferson Street—Simple two story brick house.

1063, 1067, 1071, 1074, 1076 Jefferson Street. Five small two story houses with dormered attics.

1006, 1008, 1010 Wisconsin Avenue (formerly Water Street). Group of three fine old warehouses. The center building is thought to have been built about 1770.

1066 Wisconsin Avenue (formerly Water Street). Vigilant Firehouse. Built ca 1825 on the edge of the Canal. Now a store.

1052 and 1060 Potomac Street. Small two story houses with dormered attics.

1041 33rd Street (formerly Duck Lane). Two story house of clapboard construction with great center chimney.

PROSPECT STREET

3400—STODDERT HOUSE.

Benjamin Stoddert, first Secretary of the Navy, built this house in 1783. Regrettably altered by nondescript additions, only its southern facade shows the fine original center mass with its smaller wings. Some of the boxwood in the southern terrace is over 150 years old, and the view of the river is unequalled.

3425—WORTHINGTON HOUSE.

This notable brick house of ell shape with fine doorway and cornice was built by John Thomson Mason in 1798 and was sold to John Teakel in 1807. Bought by Dr. Charles Worthington in 1810 and named "Quality Hill," it was transferred to James Kearney in 1840. Unoccupied for many years it is now being restored.

3508—TEMPLEMAN HOUSE.

Built overlooking the river in 1788 by John Templeman and later the home of Lt. Comdr. Geo. Upham Morris, the house is beautifully restored. The front has fine Georgian detail and the octagonal watchtower at the rear is unique. The galleries above the terrace, with their leaf and grape design, are later additions.

N STREET

(Formerly Gay and First Streets)

2721, 2723, 2725—Two story houses of ell-shape with dormered attics. The first and last are much altered.

2806—(See detailed account, page 24).

2808—JOHN STODDERT HAW HOUSE. (See detailed account, page 30).

2811—A fine two story and attic house of frame construction with gambrel roof. ca 1795.

2812—DECATUR HOUSE. (See detailed account, page 36).

2823—ADMIRAL WEAVER HOUSE.

(Supposed to be pre-Revolutionary) with the exception of the south front built about 1835.

2900—Built ca 1810, this house of three stories with attic dormers was once the residence of Mrs. Williamson, daughter of Rev. Stephen Bloomer Balch. It has a fine doorway and is slightly altered by a Palladian window to the left of the doorway.

2908—FOXALL HOUSE. (See detailed account, page 44).

3014—LAIRD-DUNLOP HOUSE. 1799. (See detailed account, page 48).

3017—THOMAS BEALL HOUSE. 1794.

Built as an investment, and oddly enough typical of New England seacoast mansions of the Federal era, Major George Peter purchased it in 1811 and it was later owned by John Laird, Wm. Redin and John D. Smoot. It was the residence of Newton D. Baker when he was Secretary of War.

3033—GEORGE BEALL HOUSE.

The central portion, which is asserted to have been built by Colonel George Beall before the Revolution, presently shows no characteristics of such early date. It is composed of a twelve foot hall with two twenty foot square rooms opening on it from the east. The second story is the same and the dormered third floor was finished as two rooms. The east wing was added in 1871 and the west wing and veranda were added later. George Beall (died 1780) and his wife (died 1748) were once buried in a family plot formerly to the east of the house. Thomas Beall is thought to have inherited this house in 1780, and it was subsequently the home of Mrs. Robert Peter and John Cox.

3038—RIGGS-RILEY HOUSE. ca 1805. (See detailed account, page 50).

3241—Probably built about 1820 this ell-shaped dwelling is somewhat neglected and greatly altered by a mansard roof and other victorian additions.

3249—Built ca 1820, this house, although marred by victorian alterations, has a fine arched doorway with semicircular transom and one unusual side light.

3255 to 3263—COLONEL JAMES SMITH ROW. ca 1805.

Fine examples of the Federal type of row house with classic dormers and recessed panels relieving the facade, built by Colonel Smith about the same time as Cox's Row.

3265, 3267—These identical houses were built by John Marbury, and are of three stories with attic dormers. Considerably altered.

3302—BALCH HOUSE. ca 1820.

This house, with rear wing and gallery, was the last residence of Rev. Stephen Bloomer Balch, beloved and militant Presbyterian minister of early Georgetown.

3304—A duplicate of the Balch House. ca 1820.

3308, 3310, 3312, 3314, 3316, 3318, 3320—Two "rows" of three and four houses respectively, built about 1820 of three story and attic dormer type. Numbers 3314 and 3320 have been regrettably altered by victorian additions.

3309 and 3311—Two houses, ca 1810, much changed by victorian alterations.

3331 to 3339—Cox's Row. ca 1805. (See detailed account, page 58).

3402—Small two story frame house with great center chimney and plaster front.

3525—CONVENT OF MERCY.

Built 1787-1792 as Trinity Church, the first Catholic Church in the District of Columbia.

3700—OLD NORTH BUILDING, Georgetown University, erected ca 1790. From its steps George Washington made a brief address in 1796.

DUMBARTON AVENUE

2613—A simple two story house.

2801—A simple house of brick and frame construction, ca 1810, now a store.

3040—Once the home of Jeremiah Williams and later of the Edes and Mackall families. Originally of two story and dormer type, now considerably enlarged and altered.

3100—BERRY HOUSE.

This house, erected in 1810, was the home of Philip Taylor Berry in 1820. It survived a bad fire about 1900 and with the fine rear gallery cut off, is now divided into apartments.

3123—McKENNEY HOUSE. (See detailed account, page 62).

3139—The rear portion was built about 1810, but it has been greatly enlarged by subsequent additions.

3143, 3145, 3147—Originally simple two story and attic dwellings.

O STREET

(Formerly Beall and Second Streets)

3010—WILLIAM H. TENNEY HOUSE. (See detailed account, page 66).

3017—COMMODORE CASSIN HOUSE. ca 1810.

This tall three story house has a fine doorway with side lights and arched overdoor, and a gallery to the east. It has a small door yard with fine old box and is altered only by victorian grills at the lower windows.

3112—A brick two story dwelling with attic dormers. ca 1810.

3114—A two story house with dormers. Probably built about 1810 and altered.

3122—A three story house—late Eighteenth Century.

3125—A three story house originally of two story and dormer type. ca 1805.

3126—Greatly altered, this house built in 1810 was the old Lancastrian School, later known as the Osborne house.

3130, 3132—Probably built about 1820, these houses of three stories have good attic dormers.

3131—A small two story house, ca 1805.

3213, 3216—Simple brick two story houses.

3240—SAINT JOHN'S EPISCOPAL CHURCH.

This church was completed in 1809 from plans by Dr. William Thornton, architect of the Capitol by subscribers headed by Thomas Jefferson. It is now considerably changed by a reduction in height of the octagonal steeple, stained glass, plastered walls and other neo-Gothic additions.

3245—GREGG HOUSE.

This small house, built before 1820, is of extremely simple style and has been well restored.

3322—BODISCO HOUSE. ca 1805. (See detailed account, page 74).

3328—A low two story brick house set back from the street. Probably built about 1820.

P STREET

(Formerly West and Third Streets)

2811—A three story and attic house with dormer, built about 1820 and slightly altered by an early victorian doorway and entrance stair.

2928—A three story house with good doorway. ca 1820.

3019—LINTHICUM HOUSE. 1826. (See detailed account, page 80).

3021—Built ca. 1800, this two story brick house with dormered attic was once the home of Horatio Berry. The doorway has been altered.

3023—A two story dwelling with attic dormers similar to 3021. ca. 1800.

3025—A two story brick house built about 1825. (See detailed account, page 76).

3022-3026—Two houses, three stories, part of a row of five, built ca. 1810, and at various times homes of the Magruder, Kenyon, Yarnell and Fowler families. These were rebuilt after a fire in 1860.

3028, 3030, 3034—Three houses, part of the same row, built ca. 1810, in original condition.

3033, 3035—A brick double house with greatly altered attic dormers, built about 1810.

3044—A simple two story brick house, probably built about 1820.

3101—Once the home of General Otho Holland Williams, built ca. 1800—now an apartment building and greatly changed.

3103—An interesting brick structure, one room deep; part of the Williams house. The doorway with side and fan lights opens onto a small walled garden at the side.

3108—MORSELL HOUSE. ca. 1815.

Built by Judge Morsell, this house of three stories with attic dormers, was successively the home of the Barnards, of the Marquis de Podestad, the Spanish Minister, and of General George C. Thomas.

3116—Three story brick house. ca. 1820.

3122—A two story brick house with attic dormers, built about 1810.

3142—TENNEY HOUSE. ca. 1810.

This handsome dwelling of two stories with dormered attic and wings, has been ably enlarged and restored. It incorporates the old house of the Rev. Mr. Stephenson and has a lovely garden to the rear.

3232—A small tenement of two stories.

3267—A simple house of ell shape—originally of two stories—much altered.

3270—A small house of three stories and ell shape, with excellent detail, probably built about 1810.

3323—Probably built about 1810, with a full third story and long ell added later. Now badly defaced by Victorian alterations.

3327—Built about 1820, this tall house of four stories and plaster front has a fine doorway with sidelights and fan.

3512—A two story brick house with dormered attic. ca. 1798.

Q STREET
(Formerly Stoddard and Fifth Streets)

2715—BELLEVUE, now DUMBARTON HOUSE. Built ca. 1750; enlarged 1805. (See detailed account, page 102).

3124—BOWIE HOUSE, now SEVIER PLACE. Built 1805, enlarged 1890. (See detailed account, page 86).

R STREET
(Formerly Road and Eighth Streets)

3101—DUMBARTON OAKS.

The main house was built in 1801 by William H. Dorsey, appointed first Judge of the Orphans Court by President Jefferson. It was sold in 1805 to Robert Beverley whose son James transferred it as "Acrolophos House" to James E. Calhoun in 1823. Lafayette was entertained here and it became the home of John C. Calhoun during his term as Vice President. It was bought by Brooke Mackall in 1826 and by Edward Linthicum, who named it "Monterey" in 1846. Its next owner, Col. Henry M. Blount, renamed it "The Oaks." The exterior is altered by a mansard roof and by two new wings, and the interior is similarly changed. Until recently the home of Robert Woods Bliss, former Minister to Argentina; since 1940 it has been the property of Harvard University. Given by the Blisses as a research center and enriched by their great collection of Byzantine Art, it stands among great trees surrounded by 16 acres of noteworthy gardens.

3406—MACKALL-WORTHINGTON HOUSE.

Built by Leonard Mackall in 1820 and later owned by the Worthingtons. It has a lovely garden, but has been altered by a mansard roof, bracketed cornice, etc.

28th STREET
(Formerly Montgomery Street)

1222—A tiny clapboard cottage now much below street level. Its roof is of steep pitch with dormers. Probably built before the Revolution.

1301—This house, although well restored, is much altered. It is of two stories with dormered attic. ca. 1800.

Southeast Corner of Dumbarton Avenue. OLD AUGUR HOUSE, ca. 1795. Now regrettably altered.

1314-1318—Two simple types of three stories with dormered attics, built about 1810. The first has been restored.

1352 and Southwest Corner of O Street. Two simple three story houses of ell shape. **ca. 1820.** Much altered by Victorian additions. Originally they were of two story and dormer type.

1524—MILLER HOUSE. ca. 1830. (See detailed account, page 84).

1623—EVERMAY. 1792. (See detailed account, page 94).

29th STREET
(Formerly Greene Street)

1308—A small brick dwelling, restored and much enlarged. Of two stories and attic it has dormers, brick corbel table, and a doorway with side lights and arched transom.

1332—A very small house of two stories.

1633—MACKALL SQUARE.

The main portion of this old house, (only one room in depth) set among fine old trees, was built ca. 1820 by Benjamin Mackall. The classic portico was built at the same time and is similar to Latrobe's at Dumbarton House. The wing to the rear terminates in a very old one story clapboard cottage with attic dormers, small six light windows, roof of steep pitch and great fireplace, is apparently of mid-Eighteenth Century construction.

30th STREET
(Formerly Washington Street)

1204-1204½-1208-1210—The first two of these four houses (three of them of the three story and dormered attic type) were probably built about 1770, the others about 1800. Both number 1208 and 1210 have fifteen light windows and the former has been well restored. The other two houses have been somewhat altered. Number 1204½ has a unique wide 12 light dormer.

1241—A New England type with great center chimney, probably built about 1815. The first story is of brick, the second frame, and it is set with its gable to the street.

1300—A three story house of ell shape altered by a mansard roof.

1302—Once a duplicate of 1300, it is badly altered by a Victorian mansard and tower.

1305-1315—COLONIAL APARTMENTS.

Considerably altered, this building was once part of Miss Lydia English's Female Seminary, built ca. 1820. It was a union hospital during the Civil War.

1319—MATTHEW HYDE HOUSE. ca. 1798. (See detailed account, page 106).

1325-1327—Originally one low house of two stories with great center chimney and two dormers. Lintels have raised end blocks. Built about 1820.

1330—DE LA ROCHE HOUSE. Built ca. 1820 this frame house was the residence of Captain De la Roche, early architect and is much altered.

1344—This beautiful dwelling has been reconstructed from three old houses built about 1810. It is greatly altered but has handsome gardens.

1647—BEALL-WASHINGTON HOUSE.

This house, facing R Street and set in fine grounds, was built by Thomas Beall, ca. 1784. Successively the home of his sons-in-law Col. George Corbin Washington, great nephew of the President and of Eliah Riggs and Senator Bright. It is now altered by a mansard roof and victorian detail.

31st STREET
(Formerly Congress Street)

1226—Small two story and dormered attic dwelling of brick and frame construction.

1644—TUDOR PLACE. 1802-1816. (See detailed account, page 88).

POTOMAC STREET

1217, 1219, 1220, 1221, 1222, 1223, 1225—Simple brick two story dwellings. ca. 1820.

33rd STREET
(Formerly Market Street)

1430—THE YELLOW HOUSE.

According to legend some part of this two story and attic structure, which is most apparently of early Nineteenth Century construction, was built on "Knaves Disappointment" before 1733 when it was willed to John Gordon. With a small garden to the left the door opens into a stair hall with two generous rooms to the right. To the rear, rooms extend on different levels. Several doors are of early type; flat on one side and full paneled on the other.

1501—A two story and dormer house. ca. 1810. Much altered in restoration.

1511-1513-1515-1517—Four small brick houses of two stories and dormered attic. Built ca. 1820. Restored.

1516—Same type as the above. Interesting ornate door. ca. 1820. Restored.

1520—A small two story brick house.

1524—THE YELLOW TAVERN. ca. 1795.

Also known as "The White House" this small house built of Flemish bond with white trim has a fine doorway probably taken from another dwelling and added later.

1540—A tiny two story brick house. ca. 1810.

1562-1564—Two small brick houses of two stories with attic dormers. Probably built about 1810.

1616-1620—Small brick houses somewhat altered in restoration.

34th STREET
(Formerly Frederick Street)

1310—Small brick house, probably ca. 1820, considerably enlarged when restored.

1314—Small frame house, probably ca. 1820.

Southwest corner of O Street. Originally a fine square house built about 1800—now a store, it is enlarged and regrettably altered.

1406—A handsome brick house built before 1820 of ell shape, somewhat altered in restoration.

1411—A two story dwelling with dormered attic. It is enlarged and restored with a lovely walled garden. ca. 1810.

3410—VOLTA PLACE.

Slave quarters converted into two tiny frame cottages.

35th STREET
(Formerly Fayette Street)

1307—A simple two story dwelling.

1404—A three story and attic house, ca. 1800. Recently restored.

The Church—Convent of the Visitation, ca. 1800.

RESERVOIR ROAD
(Formerly Seventh Street)

3330—A simple two story frame house with dentiled cornice. Built ca. 1800, and now much enlarged.

*　　*　　*　　*　　*

BIBLIOGRAPHY
(Selected from over 500 References)

Adams, James Thurlow, The Epic of America.

Bayard, Margaret, A Winter in Washington, or Memoirs of the Seymour Family, published in 1824.

Brown, Glenn, Papers on the Improvement of Washington City.

Bryan, W. B., A History of the National Capital—Library of the National Archives F 194, B9 VI.

Century Magazine, April 1897, pp. 803-920. Article entitled "Old Georgetown—A Social Panorama."

Clark, Allen C., Life and Letters of Dolly Madison.

Columbia Historical Society Records, V18, pp. 70-92:
　　1—Old Homes on Georgetown Heights by William A. Gordon.
　　2—Mackall Square.
　　3—Doctor and Mrs. William Thornton by Allen C. Clark, p. 144.

Columbia Historical Society Records, V33-34, pp. 133-162.

Columbia Historical Society Records, V8, p. 195. An Article on the Question of imported bricks, by George Alfred Townsend.

Cunningham, Younger & Smith, Georgian Architecture in the District of Columbia.

Ecker, Grace Dunlop, A Portrait of Old Georgetown.

Evans, Henry R., Old Georgetown on the Potomac.

Frary, I. T., They Built the Capitol.
　　Lib. Cong. NA 4411. F7. (A valuable chronology of Events through the building of the Capitol, beginning with the earliest plans.)

Great Georgian Houses of America, Vols. I and II.

Jackson, Richard P., The Chronicles of Georgetown, D.C., from 1751 to 1878.

Kimball, Fiske, Regional Types in Early American Architecture.

Leech, Margaret, Reveille in Washington.

Morris, Gouverneur, Diary.

National Geographic Magazine, April 1937. Article by Dr. W. A. R. Goodwin, Rector of Bruton Parish. "The Restoration of Colonial Williamsburg" (Problems and solutions parallel to those in other Tidewater restorations.)

Smith, Wilmer J., Measured Drawings of Georgian Architecture in the District of Columbia.

BIBLIOGRAPHY (Continued)

Taggart, Hugh Thomas, Old Georgetown.

The Restoration of Colonial Williamsburg in Virginia.

Tolbert, Alice Coyle, Doorways and Dormers of Old Georgetown.
    Lib. Cong. F202 Gs T67. (Guide book, with interesting map locating old houses.)

U. S. Catholic Historical Society, George-Town-on-the-Potowmack, 1931. Historical records and studies. V20, pp. 158-165.

Washington, D. C., A Guide to the National Capital (WPA American Guide Series.)

Washington, George, Diary.

Washington, George, Letters.

Waterman, Thomas Tileston, English Antecedents of Virginia Architecture.
    Lib. Cong. NA 730, V8 W3 Pamphlet Form.

Waterman, Thomas Tileston, Domestic Architecture of Tidewater Virginia.
    Lib. Cong. NA 7235 V5 W3 fol. Descriptions of houses.

Wilsbach, Paul, Tidewater Maryland.

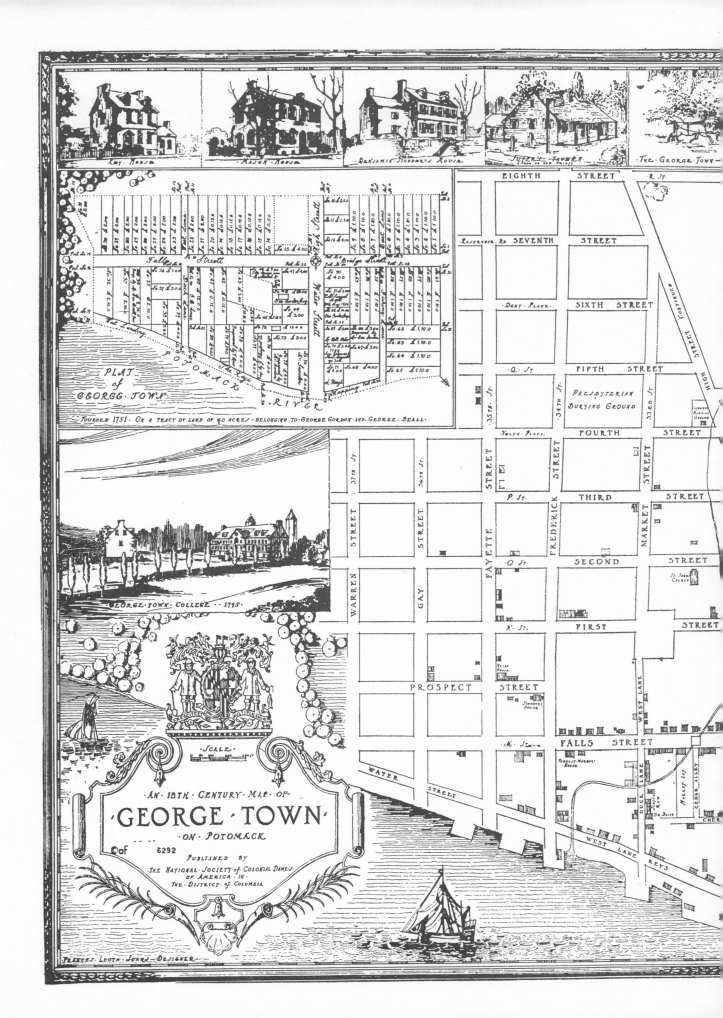

IVY HOUSE   MAJOR HOUSE   BENJAMIN STODDERT'S HOUSE   SUTER'S TAVERN (NOW AN OLD PRINT)   THE GEORGE TOWN

PLAT of GEORGE TOWN

POTOMACK RIVER

FOUNDED 1751 · ON A TRACT OF LAND OF 60 ACRES · BELONGING TO · GEORGE · GORDON · AND · GEORGE · BEALL ·

EIGHTH STREET

SEVENTH STREET

SIXTH STREET

FIFTH STREET

PRESBYTERIAN BURYING GROUND

FOURTH STREET

THIRD STREET

SECOND STREET

FIRST STREET

PROSPECT STREET

FALLS STREET

WATER STREET

WEST LANE

GEORGE TOWN COLLEGE · 1795

·SCALE·

AN · 18TH · CENTURY · MAP · OF

·GEORGE · TOWN·

· ON · POTOMACK ·

6292

PUBLISHED BY

THE · NATIONAL · SOCIETY · OF · COLONIAL · DAMES ·
OF · AMERICA · IN ·
THE · DISTRICT · OF · COLUMBIA